Somatization and Psychosomatic Symptoms

Kyung Bong Koh
Editor

Somatization and Psychosomatic Symptoms

Springer

Editor
Kyung Bong Koh
Department of Psychiatry
Yonsei University College of Medicine
Seodaemun-gu, Seoul, Korea

ISBN 978-1-4614-7118-9 ISBN 978-1-4614-7119-6 (eBook)
DOI 10.1007/978-1-4614-7119-6
Springer New York Heidelberg Dordrecht London

Library of Congress Control Number: 2013939727

Printed on acid-free paper

Springer is part of Springer Science+Business Media (www.springer.com)

Preface

After working successfully as chairperson of the Organizing Committee at the 21st World Congress on Psychosomatic Medicine held in Seoul in August 2011, I planned to write a book entitled *Somatization and Psychosomatic Symptoms* with my distinguished colleagues from all around the world. Most of them who have been interested in the field of psychosomatic medicine and actively involved in the academic as well as clinical activities for a long time accepted my proposal for publishing this book. Over a period of one and a half years, our efforts finally bore fruit in the form of this book. I am very proud of this book because it is not only a collection of up-to-date knowledge by many international professionals as the product of our collaboration, but it reveals the vision for the future of psychosomatic medicine. Furthermore, this book deals with a variety of interesting and controversial issues relevant to psychosomatic medicine.

Psychosomatic medicine has tried to integrate biopsychosocial factors in assessment and treatment of illnesses or diseases and played a central role in leading medicine to "personhood." This field has also provided a theoretical framework for effective and desirable clinical practice and helped physicians to overcome obstacles to the development of medicine, such as dualism and reductionism.

Currently, there are many patients distressed by a variety of somatic symptoms along with psychosocial problems. In particular, although the number of patients with medically unexplained somatic symptoms is increasing, a considerable number of patients are still wandering without seeking appropriate management. In addition, a number of patients with serious diseases, such as cancer, are surviving longer than before with the development of cutting-edge therapeutic modalities. Thus, they are struggling to live with chronic poor quality of life.

Somatization is a process in which there is inappropriate focus on physical symptoms which are medically unexplained. Somatization is highly prevalent in primary care. Somatoform disorders are representative of somatization. These disorders tend to be chronic and can cause significant personal suffering and social problems as well as financial burden. Treatment of somatoform disorders is challenging because they cannot be effectively treated according to the existing biomedical model. Psychosomatic symptoms refer to physical symptoms of physical diseases affected by psychosocial factors. Both patients with somatization and those with psychosomatic symptoms tend to show resistance to psychiatric or psychological assessment and treatment in common. These patients are good models for medical students and health-care professionals, such as physicians, nurses, psychologists, and social workers, to learn about the biopsychosocial approach to patient-centered care because their symptoms cannot be biomedically explained. Therefore, the professionals need to learn specific assessment skills and treatment techniques in order to deal with these patients more effectively. This book deals with a variety of issues relevant to mechanisms, education, assessment, and treatment of such disorders in terms of biopsychosociocultural perspectives. The book consists of 22 chapters. Twenty-three distinguished experts from different countries participate in this project as contributors.

The book is composed of seven parts: I. Basic understanding of somatization, II. Theoretical approaches to mind and body, III. Biopsychosociocultural mechanisms in psychosomatic medicine, IV. Practical approaches to patients and family, V. Specific psychosomatic symptoms, VI. Specific psychosomatic disorders, VII. Specific therapeutic interventions and biological effects of interventions. The first part deals with the identity of somatoform disorders because, currently, there is an identity crisis related to the survival of the terms of some subgroups as well as "somatoform disorders." In the second part, evolution of philosophy underpinning personhood in medicine is reviewed. Moreover, the recent trend of reductionism in medicine calls for such philosophy. The third part deals with genes, memes, alexithymia, culture, and the molecular mechanism of sleep-wake regulation. In particular, the relationship between memes, stress, and psychosomatic disorders is explored and meme-oriented therapies are introduced in treatment of stress-related disorders. On the other hand, our understanding of molecular aspects of sleep-wake regulation will help expand areas of traditional psychosomatic medicine.

In the fourth part, the need for psychosomatic assessment and approach to clinical practice is emphasized in terms of cost-benefit, especially in chronic diseases. The effect of assessment of alexithymia and emotional intelligence on the quality of the doctor-patient relationship is reviewed. How to integrate cognitive therapy into medical care and how to refer medically unexplained patients are presented. Differences between Western medicine and Oriental medicine and the role of complementary and alternative medicine in psychosomatic medicine are discussed. In addition, a variety of family assessment tools are introduced and problem-centered systems therapy of the family is described in detail.

The fifth part includes psychosomatic symptoms, especially pain: "pain as a common language of human suffering," "fibromyalgia," and "a psychosomatic approach to difficult chronic pain patients." In the sixth part, specific psychosomatic disorders such as "stress-induced cardiomyopathy"; "cancer," especially "breast cancer"; and "poststroke depression" are reviewed. In the past, the mechanism of stress-induced cardiomyopathy was not addressed in books related to psychosomatic medicine. This topic will help medical students to understand the relationship between stress and heart problems. In the chapter related to breast cancer, a variety of therapeutic modalities, including cognitive behavioral therapy and psychopharmacotherapy, are presented. Poststroke depression can be a good candidate for an integrative or biopsychosocial approach. Herein, mechanisms and management of poststroke depression are mainly addressed, focusing on biological and psychological therapies (including cognitive behavioral therapy).

The last part deals with "motivational interviewing," "wisdom and wisdom psychotherapy," and "advanced psychopharmacology" as therapeutic interventions in psychosomatic medicine. Motivational interviewing is reviewed as a cost-effective and culturally sensitive intervention for domestic violence victims. The usefulness of wisdom therapy in coping with stress is addressed as a way of strengthening resilience. In addition, the effects of interventions, such as relaxation, mindfulness-based stress reduction, and cognitive behavioral therapy, on immunity are reviewed. These results will provide a rationale for clinical applications of these interventions to improve immunity in patients with immune-related disorders.

I believe this book will be a good guide for medical students, nurses, psychologists, social workers, as well as psychiatrists and physicians who want to learn about psychosomatic medicine or an integrative approach to medicine.

First and foremost, I wish to thank my contributors for sharing their clinical experience, research, and insights. I am truly grateful to Ms. Janice Stern, senior editor, and Ms. *Christina Tuballes*, editorial assistant, for their assistance throughout the process of editing and publication of this book. In addition, I thank my wife, Sungsook Cho, for her constant encouragement and emotional support. I also thank God for enabling me to finish this hard work without giving up.

Seoul, Korea — Kyung Bong Koh

Contents

Part VII Specific Therapeutic Interventions and Biological Effects of Interventions

Contributors

Matteo Bruscoli, M.D. Societa Italina Medicina Psichosomatica, Italy, Affiliated to Institute of Psychosomatic Medicine, Sweden

Sung Hee Cho, Ph.D. Christian Studies Division, Baekseok University, Cheonan, Chungnam Province, Korea

Byung-il William Choi, M.D. Division of Cardiology, Medical College of Wisconsin, Milwaukee, WI, USA

Sae-il Chun, M.D. Department of Integrative Medicine, The Graduate School of Integrative Medicine, CHA University, Sungnam City, Kyeonggi Province, Korea

Giovanni Andrea Fava, M.D. Laboratory of Psychosomatics and Clinimetrics, Department of Psychology, University of Bologna, Bologna, Italy

Department of Psychiatry, State University of New York at Buffalo, Buffalo, NY, USA

Arnstein Finset, Ph.D. Department of Behavioural Sciences in Medicine, Institute of Basic Medical Sciences, Faculty of Medicine, University of Oslo, Blindern, Oslo, Norway

Gabor I. Keitner, M.D. Department of Psychiatry, Rhode Island and Miriam Hospitals, Brown University, Providence, RI, USA

Woesook Kim, Ph.D. Clinical Psychology, College of Nursing Art and Science, University of Hyogo, Akashi, Hyogo, Japan

Kyung Bong Koh, M.D., Ph.D. Department of Psychiatry, Yonsei University College of Medicine, Seodaemun-gu, Seoul, Korea

Gen Komaki, M.D., Ph.D. School of Health Sciences at Fukuoka, International University of Health and Welfare, Ohkawa, Fukuoka, Japan

Jun-Won Lee, M.D. Division of Cardiology, Department of Internal Medicine, Yonsei University Wonju College of Medicine, Gangwon Province, Korea

Hoyle Leigh, M.D. Department of Psychiatry, University of California, San Francisco, USA

UCSF Fresno, Fresno, CA, USA

Michael Linden, M.D. Research Group Psychosomatic Rehabilitation at der Charité University Medicine Berlin

Department of Behavioral and Psychosomatic Medicine at the Rehabilitation Center Seehof, Lichterfelder Allee 55, Teltow/Berlin, Germany

Sung Kil Min, M.D., Ph.D. Yonsei University College of Medicine, Seoul Metropolitan Eunpyeong Hospital, Eunpyeong-gu, Seoul, Korea

Masato Murakami, M.D., Ph.D. Department of Psychosomatic Internal Medicine, Nihon University Hospital, Itabashi-ku, Tokyo, Japan

Michael Alan Schwartz, M.D. Departments of Humanities in Medicine and Psychiatry, Texas A&M Health Science Center College of Medicine, Round Rock, TX, USA

Amarendra N. Singh, M.D. Psychopharmacology, Department of Psychiatry, Pharmacology and Neurosciences, Queen's Univeristy, Kingston, ON, Canada

Tatjana Sivik, M.D., Ph.D. Department of General Medicine, Institute of Psychosomatic Medicine, University of Göteborg, Fridkullagatan, Göteborg, Sweden

Jon Streltzer, M.D. Department of Psychiatry, University of Hawaii at Manoa, John A. Burns School of Medicine, Honolulu, HI, USA

Eliana Tossani, Ph.D. Department of Psychology, University of Bologna, Bologna, Italy

Yoshihiro Urade, Ph.D. Department of Molecular Behavioral Biology, Osaka Bioscience Institute, Osaka, Japan

Adriaan Visser, Ph.D. Knowledge Center Innovations in Care, Rotterdam University of Applied Sciences, Rotterdam, The Netherlands

Osborne P. Wiggins, Ph.D. Philosophy Department, University of Louisville, Louisville, KY, USA

Part I
Basic Understanding of Somatization

Chapter 1
Identity of Somatoform Disorders: Comparison with Depressive Disorders and Anxiety Disorders

Kyung Bong Koh

1.1 Introduction

Somatoform disorders are among the most prevalent psychiatric disorders in general practice. Somatoform disorders were diagnosed in 16.1 % of consecutive consulting patients [1]. Patients with somatoform disorders are often referred to as "medical orphans" [2], because correct diagnosis is not made by physicians and the patients end up "shopping" for diagnoses by visiting many physicians.

The term "somatoform disorders" was introduced in the third edition of Diagnostic and Statistical Manual (DSM) in recognition that many patients present with somatic distress that does not fit in the rubric of physical diseases, anxiety, mood, or psychotic disorders. Somatoform disorders represent heterogeneous subgroups of patient presentations, ranging from conversion disorder to hypochondriasis to somatization disorder to pain disorder [3].

1.1.1 How to Get Labeled as Misdiagnosed Somatoform Disorder

The diagnosis of somatoform disorders relies on the presence of subjective distress in the absence of objective findings. As a result, there is always the possibility that a diagnosis will be missed or altered later. In addition, patients are sometimes misdiagnosed with somatoform disorders, because the doctor has simply missed the diagnosis by insufficient attention to the history, physical examination, or laboratory tests and by not relying on contemporary diagnostic techniques. In addition,

K.B. Koh, M.D., Ph.D (✉)
Department of Psychiatry, Yonsei University College of Medicine,
50 Yonsei-ro, Seodaemun-gu, Seoul 120-752, Korea
e-mail: kbkoh@yuhs.ac

K.B. Koh (ed.), *Somatization and Psychosomatic Symptoms*,
DOI 10.1007/978-1-4614-7119-6_1, © Springer Science+Business Media New York 2013

symptoms have the potential to be worsened by iatrogenic factors. New diseases, unknown in past years, have also come to light (e.g., hepatitis C with fatigue and depression) [3]. However, the rate of misdiagnosis for somatoform disorders (less than 10 %) is not as high as expected, because it is in the range of misdiagnoses that are found for other mental disorders or physical diseases [4].

1.1.2 Shortcomings of Somatoform Disorders as Diagnoses

Although retained and enlarged in the DSM-IV, somatoform disorders have been the subject of continuing criticism by both professionals and patients [5]. Many clinicians believe that the current terminology and classification system performs poorly in respect to the functions of diagnosis [5]. First, the terminology is unacceptable to patients. Second, the category is inherently dualistic. Third, somatoform disorders do not form a coherent category. Fourth, somatoform disorders are incompatible with other cultures. Fifth, there is ambiguity in the stated exclusion criteria. Sixth, somatoform disorders are unreliable. Seventh, somatoform disorders lack a clearly defined threshold. Finally, somatoform disorders cause confusion in disputes over medical-legal and insurance entitlements.

1.1.3 Shortcomings of the Specific Somatoform Disorder Subcategories

Many of the diagnostic subcategories currently housed within the somatoform disorders either lack validity as separate conditions or may be better housed elsewhere [5]. Shortcomings of the specific somatoform disorder subcategories have already been outlined in previous studies. In somatization disorder, doubts have been expressed about both its clinical value and conceptual basis [6] because it has substantial overlap with personality disorders, particularly borderline personality disorder [7]. This diagnosis has shown a low stability in longitudinal surveys, because the diagnosis relies on a lifetime history of symptoms, that is, patients' recall of past symptoms [8]. Moreover, the diagnosis is based simply on counting the number of "unexplained" somatic symptoms. Such diagnosis merely represents an extreme of severity on what appears to be a continuum of distress [9]. As such, the threshold of the criteria for somatization disorder is too high, and patients with this diagnosis are so rare. Therefore, somatization disorder has little clinical validity. Hypochondriasis also remains controversial as a diagnostic category. Although there is good evidence of the co-occurrence of the triad of disease conviction, associated distress, and medical help-seeking, these symptoms are better conceived of as a form of anxiety that happens to focus on health matters and is closely related to other forms of anxiety disorder [10, 11]. Conversion disorder has long been a problem for diagnostic classification. DSM-III placed this disorder with other diagnoses in the somatoform section because of the shared characteristic of somatic symptoms that are not intentionally produced [12]. However, the DSM-IV workgroup recognized it has a close relationship with dissociative disorder [13]. The prevalence of undifferentiated somatoform disorder is high, ranging from 10 % to 30 % [1, 14, 15]. However, there have been few studies on undifferentiated somatoform disorder. Its existence represents the need to have a diagnosis for a very large group of patients not easily classified elsewhere, even though this diagnosis is not widely used in clinical practice [5]. Despite revision of pain disorder between DSM-III and DSM-IV, there remain problems both in its definition and in establishing it as a separate disorder [16]. Body dysmorphic disorder might be better grouped with obsessive-compulsive disorder [17].

The heterogeneous classification of somatoform disorders according to the DSM-IV and the International Classification of Diseases (ICD-10) has been found to be insufficiently useful for therapeutic and scientific purposes [18–22]. Therefore, the identity of somatoform disorder is confusing. Currently, there is an identity crisis related to the survival of somatoform disorders. Some scientists have proposed that these diagnostic categories should be abolished and that a new term for somatic symptoms be adopted [5].

The diagnostic group should be made more homogeneous and its biopsychosociocultural characteristics should be elucidated in order to resolve the identity confusion. For this purpose, the author compared somatoform disorders with other major mental disorders, such as depressive disorders and anxiety disorders in terms of biopsychosociocultural perspectives, including incidence and specificity of psychosociocultural and behavioral features and biological features. Therefore, the similarities and differences in these biopsychosociocultural aspects between the three disorders will help to clarify whether somatoform disorders are independent.

1.2 Incidence and Specificity of Psychosociocultural and Behavioral Features in Patients with Somatoform Disorders

1.2.1 Severity of Somatic Symptoms, Depression, and Illness Anxiety

Patients with depressive disorders have higher levels of depression, illness anxiety, and somatic symptoms than patients with somatoform disorders. Patients with anxiety disorders have higher levels of illness anxiety than patients with somatoform disorders. However, there are no differences in the severity of somatic symptoms and depression between patients with anxiety disorders and somatoform disorders [23]. In this study, diagnoses of mental disorders were made by general practitioners. In another study [29], patients with depressive disorders have higher levels of depression than patients with somatoform disorders or anxiety disorders, but there are no significant differences in the levels of somatic symptoms and anxiety among the three disorders. These diagnoses were made by psychiatrists. Therefore, somatoform disorders are similar to anxiety disorders in the severity of somatic symptoms and depression, but both disorders are different from depressive disorders in the levels of depression.

1.2.2 Attribution

Patients with somatization report fewer normalizing symptom attributions than nonclinical subjects [24]. Somatization patients have more organic attributions than depressed patients [24, 25], but they usually do not have monocausal simplistic explanations [24].

1.2.3 Health Anxiety/Illness Worry

Somatization patients show elevated health anxiety scores [26]. It has been shown that different chronic pain syndromes share health anxiety as a common feature [27]. Health anxiety is elevated in somatization and hypochondriasis as compared to mixed clinical controls [26]. However, it is possible that the content of worry is different in somatization versus hypochondriasis [28].

1.2.4 Anger and Anger Management Style

Patients with somatoform disorder scored significantly higher on the Stress Response Inventory (SRI) anger subscale than normal controls [29]. Somatoform disorder or anxiety disorder patients are less likely to have high levels of anger than depressive disorder patients [29]. Somatic symptoms in anxiety disorder [30] and somatoform disorder [31] patients are associated with anger suppression, whereas somatic symptoms in depressive disorder patients are more associated with anger expression [31] (Figs. 1.1, 1.2, and 1.3). Therefore, in terms of anger levels and the relationship between anger management style and somatic symptoms, somatoform disorders are similar to anxiety disorders but are different from depressive disorders.

1.2.5 Alexithymia

Alexithymia is significantly more prevalent in somatizers without organic pathology than in healthy subjects [32]. Adolescents with persistent somatoform pain disorder have higher levels of alexithymia than healthy adolescent controls [33].

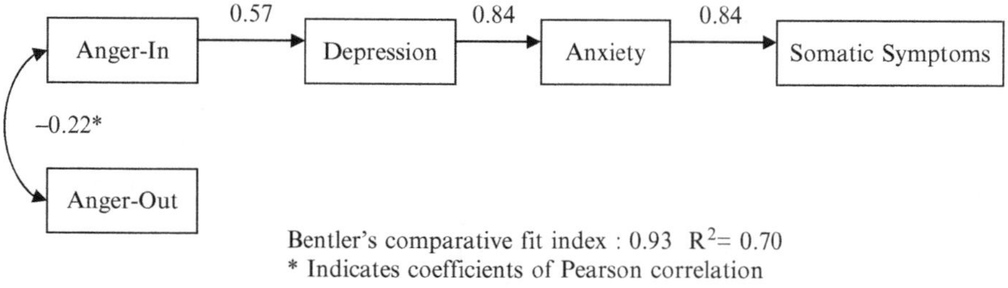

Fig. 1.1 The relation between anger management style, mood, and somatic symptoms in anxiety disorders (From Koh et al. [30])

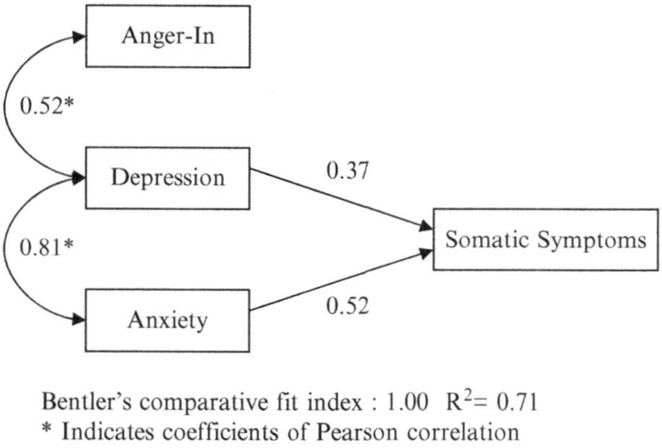

Fig. 1.2 The relation between anger management style, mood, and somatic symptoms in somatoform disorders (From Koh et al. [30])

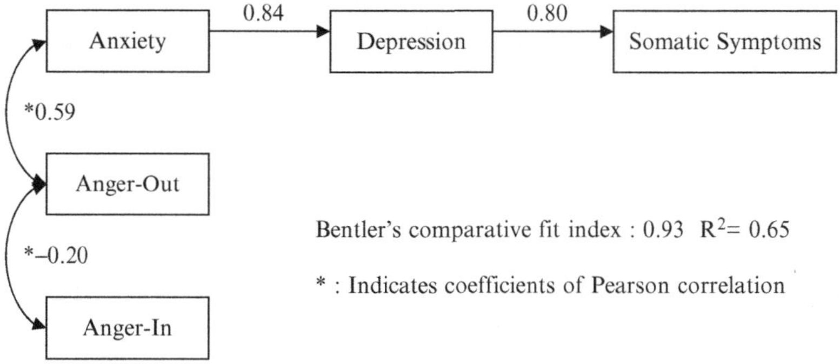

Fig. 1.3 The relation between anger management style, mood, and somatic symptoms in depressive disorders

In patients with somatoform pain disorder, alexithymia was negatively correlated with quality of life [34]. Patients with tension headache were significantly more alexithymic than patients with anxiety disorders and depressive disorders [35]. However, the correlation between alexithymia and somatization has not been established [32].

1.2.6 Cognitive Factors

Somatization patients over-interpret minor physical symptoms as possible signs of illness and have a self-concept of being "weak" [26]. The catastrophizing of physical symptoms is specific to somatization and hypochondriasis but is not seen in patients with depressive and anxiety disorders. The self-concept of being "weak" is a distinguishing characteristic between somatoform disorder patients and patients suffering from other mental disorders [26].

1.2.7 Somatosensory Amplification

Increased somatic symptom reports are associated with higher somatosensory amplification [24, 36]. However, there are contradictory results regarding the specificity of somatosensory amplification in somatoform disorders, especially concerning the differentiation from patients with anxiety disorders and depressive disorders [24].

1.2.8 Illness Behavior

Increased health-care use in somatization [24, 37] and significant differences in somatization patients compared to controls were found in various aspects of illness behavior (e.g., body scanning, expression of symptoms) [38]. In addition, chronic pain syndromes are associated with reassurance-seeking behavior [27]. Increased health-care use also occurs in hypochondriasis, depressive disorders, and anxiety disorders [36]. However, evidence of the ability of single aspects of illness behavior to differentiate between patients with somatization, depressive disorders, and anxiety disorders is still inconclusive [38].

1.2.9 Culture

Sociocultural restraints may play a role in the somatic symptoms of somatoform disorders by blocking emotionally charged feelings or ideas from being expressed [39]. *Hwabyung*, an anger syndrome specific to Korean culture and characterized by a variety of somatic symptoms, is associated with anger suppression [40–43].

In East Asian societies, the Westernized "medically unexplained" concept of the somatoform disorders is not easily accepted due to the strong influence of the non-dualistic and syndromal approach of traditional medicine [44]. *Hwabyung* is not considered to be "medically unexplained" in traditional medicine practitioners in Korea. Therefore, we need to address the future diagnostic utility of somatoform disorders in a broader cross-cultural conceptual and contextual framework [45].

1.3 Why Are Biological Findings Important in Establishing the Identity of Somatoform Disorders?

A better understanding of the underlying neurobiological underpinnings of frequently co-occurring disorders may help to determine whether they are independent entities [46]. In particular, biological findings may be helpful to address the limit of self-reporting when diagnosing somatizing patients. Such biological findings include neural imaging, along with neural immune and genetic studies.

1.3.1 Incidence and Specificity of Biological Features in Patients with Somatoform Disorders

1.3.1.1 Brain Imaging

Somatoform disorder patients showed hyperperfusion in the left hemisphere at the superior temporal gyrus, inferior parietal lobule, middle occipital gyrus, precentral gyrus, and postcentral gyrus and in the right hemisphere at the superior temporal gyrus, as compared to the healthy controls. Hyperperfusion in the left superior temporal gyrus and hypoperfusion in the right parahippocampal gyrus were found in patients with undifferentiated somatoform disorder and panic disorder when compared to healthy controls [47]. Together, these findings suggest that two disorders share neural activities (Fig. 1.4). In addition, in pain disorder patients, when compared with healthy controls, there was reduced gray matter in the anterior cingulate cortex, posterior cingulate cortex, lateral prefrontal cortex, ventromedial prefrontal cortex, and anterior insular cortex [48].

Another study also found that panic disorder patients showed increased gray matter in the left superior temporal gyrus when compared with healthy controls [49]. However, another report found that the gray matter in the right middle and superior temporal gyrus regions was reduced in anxiety disorder patients when compared with healthy controls [50]. In contrast, increased cerebral blood flow in the amygdala and medial orbital areas was found in major depressive disorder patients when compared with healthy controls. In addition, major depressive disorder patients showed reduced metabolism in the prefrontal cortex [51], as well as reduced gray matter in the right inferior frontal gyrus [50] when compared with healthy controls. Therefore, major depressive disorder is likely to differ from somatoform disorders and anxiety disorders in terms of neural activity.

1.3.1.2 Genetic Findings

One study examined serotonin-related gene polymorphisms in patients with undifferentiated somatoform disorder and healthy controls. However, no significant differences were found in serotonin-related gene polymorphisms between the two groups.

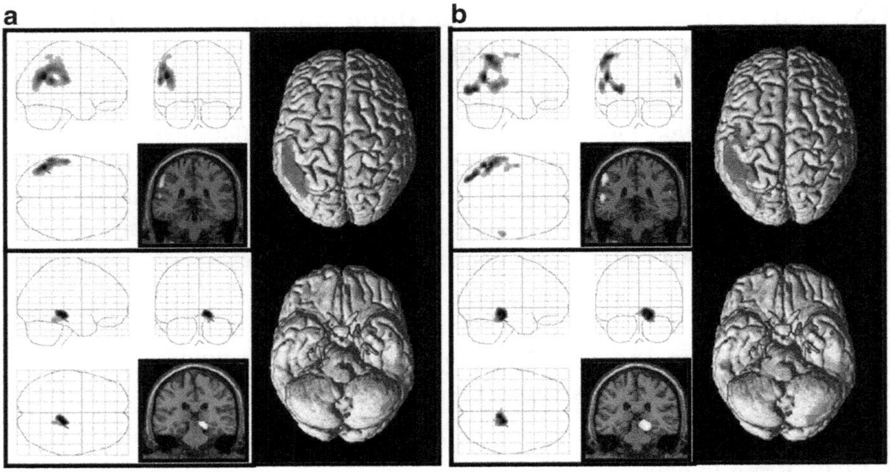

Fig. 1.4 Hyperperfused (*red/gray*) or hypoperfused (*green/white*) brain regions in panic disorder (**a**) and undifferentiated somatoform disorder (**b**) patients compared with healthy controls From Koh et al. [47]. Adapted and Reprinted by permission of Physicians Postgraduate Press

Therefore, serotonin-related gene pathways are unlikely to be genetic risk factors for undifferentiated somatoform disorder [52].

In contrast, some serotonin-related gene polymorphisms, such as tryptophan hydroxylase (TPH)1 A218C gene [53], variants of TPH2 gene [54], and serotonin receptor 2A (5-HTR 2A) gene [55], were regarded as candidate genes for major depressive disorder. In addition, a functional polymorphism located in the promoter region of the serotonin transporter gene (5-HTTLPR) has been shown to be associated with seasonal affective disorder [56].

On the other hand, it was reported that aggression in major depressive disorder patients is more susceptible to an excess of TPH1 CC homozygote than in undifferentiated somatoform disorder patients, though the two disorders are high-risk groups for aggression [53].

More than 350 candidate genes have been examined in association studies of panic disorder. However, most of these results remain negative or have not been clearly replicated. Only Val158Met polymorphism of the catechol-O-methyltransferase gene has been implicated in a susceptibility to panic disorder by several studies in independent samples and was confirmed in a recent meta-analysis [57].

1.3.1.3 Immunological Findings

There have been few studies on the comparison of immune function between somatoform disorder patients and healthy controls. One study showed reduced lymphocyte proliferation in patients with undifferentiated somatoform disorder compared with normal controls [58].

When compared with normal controls, panic disorder patients were found to have a wide range of lymphocyte proliferative response to mitogens: decreased [59], normal [60, 61], or increased [62]. However, several additional studies observed reduced blastogenic response to the mitogens PHA [63, 64] and PWM [59], as well as reduced serum IL-2 production level [64] in patients with anxiety disorders, especially panic disorder. Moreover, patients with panic disorder had significantly lower levels of CD4+ than depressive disorder patients [65].

In patients with depressive disorders, meta-analytic approaches to the literature showed statistically reliable decreases in T cell responses [66, 67], although there have been both successful and unsuccessful replication attempts.

1.4 Considerations for a New Classification of Somatoform Disorders

Converging evidence from the biopsychosocial data should be used for establishing any new classification of somatoform disorders. It is possible to consider reestablishing the relationship between somatoform disorders and psychosomatic disorders in a new classification. For example, functional psychosomatic disorders (somatic syndromes) such as irritable bowel syndrome, tension headache, and functional dyspepsia may be included in the new classification of somatoform disorders (e.g., autonomic somatoform disorder).

In addition, there may be an immediate need to specify an undifferentiated somatoform disorder, due to its high prevalence among somatoform disorders. This diagnosis may be included in somatization disorder by lowering threshold for diagnosing somatization disorder. Future diagnostic concepts and somatoform disorder criteria should be meaningful and useful in both Western and non-Western countries. Potential new classification of somatoform disorders is proposed and presented in Table 1.1.

Table 1.1 Controversial subgroups of somatoform disorders and potential new classification

DSM-IV	Potential new classification
Hypochondriasis	Anxiety disorder (e.g., illness anxiety disorder)
Body dysmorphic disorder	Obsessive-compulsive disorder
Conversion disorder	Dissociative (conversion) disorder (ICD-10)
Pain disorder	Somatoform pain disorder (DSM-III)
Somatization disorder	
Undifferentiated somatoform disorder	Somatization disorder
Functional psychosomatic disorders	Autonomic somatoform disorder (e.g., IBS, tension headache, functional dyspepsia)
Somatoform disorder not otherwise specified	Nonspecific somatoform disorder

DSM-IV Diagnostic and Statistical Manual, 4th edition, *ICD-10* International Classification of Diseases, 10th revision, *IBS* irritable bowel syndrome

1.5 Conclusions

The identity of somatoform disorder is confusing due to the heterogeneous classification of somatoform disorders according to the DSM-IV and the ICD-10. In order to resolve the identity confusion, we need to elucidate more about the biopsychosociocultural characteristics of somatoform disorders. For this purpose, somatoform disorders were compared with other major mental disorders, such as depressive disorders and anxiety disorders, in terms of biopsychosociocultural perspectives. Biological findings, as well as psychosocial findings, may help to differentiate between somatoform disorders and other mental disorders, such as depressive disorders and anxiety disorders. Somatoform disorders are biopsychosocially more similar to anxiety disorders than to depressive disorders, especially major depressive disorder. However, somatoform disorders may be more affected by sociocultural factors than anxiety disorders. Among many factors relevant to somatoform disorders, anxiety disorders, and depressive disorders, there are some factors showing clear differences between the three disorders, including psychosociocultural factors, such as attribution, anger levels, anger management style, cognitive factor, and cultural difference, as well as biological factors, such as neural activity and genetic factors. The converging evidence from the biopsychosociocultural data may help resolve the identity confusion of somatoform disorders and establish a new classification of somatoform disorders.

References

1. De Waal, M. W., Arnold, I. A., Eekhof, J. A., et al. (2004). Somatoform disorders in general practice: Prevalence, functional impairment and comorbidity with anxiety and depressive disorders. *The British Journal of Psychiatry, 184*, 470–476.
2. Aronowitz, R. A. (2001). When do symptoms become a disease? *Annals of Internal Medicine, 134*, 803–808.
3. Dimsdale, J. E., & Dantzer, R. (2007). A biological substrate for somatoform disorders: Importance of pathophysiology. *Psychosomatic Medicine, 69*, 850–854.
4. Rief, W., & Rojas, G. (2007). Stability of somatoform symptoms – implications for classification. *Psychosomatic Medicine, 69*, 864–869.
5. Mayou, R., Kirmayer, L. J., Simon, G., et al. (2005). Somatoform disorders: Time for a new approach in DSM-V. *The American Journal of Psychiatry, 162*, 847–855.
6. Bass, C. M., & Murphy, M. R. (1990). Somatization disorder: Critique of the concept and suggestions for further research. In C. M. Bass & R. H. Cawley (Eds.), *Somatization: Physical symptoms and psychological illness*. Oxford, UK: Blackwell Scientific.
7. Rost, K. M., Atkins, R. M., Brown, F. W., et al. (2003). The comorbidity of DSM-III-R personality disorders in somatization disorder. *General Hospital Psychiatry, 14*, 322–326.
8. Simon, G. E., & Gureje, O. (1999). Stability of somatization disorder and somatization symptoms among primary care patients. *Archives of General Psychiatry, 56*, 90–95.
9. Katon, W., Lin, E., Von Korff, M., et al. (1991). Somatization: A spectrum of severity. *The American Journal of Psychiatry, 148*, 34–40.
10. Barsky, A. J., Wyshak, G., & Klerman, G. L. (2003). Hypochondriasis: An evaluation of the DSM-III criteria in medical outpatients. *Archives of General Psychiatry, 43*, 493–500.

11. Salkovskis, P. M., & Warwick, H. M. (1986). Morbid preoccupation, health anxiety and reassurance: A cognitive-behavioral approach to hypochondriasis. *Behaviour Research and Therapy, 24*, 597–602.
12. Hyler, S. E., & Spitzer, R. L. (1978). Hysteria split asunder. *The American Journal of Psychiatry, 135*, 1500–1504.
13. Martin, R. L. (1992). Diagnostic issues for conversion disorder. *Hospital & Community Psychiatry, 43*, 771–773.
14. Chang, D. F., Myers, H. F., Yeung, A., et al. (2005). Shenjing shuairuo and the DSM-IV: Diagnosis, distress, and disability in a Chinese primary care setting. *Transcultural Psychiatry, 42*, 204–218.
15. LeiKeiknes, K. A., Finset, A., Mount, T., et al. (2007). Current somatoform disorders in Norway: Prevalence, risk factors and comorbidity with anxiety, depression and musculoskeletal disorders. *Social Psychiatry and Psychiatric Epidemiology, 42*, 698–710.
16. Sullivan, M. D. (2000). DSM-IV pain disorder: A case against the diagnosis. *International Review of Psychiatry, 12*, 91–98.
17. Phillips, K. A., McElroy, S. L., Hudson, J. I., et al. (1995). Body dysmorphic disorder: An obsessive-compulsive spectrum disorder, a form of affective spectrum disorder, or both? *The Journal of Clinical Psychiatry, 56*(suppl. 4), 41–51.
18. Lowe, B., Mundt, M., Herzog, W., et al. (2008). Validity of current somatoform disorder diagnoses: Perspectives for classification in DSM-V and ICD-11. *Psychopathology, 41*, 4–9.
19. Kroenke, K., Sharpe, M., Sykes, R., et al. (2007). Revising the classification of somatoform disorders: Key questions and preliminary recommendations. *Psychosomatics, 48*, 277–285.
20. Janka, A. (2005). Rethinking somatoform disorders. *Current Opinion in Psychiatry, 18*, 65–71.
21. Creed, F. (2006). Can DSM-V facilitate productive research into the somatoform disorders? *Journal of Psychosomatic Research, 60*, 331–334.
22. Smith, R., Gardiner, J., Lyles, J., et al. (2005). Exploration of DSM-IV criteria in primary care patients with medically unexplained symptoms. *Psychosomatic Medicine, 67*, 123–129.
23. Hanel, G., Henningsen, P., Herzog, W., et al. (2009). Depression, anxiety, and somatoform disorders: Vague or distinct categories in primary care? Results from a large cross-sectional study. *Journal of Psychosomatic Research, 67*, 189–197.
24. Duddu, V., Isaac, M. K., Chaturvedi, S. K., et al. (2006). Somatization, somatosensory amplification, attribution styles and illness behavior: A review. *International Review of Psychiatry, 18*, 25–33.
25. Koh, K. B., & Ki, S. W. (1997). A comparison of illness behavior among patients with somatoform disorders, depressive disorders and psychosomatic disorders. *Korean Journal of Psychosomatic Medicine, 5*, 185–194.
26. Rief, W., Hiller, W., & Margraf, J. (1998). Cognitive aspects of hypochondriasis and the somatization syndrome. *Journal of Abnormal Psychology, 107*, 587–595.
27. Aggarwal, V. R., McBeth, J., Zakrzewska, J. M., et al. (2006). The epidemiology of chronic syndromes that are frequently unexplained: Do they have common associated factors? [see comment]. *International Journal of Epidemiology, 35*, 468–476.
28. Noyes, R., Stuart, S., Watson, D. B., et al. (2006). Distinguishing between hypochondriasis and somatization disorder: A review of the existing literature. *Psychotherapy and Psychosomatics, 75*, 270–281.
29. Koh, K. B., Kim, C. H., & Park, J. K. (2002). Predominance of anger in depressive disorder compared to anxiety disorder and somatoform disorder. *The Journal of Clinical Psychiatry, 63*, 486–492.
30. Koh, K. B., Kim, D. K., Kim, S. Y., et al. (2008). The relation between anger management style, mood, and somatic symptoms in anxiety disorders and somatoform disorders. *Psychiatry Research, 160*, 372–379.
31. Koh, K. B., Kim, D. K., Kim, S. Y., et al. (2005). The relation between anger expression, depression, and somatic symptoms in depressive disorders and somatoform disorders. *The Journal of Clinical Psychiatry, 66*, 485–491.
32. Shipko, S. (1982). Alexithymia and somatization. *Psychotherapy and Psychosomatics, 37*, 193–201.

33. Burba, B., Oswald, R., Grigaliunien, V., et al. (2006). A controlled study of alexithymia in adolescent patients with persistent somatoform pain disorder. *Canadian Journal of Psychiatry, 51*, 468–471.
34. Nunez, G., Rufer, M., Leenen, K., et al. (2010). Quality of life and alexithymia in somatoform pain disorder. *Schmerz, 24*, 62–68.
35. Koh, K. B. (1994). Comparison of alexithymia among patients with psychosomatic disorders, anxiety disorders and depressive disorders. *Korean Journal of Psychosomatic Medicine, 2*, 59–68.
36. Rief, W., & Broadbent, E. (2007). Explaining medically unexplained symptoms-models and mechanisms. *Clinical Psychology Review, 27*, 821–841.
37. Kolk, A. M., Schagen, S., & Hanewald, G. J. (2004). Multiple medically unexplained physical symptoms and health care utilization: Outcome of psychological intervention and patient-related predictors of change. *Journal of Psychosomatic Research, 57*, 379–389.
38. Rief, W., Martin, A., Klaiberg, A., et al. (2005). Specific effects of depression, panic, and somatic symptoms on illness behavior. *Psychosomatic Medicine, 67*, 596–601.
39. Guggenheim, F. G. (2000). Somatoform disorder. In B. J. Sadock & V. A. Sadock (Eds.), *Comprehensive textbook of psychiatry* (7th ed.). Baltimore, MD: Lippincott Williams & Wilkins.
40. Koh, K. B. (2002). *Stress and psychosomatic medicine* (pp. 231–249). Seoul, Korea: Ilchokak.
41. Mezzich, J. E., Lin, K., & Hughes, C. C. (2000). Acute and transient psychotic disorders and culture bound syndromes. In B. J. Sadock & V. A. Sadock (Eds.), *Comprehensive textbook of psychiatry* (7th ed., pp. 1264–1276). Baltimore, MD: Lippincott Williams & Wilkins.
42. Lin, K. M. (1983). Hwa-byung: A Korean culture-bound syndrome? *The American Journal of Psychiatry, 140*, 105–107.
43. Min, S. K. (1989). A study of the concept of hwabyung. *Journal of Korean Neuropsychiatric Association, 28*, 604–616.
44. Lee, S., & Kleinman, A. (2007). Are somatoform disorders changing with time? The case of neurasthenia in China. *Psychosomatic Medicine, 69*, 846–849.
45. Leiknes, K. A., Finset, A., & Moum, T. (2010). Commonalities and differences between the diagnostic groups: Current somatoform disorders, anxiety and/or depression, and musculoskeletal disorders. *Journal of Psychosomatic Research, 68*, 439–446.
46. Nutt, D. J., & Stein, D. J. (2006). Understanding the neurobiology of comorbidity in anxiety disorders. *CNS Spectrums, 11*, 13–20.
47. Koh, K. B., Kang, J. I., Lee, J. D., et al. (2010). Shared neural activity in panic disorder and undifferentiated somatoform disorder compared with healthy controls. *The Journal of Clinical Psychiatry, 71*, 1576–1581.
48. Valet, M., Gundel, H., Sprenger, T., et al. (2009). Patients with pain disorder show gray-matter loss in pain-processing structures: A voxel-based morphometric study. *Psychosomatic Medicine, 71*, 49–56.
49. Uchida, R. R., Del-Ben, C. M., Busatto, G. F., et al. (2008). Regional gray matter abnormalities in panic disorder: A voxel-based morphometry study. *Psychiatry Research, 163*, 21–29.
50. van Tol, M.-J., van der Wee, N. J. A., van den Heuvel, O. A., et al. (2010). Regional brain volume in depression and anxiety disorders. *Archives of General Psychiatry, 67*, 1002–1011.
51. Drevets, W. C. (2001). Neuroimaging and neuropathological studies of depression: Implications for the cognitive-emotional features of mood disorders. *Current Opinion in Neurobiology, 11*, 240–249.
52. Koh, K. B., Choi, E. H., Lee, Y., et al. (2011). Serotonin-related gene pathways associated with undifferentiated somatoform disorder. *Psychiatry Research, 189*, 246–250.
53. Koh, K. B., Kim, C. H., Choi, E. H., et al. (2012). Effect of tryptophan hydroxylase gene polymorphism on aggression in major depressive disorder and undifferentiated somatoform disorder. *The Journal of Clinical Psychiatry, 73*, e574–e579.
54. Zill, P., Baghai, T. C., Zwanzger, P., et al. (2004). SNP and haplotype analysis of a novel tryptophan hydroxylase isoform (TPH2) gene provide evidence for association with major depression. *Molecular Psychiatry, 9*, 1030–1036.

55. Oquendo, M. A., & Mann, J. J. (2001). Neuroimaging findings in major depression, suicidal behavior and aggression. *Clinical Neuroscience Research, 1*, 377–380.
56. Rosenthal, N. E., Mazzanti, C. M., Barnett, R. L., et al. (1998). Role of serotonin transporter promoter repeat length polymorphism (5-HTTLPR) in seasonality and seasonal affective disorder. *Molecular Psychiatry, 3*, 175–177.
57. Maron, E., Hettema, J. M., & Shlik, J. (2010). Advances in molecular genetics of panic disorder. *Molecular Psychiatry, 15*, 681–701.
58. Koh, K. B., Sohn, S.-H., Kang, J. I., et al. (2012). Relationship between neural activity and immunity in patients with undifferentiated somatoform disorder. *Psychiatry Research: Neuroimaging, 202*, 252–256.
59. Schleifer, S. J., Keller, S. E., Scotte, B. J., et al. (1990). Lymphocyte function in panic disorder. *Biological Psychiatry, 27*(suppl. 9A), 66A.
60. Surman, O. S., Williams, J., Sheehan, D. V., et al. (1986). Immunological response to stress in agoraphobia and panic attacks. *Biological Psychiatry, 21*, 768–774.
61. Brambilla, F., Bellodi, L., Perna, G., et al. (1992). Psychoimmunoendocrine aspects of panic disorder. *Neuropsychobiology, 26*, 12–22.
62. Andreoil, A., Keller, S. E., Taban, C., et al. (1990). Immune function in major depressive disorder: Relation to panic disorder comorbidity. *Biological Psychiatry, 27*(suppl. 9A), 95A.
63. Koh, K. B., & Lee, B. K. (1998). Reduced lymphocyte proliferation and interleukin-2 production in anxiety disorders. *Psychosomatic Medicine, 60*, 479–483.
64. Koh, K. B., & Lee, Y. (2004). Reduced anxiety level by therapeutic interventions and cell-mediated immunity in panic disorder patients. *Psychotherapy and Psychosomatics, 73*, 286–292.
65. Marazziti, D., Ambrogi, F., Vanacore, R., et al. (1992). Immune cell imbalance in major depressive and panic disorders. *Neuropsychobiology, 26*, 23–26.
66. Irwin, M. R., & Miller, A. H. (2007). Depressive disorders and immunity: 20 years of progress and discovery. *Brain, Behavior, and Immunity, 21*, 374–383.
67. Zorrilla, E. P., Luborsky, L., McKay, J. R., et al. (2001). The relationship of depression and stressors to immunological assays: A meta-analytic review. *Brain, Behavior, and Immunity, 15*, 199–226.

Part II
Theoretical Approaches to Mind and Body

Chapter 2
Toward a Philosophy of Life to Underpin Personhood in Medicine

Osborne P. Wiggins and Michael Alan Schwartz

2.1 Introduction

2.1.1 Modern Heritage and the Puzzle About Persons in Medical Practice

Hans Jonas has broken new ground in the history of Gnosticism [1] and modernity [2], medical ethics [3], and philosophical biology [4]. He has been embraced by people on the political left and others on the political right. Our presentation draws on his interpretation of modernity and his attempt in his philosophical biology to provide a new path out of some of the dead ends of modernity. As Jonas knew, these concerns have a direct bearing on how we think about medicine.

Modern medicine has enjoyed much success by drawing on those sciences which study the most elementary components of living beings, namely, the sciences of physics, chemistry, genetics, and others. There can be no doubt that these basic sciences do and will play large roles in helping to explain and treat diseases and injuries of various kinds. However, such sciences fall far short in providing for medical practitioners, especially clinicians, a conception of the patient as a living human self that is needed for the practical purposes of healthcare.

O.P. Wiggins, Ph.D.
Philosophy Department, 313 Bingham Humanities Building,
University of Louisville, Louisville, KY 40292, USA
e-mail: opwigg01@louisville.edu

M.A. Schwartz, M.D. (✉)
Departments of Humanities in Medicine and Psychiatry,
Texas A&M Health Science Center College of Medicine,
Round Rock Campus, 3950 North A. W. Grimes Blvd, Round Rock, TX 78665, USA
e-mail: michael.schwartz@mas1.cnc.net

K.B. Koh (ed.), *Somatization and Psychosomatic Symptoms*,
DOI 10.1007/978-1-4614-7119-6_2, © Springer Science+Business Media New York 2013

2.1.2 Approaches to This Puzzle

In its approach this chapter is divided into two main sections: historical background and conditions for life. The two sections are continuous with one another by drawing on the philosophy of living beings developed by Hans Jonas.

In historical background, we shall briefly sketch the history of modern conceptions of human life which lead to our present-day puzzlement. This sketch will lead to the recognition of the *mind/body problem* as the persistent intellectual framework from which we still have not succeeded in escaping. As the new sciences of nature emerged in the seventeenth and eighteenth centuries, a philosophical framework for trying to unify the ever-expanding multiplicity of theories and concepts took shape. This framework consisted in a *hierarchy of the sciences,* each higher level science being theoretically dependent upon the concepts and laws of sciences of the lower levels. This hierarchy of the sciences, however, gave rise to an attempt to simplify them all by proposing an all-encompassing *naturalism,* the philosophy that all the sciences would (and must) someday be reduced to physics. Reductionistic naturalism has never proven to fully satisfy the modern mind, however, and consequently the mind/body dualism persisted to thwart attempts to see living beings – human beings in particular – as unified wholes. Present-day efforts in medicine to make overall sense of the patient as a *person* thus encounter road blocks.

2.2 Historical Background

2.2.1 The Modern Hierarchy of the Sciences and Reductionism

By placing its confidence in the ability of physics, chemistry, and other such fundamental sciences to furnish its conceptual base, medicine adheres to an understanding of the relations among the sciences that is at least a century and a half old. In the middle of the nineteenth century, Auguste Comte was the first thinker to explicitly set forth an ordering of the sciences into a hierarchy that is tacitly taken for granted today [5]. According to this hierarchy mathematics is the most fundamental of the sciences. It is the most fundamental because it articulates the formal relations of the elements of any science whatsoever. Founded on mathematics and logically presupposing it is physics. Based on physics and presupposing it is chemistry. Based on chemistry and logically rooted in it is biology. Founded on all of these natural sciences are the social sciences, such as psychology and sociology. The social sciences differ from the natural sciences because the social sciences fall into no particular rank ordering among themselves; logically and conceptually they seem to reside on the same level. Comte claimed that this hierarchy followed two principles: (1) a science was more basic if it was more comprehensive or more inclusive and (2) a science was more basic if its components were simpler. Hence, to illustrate the first principle, physics was more comprehensive than chemistry because all chemical realities are physical, but not all physical realities are chemical. And, to illustrate the second principle, the constituents of physical realities that physics studies are simpler in their makeup than are the constituents of chemical realities; the elements of chemistry include elements of physics plus something more, something that renders them distinctively chemical.

This conception of the hierarchical dependencies among the sciences continues to dominate our thinking to the present day. Because the hierarchy entails that the higher level sciences are conceptually based on the lower level ones, repeated attempts have been made to simplify the overall picture of the universe by showing how the higher level sciences can be *reduced to* the lower level ones.

Now "reductionism" in the sciences can be understood in different senses. The way in which we understand it here is that a higher level science is reduced to a lower level one if the higher level science can be logically derived from the concepts and laws of the science just below it. Ideally such a reductionism implies that *all* the concepts and laws of all the sciences should be reducible to the concepts and laws of mathematical physics.

A less stringent notion of reductionism is very prominent today. It is called "naturalism." It stipulates that any entity that is not physical, chemical, or biological will ultimately be logically explainable in terms of these natural sciences. In other words, all realities that are not yet considered natural realities will be in the future fully explained by the natural sciences. In other words, the natural sciences will ultimately provide the concepts and laws that explain the whole of reality, even those parts that are now studied by the social sciences and humanities. Moreover, it is incumbent on scientists at work today to search for possible reductionistic connections. For example, neuroscience is today thought to hold out the hope for a reduction of mental processes of all sorts to brain structures and processes, a reduction that would ideally eliminate all need to even use the terms "mental" or "psychological."

Much of the resistance to such a reductionism arises from the fact that thinkers in the social sciences and humanities persist in talking about realities and events that seem to be irreducible. For social sciences to speak of mental processes such as ideas, emotions, purposes, or moods is for them to use a terminology not derived from the natural sciences. Modern-day naturalism has a response to such an "unscientific" way of speaking. Talk about mental events of all sorts is thought by naturalists to be merely a holdover from "folk psychology." Folk psychology is simply a prescientific, commonsensical way of speaking. As genuine science develops, it will progressively eliminate the need to resort to such nonscientific terms, and in their place we can refer to events and structures in the brain. In other words, the vocabulary of neuroscience will entirely replace the words of everyday speech, "folk psychological" words.

2.2.2 The Mathematization of Nature and Mind/Body Dualism

The depositing of all words and concepts of mental events into the despised category of "folk psychology" illustrates merely the most recent case of having to find some separate sphere for mind. Since we cannot avoid referring constantly to mental processes, we seek to circumvent our dependence on them by drawing strict lines of demarcation between mental events and "true reality," that is, natural reality. We are historically familiar with these determined attempts at strict separation through our troubled heritage of "the mind/body problem."

From the moment Descartes sought to define the external world as *res extensa,* he had to admit that it bore little resemblance to that other, equally real "reality," *res cogitans* [6]. Thus began the dualism of the two metaphysically different realms, physical body and nonphysical mind. And, according to some philosophers of the seventeenth and eighteenth centuries, not only were the physical and the mental fundamentally different but also they were completely separate in their operations and laws. For these thinkers, mind did not determine matter, and matter did not determine mind. On the other hand, some writers sought to locate a point of mutual interaction – Descartes' "pineal gland" being the most well known – while still others recognized the hopelessness of the attempt.

Descartes also defined the model of *pure* nature that the new science of nature would study. By defining the metaphysical basis of the physical realm as *res extensa,* Descartes strips it of all properties except its mathematizable ones. *Res extensa* means "extended thing" or "extended substance." By categorizing physical matter as exclusively extended, Descartes defines it as possessing solely geometrical properties. No other properties belong to it. The mathematization of reality had at first to take the form of geometrization because analytical geometry was the most advanced mathematics of Descartes' time. In other words, what Descartes was saying was that true nature possesses solely mathematical properties. The laws of nature must then be formulatable as algebraic equations and geometrical figures. This set the program for future natural science; one can arrive at the ultimate truth about nature when one can conceptualize its movements and constituents with mathematical formulae alone. All other properties of nature were abstractly disregarded. What happens to these abstractly discarded properties? Do they simply vanish? No, they stubbornly remain in some form that has now, with the abstraction, been rendered mysterious. But at this juncture the usefulness of positing a separate domain of *res cogitans* becomes clear; everything that was excluded from the sphere of nature can be conveniently deposited in the sphere of mind.

Let us cite just two examples of the abstractions that were necessary to constitute the domain of "pure matter," that is, matter stripped of all properties except mathematical ones. Our first example of disregarded features is *teleology* and, with the exclusion of goal-directed behavior, the discarding of teleological explanations. All changes in nature, including alterations in biological organisms, must be explained as the results of antecedent causal conditions. Already Francis Bacon had branded teleological explanations as *anthropomorphic* fallacies: human investigators were all too prone to understand natural events in terms of the human mind. To avoid this, scientists must carefully check this human weakness in themselves and systematically refrain from seeing goal-directed behavior in things. The appearance of teleology was an anthropomorphic illusion [7].

Our other example is the abstraction that systematically disregards values and norms. The *fact/value distinction* was firmly in place at least by the time of David Hume (1711–1776). Science was "empirical" only to the extent that it studied a nature of *pure facts* [8]. At this stage, the time of the European Enlightenment, values were not banished; they were simply confined to other disciplines such as moral or political philosophy.

The usefulness of this modern dualism cannot be overestimated for the early development of the natural sciences. It allowed these natural scientists to abstract from everything mental, social, political, economic, and religious and to attend exclusively to what remained, matter and the physical forces that determined it. Moreover, natural scientists could apply various *idealizations* to this matter if applied to the mind and its workings. The most obvious example here is *the idealization of strict causal determination.* If we assert that the changes in matter are strictly determined by antecedent causal events, we can proceed to seek out these prior events and their law-governed relations to the ensuing changes. However, if we apply this idealization to the investigation of mental changes, we implicitly – if not explicitly – deny any freedom to the will. If, on the other hand, we conceive of the will as a faculty of the mind alone, then our dualism of mind and matter allows us to place free will in the mental realm and strict causal determinism in the physical.

Human thinkers seem, however, to remain unhappy with dualistic systems which so sharply divide reality into metaphysically different spheres. The thinking intellect appears to long for a *monism,* a single unified system into which all of reality can at least potentially fit. And therefore as dissatisfactions grew more troubling in the early modern period, monisms were proposed: idealism, the monism of mind, and materialism, the monism of matter. But a monism satisfies finally only if it can absorb the other reality into itself. So idealism must explain our persistent experiences of matter as somehow ultimately a mental reality itself. And similarly, materialism works only if it can successfully account for the persistence of our own subjective experiences with purely physical concepts. Each, of course, has proven itself unable to prevail over the other. But it should be remembered that there are versions of "naturalism" prominent today which still strenuously aspire to a monism and seek to account for our subjective experiences as somehow or other merely natural processes in the brain.

2.2.3 Darwinism and the Need to Rethink Life

In the middle of the nineteenth century, Darwin's theory of evolution disturbed the peace that metaphysical dualism had sought to establish [9, 10]. The Darwinian approach explained the human mind as having evolved through the same regular processes of chance mutation and natural selection that had produced all other living beings. Hence, the human mind was incorporated back into the physical domain, and as a consequence the mind required no other explanation than that which natural science could now offer. Natural science was thereby seen as *universal: all of reality* could be understood in the same basic scientific terms and laws [4].

This universalizing of scientific conceptualization seemed to betoken the victory of *metaphysical materialism*. If all of reality could be explained by science, then all of reality could ultimately be explained in terms of the most basic constituents that science had uncovered, namely, inorganic matter. Hence, we need not speak of "mind," "spirit," or "soul" anymore except to demonstrate how even these phenomena could be accounted for fully by a law-governed physical causality.

Such a metaphysical materialism, if it could be developed, would signal the victory of what Gabriel Marcel has called "the spirit of abstraction" and what Alfred North Whitehead labeled "the fallacy of misplaced concreteness" [11–13]. The "spirit of abstraction" consists in mistaking parts of reality that have been *intellectually separated out* from other parts of the same reality and treating the abstract parts as *actually existing as separate* from the other parts. The fallacy of misplaced concreteness goes one step further and seeks to explain all the other parts of reality as produced or caused by this privileged part. The intellectually abstracted part is thus treated as the most "concrete" dimension of reality from which the other dimensions are derived. In metaphysical materialism this is precisely what has happened; the part of reality which is inorganic, purely physical matter, the part studied by physics, has been intellectually abstracted from the other parts of reality and deemed the primary, fundamental, or basic part.

Hans Jonas' approach opposes such a privileging of one part of reality and deeming it the most "concrete" or formative part. Indeed, he opposes all forms of reductionism. And he does this precisely by interpreting the Darwinian breakthrough in a different way. If, in this post-Darwinian age, we must now account for everything living and nonliving in a unified system of thought, then we should be able to draw on everything we know about the living and nonliving in our account of reality. In other words, the Darwinian victory reincorporates into our understanding of living beings *the entire human realm* which materialism had excluded, and it does so with the demand that we now see the living world as a unified whole. Hence, we seem to be called on to develop a theory of this unitary whole which is life in both its mental and physical dimensions.

Still it seems we cannot heed this call. We cannot because we in the West have inherited a centuries-long understanding of life that is dualistic, and this heritage is not easily discarded. Just as in the past, the unacceptability of dualism has led merely to the reduction of one side to the other, to either materialism or idealism, so today the most popular attempt to construct a monism is *naturalism* which is nothing other than materialism in a new guise.

This leaves the reality of life, most obviously human life, inconceivable except by reducing it to one monism or the other. And it is human life, in illness and health, which centrally concerns medicine. What medicine needs is a non-dualistic, a post-dualistic, theory of life.

Hence, the question arises of how to develop such a theory. Obviously we must fully appreciate what the separate sciences have taught us, but we should view them all, the natural sciences, the social sciences, and the humanities, as equally important contributions to the general theory. And yet it is the sprawling multiplicity of these disciplines that must be overcome. Overcoming it will require overcoming the one-sidedness and exclusivity that limits each.

What should be the starting point of our inclusive, unified philosophy of life? Beyond abstract theories, an indispensable beginning for the development of a non-dualistic philosophy of life can be found *in the directly and constantly felt reality of being alive in ourselves.* This determines our starting point because here we can claim *privileged access: since we are living beings ourselves, we know what it means to be alive from our own first-hand experience.* Every moment of our lives we directly experience life, life in ourselves and in others. Our most intimate experience of life is in our own individual lives. But this constant experience of our own being alive makes it possible for us to make sense of the being alive of other people and, to some extent, of animals. We move beyond abstract theories here because we cannot imagine a datum more *concrete* than the experience of ourselves in our constant living reality. Direct reflection on this experience reveals to us the basis of any other experience of life. And such a concrete given is certainly more basic than any of our theorizing about life [14].

Quite independently of Jonas, the zoologist Adolf Portmann has put forward the same idea. In order to develop a non-reductionistic view of all forms of life, Portmann writes,

> … we must, then, also emphasize – more than is usually done –what we owe to the knowledge of our own inner life for the understanding of all animal existence. There is also a continuous stream of interpretation flowing from our own experience into our biological work with animals, a stream that can only come from that special wellspring of our own experience. This subjectivity should not be perfunctorily deemed suspect for being all too human, but, rather, should be made use of in a meaningful way. The vision of life looking down from above, from the point of view of the human being is a necessary complement to the attempt at building from beneath, to proceeding from the simplest forms. [15]

Hence, we should be able to start from both sides – from the side of what science can tell us about inorganic, organic, psychological, and social realities and from the side of our own direct experience of life in ourselves and in others – and show how these realities meet in the living being. If dualism is to be discarded, then we must strive for a unified understanding of life, an understanding that fully appreciates both the natural processes of the organism and the inward-felt experiences of being alive. Hence, aiming at their intersection, we shall reason from both directions.

We do this in the confidence that life is ultimately *one* reality, however complex. Human beings are *psychosomatic wholes,* and therefore, a theory that reintegrates *psyche* with *soma* can be developed as long as no component of the whole is short changed. We shall search for features that characterize *life as such,* whether "objective" or "subjective." These features of living beings in general emerge, in our view, as *conditions for being alive.* If the organism ceases to meet the conditions we shall outline, it will cease to live. Hence, they might be called "necessary conditions of life." We shall now, drawing on Jonas, attempt to describe some of these vital conditions [4, 11].

2.3 Conditions for Life

In this second part of this chapter, we employ the method sketched just above and seek to lay out conditions for being alive that are found in both the mental and the more physical dimensions of life. These conditions are the following: (1) the necessity for living individuals to *constantly act* in order to sustain their ongoing existence; (2) the *separateness* of the individual living being from its environment while at the same time maintaining an *openness* to the environment and engaging in *transactions* with it; (3) the necessity for the organism to undergo constant change while always making a sameness of self throughout this change; (4) the directedness of the organism's activity toward its own future being, hence the teleological orientation of organic processes; (5) the origin of feelings in higher life forms. These five conditions of life can serve as a framework within a unified conception of the person which for the purposes of medicine includes both the more physical and the more mental dimensions of patients.

2.3.1 *The Need for Self-Preservation*

The existence of every living being is sustained through metabolism. Unlike inorganic matter, the very being of a living entity is contingent upon its own ceaseless *activity.* As a result the existence of the organism from moment to moment is its own *dynamic achievement.* Inorganic matter need not *actively do* anything in order to endure as the being it is, but organisms must. This inescapable need to persistently bring about their own continuation through their own metabolic functioning proves that organisms are *threatened* beings: if they do not actively achieve and repeatedly re-achieve their own reality, they die. Ceaselessly dependent on their own functioning for their survival, organisms hang suspended over the abyss of nonbeing. Hence, we can acknowledge one of the conditions that necessarily define life: *always threatened by nonbeing, the organism must constantly reassert its being through its own activity* [2, 4].

2.3.2 *Enclosed Within the Self and Open to the World*

This activity, however, must be an *organized* activity. Metabolic processes are structured processes, and it is this very structure of the processes of the organism that must be maintained as such. When the structure fails to determine the direction of the processes, the organism dies. Accordingly, the identity of the organism depends on the maintenance of its internal structure. We might even say that the identity of the organism is the identity of the structure. This becomes even more obvious when we note that the components that constitute the organism are constantly changing. The material components of the organism come and go, but it is important that the organism remains as the same one. To "remain as the same one" is to maintain the same structure even in the midst of constant change of components. In order to maintain this constant change of its components, however, the organism must to some extent be *open* to its environment, the ultimate source of the components. We are now in a position to appreciate another one of the distinctive conditions of being alive. *Living beings are both enclosed within themselves, defined by the boundaries that separate them from their environment, while they are also ceaselessly reaching out to their environment and engaging in transactions with it.* This vital feature is found even in the single cell [2], and it continues in different forms all the way up to social institutions.

On the one hand, the cell membrane determines the cell's boundaries: the reality of the cell extends no farther than this membrane. And indeed these boundaries must be maintained if the cell is to continue to be. Hence, the membrane must maintain the separation of the cell from the rest of reality. Death consists in the loss of this separation. This need to remain bounded and distinct from that which is outside is observed at all levels of life. From the single cell, through the different organs of animal bodies, to the level of human beings as whole persons, "self" and "other" are definitely distinguished. This distinction between self and other is demonstrated most clearly, of course, in the immune system. The immune system is geared to detect what is nonself, and once this detection of otherness occurs, the immune system actively opposes the invader.

On the other hand, the membrane is semipermeable so that the cell may continually exchange its material with realities outside of it. Literally *through* its membrane the cell metabolically carries on transactions with that which is not itself. Indeed, this transaction with other entities is necessary if the cell is to maintain its existence; the cell is physically dependent upon the outside for its continuation in being. This dependency on what is not itself in order to survive evinces the organism's *neediness;* lacking self-sufficiency, the living being must of necessity acquire the means for its existence from its environment. However, this unavoidable exposure to the environment, born out of need, manifests again the riskiness of organic existence. The environment can prove harmful and even deadly. Moreover, the unfamiliar and uncontrollable nature of the environment poses an additional threat to the already precarious venture, that is, organic life. Hence, the cell is enclosed within its own boundaries in order to maintain its separate and autonomous being while it is also open, constantly engaging in transactions with outside realities and indeed even exchanging its own matter with them.

2.3.3 Change and Sameness

Through the metabolic exchange of material components, the cell undergoes ceaseless change in its physiochemical makeup. But this change is, as we have seen, an organized change: it is determined by the *internal structure* of the cell. Through the change, then, the cell maintains its own separate identity while it also changes the physicochemical parts that compose it. It is both in flux and stable. Maintaining its stable identity through constant turnover in its material constituents, the being of the organism is both independent of and dependent on these constituents. *Some* material constituents are always necessary for the existence of the organism, hence the *dependence* of the organism. But since these constituents will eventually be exchanged for others as the organism continues to live, the organism is *independent* of precisely *these* constituents, that is, of whichever constituents compose it at any given time. We can therefore recognize one of the other conditions of life in organisms: *they are both dependent on the material components that constitute them at any given moment and independent of any particular groupings of these components across time.* These conditions of dependence and independence always define organic existence [2].

2.3.4 The Organism's Teleology and the Basis for Value

As we have said, the metabolic activity of the organism is geared toward sustaining the existence of the organism. This being geared toward the sustaining of its own being shows that the metabolism of the organism is "for the sake of" its own continuation in being. The being that the transactions are geared toward preserving is the organism's *future* being. The metabolic functioning is for the sake of bridging the temporal gap that separates the organism in the present from its own existence in the future. In slightly different terms, metabolic activity serves the *temporal enduring* of the organism. Hence, it is temporal duration that poses the main threat to the organism's contingent existence; the question of whether the organism will endure from moment to moment remains unanswered until the future becomes the present and the organism still lives. And the threat can be defeated only if the activity of metabolism is sustained. Life is thus *teleological*: the present activity of the living being *aims at* its own future being [10, 16].

If we can speak of the metabolic transactions of the organism as occurring "for the sake of" the organism's future being, this means that at some fundamental level the organism posits its own continuation in reality as "good." In other words, the organism posits its own existence as having a positive value. Value is thus built into the reality of being alive; it is organic life itself that places value there. It is not human beings and certainly not human agency that introduces value into an otherwise value-free universe. Living beings themselves, by striving to preserve themselves, already signal that, at least for the being involved, its own life is good [3, 4, 17].

We can see, then, that the values that motivate medical practice are grounded in organic life itself. While only human beings can develop and practice medicine, it is not human beings who introduce into the world the values that call for and justify it. The same would be true for suffering and pain, at least for those organisms that can *feel*. *Felt* suffering and pain are posited by the organism feeling them as bad. Hence, the moral need to relieve and even eradicate pain through medical treatment arises at the most basic levels of life, even if only human beings can recognize this value as a moral requirement and develop the medical techniques to respond to it [3, 4].

2.3.5 The Origin of Feeling in Higher Life Forms

Since we have mentioned *feeling,* we would like to conclude by indicating its importance for any philosophy of life. Although it is difficult to pinpoint the precise level, at some level of life, the organism's relationship with the world becomes a relationship of *feeling;* many organisms are *sensitive to* elements in their environments. Again this applies to individual cells as well as to conglomerates of cells and whole organisms. Sensitivity is the first glimmering of *subjectivity* in organisms, if we may apply the word "subjectivity" to even the most primitive and elemental kinds of feeling. Moreover, as we move up the living kingdom to more and more complex organisms, sensitivity too becomes more complex, and at a certain point we can speak of organisms *perceiving* items composing the environment. It would, of course, be difficult to mark the progressive difference between an elemental *sensitivity* to the outside and an actual *perception* of it, for any form of felt sensitivity may already count as an *experience,* at least of a very basic sort. Our point here is, however, that the first glimmerings of subjectivity arise relatively early in the phylogenetic scale. And once subjectivity appears, it grows in complexity, refinement, and acuity. "Mind," then, is certainly not the exclusive privilege of human beings. It is not even the exclusive possession of the higher animals. Mental life begins where sensitivity to the outside is felt [3].

This birth of subjectivity marks another aspect of the selfhood of living beings. For as subjectivity grows and becomes more complex, the organism is able to sense its environment across spatial distances and to feel a desire for things across time. If we add to this subjectivity the movement of the organism's body, then the living being can move across the spatial distances and pursue objects as long as desires for them are felt. With growing experience and motility, then, living beings confront a world that grows in its spatial extent and its temporal duration. Mind renders organic world-relatedness richer and more encompassing, even if this larger exposure to the outside also expands the realm from which threats to life can emerge [3].

2.4 Conclusions

Medicine's laudable attempt to orient its activities toward the patient as a person encounters the problem that confounds all such attempts in the modern era; the centuries-long persistence of mind/body dualism renders it extremely difficult to conceive of persons as integral wholes. Obviously if such reconceiving of patients is to serve medicine, it must incorporate what we know from present-day biology and other natural sciences as well as what we know about persons as psychological and spiritual beings. The way we have suggested for incorporating the two facets is to reason from both points of view at once and to thereby uncover conditions for life found in each. This integral view supports a medicine that is able to comprehend the personhood of a patient as well as his or her biological being.

References

1. Jonas, H. (1958). *The gnostic religion: The message of the alien God and the beginnings of Christianit*. Boston: Beacon Press.
2. Jonas, H. (1974). *Philosophical essays: From ancient creed to technological man*. Chicago: University of Chicago Press.
3. Jonas, H. (1984). *The imperative of responsibility: In search of an ethics for the technological age*. Chicago: University of Chicago Press.
4. Jonas, H. (1966). *The phenomenon of life: Toward a philosophical biology*. Chicago: University of Chicago Press.
5. Comte, A., & Ferré, F. (1988). *Introduction to positive philosophy*. Indianapolis, IN: Hackett Publishing Company.
6. Gurwitsch, A. (1974). *Phenomenology and the theory of science*. Evanston, IL: Northwestern University Press.
7. Bacon, F. (2009). In L. Jardine, M. Silverthorne (Eds.), *The new organon*. Cambridge University Press, Cambridge.
8. Putnam, H. (2004). *The collapse of the fact/value dichotomy and other essays*. Boston: Harvard University Press.
9. Darwin, C. (1897). *The origin of species by means of natural selection*. New York: D. Appleton and Company.
10. Jonas, H. (1996). *Mortality and morality: A search for the good after Auschwitz*. Chicago: Northwestern University Press.
11. Schwartz, M. A., & Wiggins, O. (1985). Science, humanism and the nature of medical practice: A phenomenological view. *Perspectives in Biology and Medicine, 28*, 331–361.
12. Marcel, G. (1962). *Man against mass society* (G. S. Fraser, Trans.). Chicago: Regnery.
13. Whitehead, A. N. (1948). *Science and the modern world*. New York: New American Library.
14. Schwartz, M. A., & Wiggins, O. P. (2010). Psychosomatic medicine and the philosophy of life. *Philosophy, Ethics, and Humanities in Medicine, 5*, 2.
15. Portmann, A. P. (1990). *A zoologist looks at humankind*. New York: Columbia University Press.
16. Thompson, E. (2007). *Mind in life: Biology, phenomenology, and the sciences of mind*. Boston: Harvard University Press.
17. Grene, M. (1974). *The understanding of nature: Essays in the philosophy of biology*. Heidelberg: Springer.

Part III
Biopsychosociocultural Mechanisms in Psychosomatic Medicine

Chapter 3
Genes, Memes, Culture, and Psychosomatic Medicine: An Integrative Model

Hoyle Leigh

3.1 Evolution of Memes from Memory

The brain evolved as a specialized organ dedicated to processing information. Information is stored as memory, which may be a result of learning, or may be intrinsic, derived from genes. The evolution of the brain facilitated learning, survival, reproduction, and further enlargement of the brain. Learning through trial and error created information that facilitated individual and species survival, but the information contained in the memories died with the organism until the brain developed imitation as a learning tool [1].

With imitation, which is robustly in evidence in primates and in songbirds, information (memory) could be transferred from one brain to other brains in the form of *memes* (which is a term coined by Dawkins, which I use here to denote any portable memory, i.e., information).

Prior to the advent of language, however, most memes residing in individual organisms died with the organisms. Chimpanzees could observe a bright chimpanzee cracking a nut with a stone, and this information could spread, but only to a limited degree. First, they had to be in visual contact with the bright chimpanzee, and second, the bright chimpanzee must engage in the behavior for the meme (how to crack a nut) to spread, and this presupposes that there are nuts and stones around. If chimpanzees had language, one who observed the behavior could describe it even when there were no nuts and stones, and such a meme could spread much faster and wider. Such was the case with humans.

H. Leigh, M.D. (✉)
Department of Psychiatry, University of California, San Francisco, CA, USA

UCSF Fresno, 155 N. Fresno St, Fresno, CA 93701, USA
e-mail: hoyle.leigh@ucsf.edu

K.B. Koh (ed.), *Somatization and Psychosomatic Symptoms*,
DOI 10.1007/978-1-4614-7119-6_3, © Springer Science+Business Media New York 2013

With the development of the written word, memes found an abode outside of brains. Now they could reside in patterns of indentations in clay, stone, and ink in paper, and eventually as electronic signals in magnetic tapes and optical media. Now, more memes reside outside of human brains than inside them, in printed form in libraries and homes, in electronic media, and in digital form in computers, CDs and DVDs, and in the cloud. The acquisition of language by *Homo sapiens* was instrumental in memes' attaining dominance over genes for the first time on planet earth. In fact, memes in the form of moral codes have suppressed gene-derived sexual drive in many cultures, and memes in the form of scientific knowledge provides humans with the ability to control gene propagation.

3.2 Neural Memes and Natural Selection

Kandel described a sequence of events in long-term memory formation in *Aplysia*. With repeated stimulus of a neuron, a sequence of chemical reactions causes gene activation in the nucleus of the neuron, resulting in release of messenger RNA in a dormant form. Further stimulation of the neuron causes a prion-like protein, cytoplasmic polyadenylation element-binding protein (CPEB), which is present in all synapses, to become activated to an infectious form, which in turn activates the dormant messenger RNA, which in turn makes protein to form a new synapse. The prion-like infectious form of CPEB infects adjacent CPEB and thus perpetuates itself and the protein synthesis, maintaining and reenforcing the new synaptic connection [2].

In higher organisms, the stimulus that reaches a neuron resulting in this series of events is itself modified in several interneurons which have their own connections, that is, stimulus (perception) is modified by existing memory (memes). Furthermore, neurons are capable of generating impulses without external stimulus, which may stimulate and reinforce connected neural clusters. A reinforced neural cluster may be represented as a binary neural code [3, 4], which represents a meme complex, that is, information that is connected and potentially processed as a unit.

An important aspect of the concept of memes as proposed by Dawkins is that memes are replicators. Originally, Dawkins pointed out that memes are replicated in the brains of those who learn by imitation. As these replications are not always exact, memes undergo Darwinian natural selection and evolution. How about the memes within the brain?

Edelman described Darwinian natural selection of certain clusters of reinforced neurons in the brain in somatic time [5]. *Neuronal groups may be reinforced by signals from other similarly firing neuronal groups (forming memes) and thus gain survival advantage*. One might say that neurons thrive on memes. When a competing meme becomes dominant, neural clusters underlying it are enhanced, that is, better fed, with more synapses. Thus, some memes will become dominant with repeated exposure and rehearsal and proliferate, that is, recruit other neuronal groups; others will become dormant, not forming new connections or recruiting others. The process resulting in new parallel connections may be seen to be a process of replication of the meme, a prion-like replication by contact through synaptic and/or dendritic connection. This is not to imply that one neuron serves only one meme. In fact, a neuron has many connections and may be a component of a number of different memes and memetic connections. Meme replication in the brain, therefore, does not necessarily involve reproducing new neurons, but rather occurs through recombination of component memes in existing neuronal groups. Such replication may occur through meme-processing mechanisms such as cognition, often stimulated by the entry of new memes into the brain.

3.3 Memeplexes, Development, and Psychopathology

Why are our brains full of thoughts? According to Blackmore [6], the answer lies in the fact that memes are replicators, and the thoughts we have are expert replicators that survived Darwinian selection.

While most of the memes in our brains come from outside of the brains, some memes are created or cobbled together in new combinations within our brains in the form of new memeplexes. Our brain is full of memes and memeplexes that we have acquired over time. Some examples of memeplexes include the following: "I am intelligent," "good," "evil," "health," "God," "Devil," "socialism," and "psychosomatic medicine." Memeplexes may be complexes of ideas, sounds, and other perceptual memories, for example, songs, scenes, posters, and jingles.

Humans live in niches of memes called culture. Culture consists of memes such as language, rules, morals, religion, beliefs, traditions, and esthetics. It also consists of matter-meme complexes like food, buildings, and edifices. In any meme pool we call culture, there are prevalent or dominant memes and non-prevalent, recessive, and/or latent memes.

Niches, by definition, tend to be stable habitats, and memes that form a particular niche are those that made stable copies of themselves over time, that is, did not change much. Memetic niche culture, therefore, tends to be conservative, that is, resistant to change. The conservative meme pool incorporated, over time, memetic infrastructures to support the existing gene-meme social power structure, such as hereditary caste, wealth, and access to information. Social customs, religions, rituals, and other codes of conduct are such memeplexes that support the dominant culture. Cultural artifacts such as books, scripture, churches, and tombs all embed such memes.

The environment consists of memes and potential memes like a culture medium in a Petri dish. The culture medium consists of molecules, some of them nutrients, others toxins, and yet others inert. Some enter the organism and become part of it or give it energy. Others may simply enter and stay without much effect. Under certain conditions, such as an increase in the concentration of the toxic molecules, some such molecules will penetrate the protective barrier of the organism and cause a reaction in the host – perhaps an immune reaction that gets rid of the toxic molecule, or the organism may succumb to the toxin. The shape and nature of the toxic molecule play important roles in whether it enters the host and what happens afterwards. So with memes. The shapes and other characteristics of the vehicles of memes are physical in nature such as printed words, spoken words, melodies, rhythm, scenes,

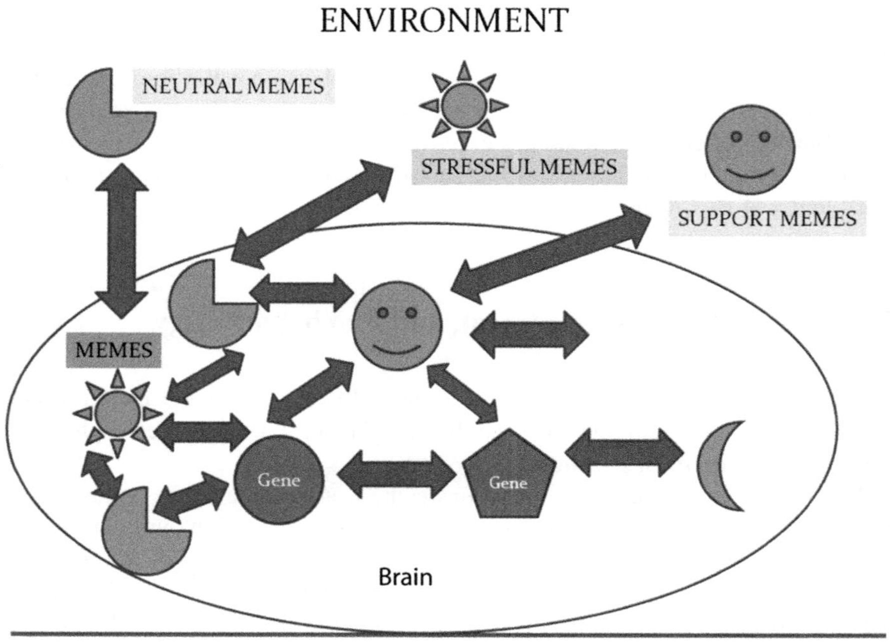

Fig. 3.1 Memes in environment and brain

movements, facial expressions, and touch. Those memes that are endemic are the cultural memes that enter the brain in early life.

A person is the net result of gene × meme × environment interaction that we call development. Except in rare cases where the environment interacts directly with genes as with environmental toxins and climate, genes interact with memes in the brain, which may have been absorbed directly from the environment as information or may have been induced through experiential learning. Some newly introduced memes may conflict with existing memes in the brain and may either die or become dormant (unconscious). Others may combine with existing dormant memes and activate them (Fig. 3.1).

While the aggregate of these memes and memeplexes constitute our personalities, some such acquired memes are pathogens and in interaction with genes and other "host factors" may cause mental or psychosomatic illness. Treating such an infection may require the equivalents of either a pathogen-specific antibody or a broad-spectrum antibiotic therapy. Prevention may also be possible through appropriate immunization.

3.4 Gene × Meme × Environment Interaction in the Pathogenesis of Stress-Related Disorders

A single gene that codes for the vulnerability to multiple stress-related disorders is the serotonin transporter gene (SERT) and its promoter region polymorphism (5HTTLPR). SERT is highly evolutionarily conserved and regulates the entire serotonergic system

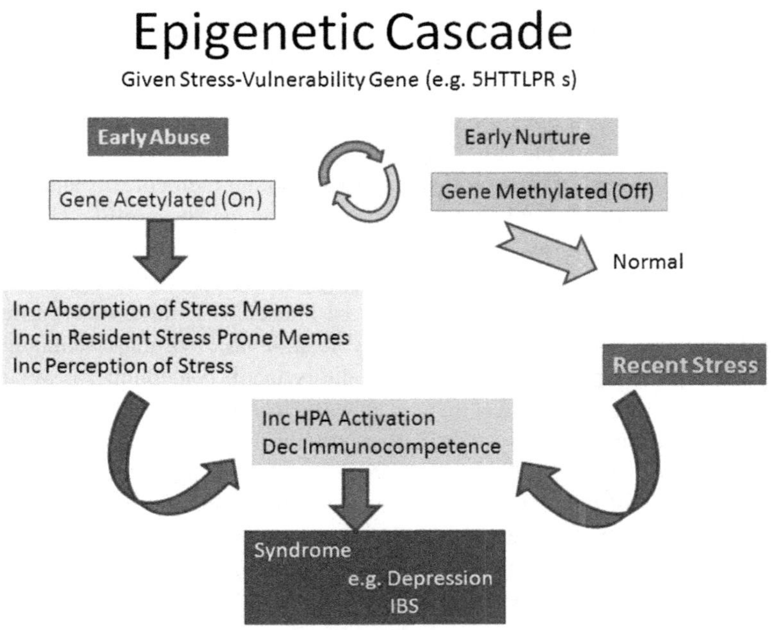

Fig. 3.2 Epigenetic cascade

and its receptors via modulation of extracellular fluid serotonin concentrations. 5HTTLPR polymorphism consists of short (s) and long (l) alleles, and the presence of the short allele tends to reduce the effectiveness and efficiency of SERT. The short allele has been identified as the underlying variation for increased anxiety, increased neuroticism, smoking behavior, especially to reduce negative mood and feel stimulated, difficulty in quitting smoking, social phobia, major depression, and irritable bowel syndrome [7–10].

Genes may create an environment in the brain that is more hospitable to certain types of memes than others. For example, in the presence of the short allele of the serotonin transporter promoter gene (5HTTLPR), the amygdala tends to be more sensitive to threatening stimuli (memes) [11, 12] In spite of the gene, if the child experiences abundant nurturance, the gene may be turned off. On the other hand, if the child is mistreated, the brain will respond with increased fear, anxiety, and helplessness, generating corresponding memes, which are likely to epigenetically activate the vulnerability gene. Such a brain would be more susceptible to infection by depressive and dysphoric memes and memeplexes coming from social interactions, learning, and even the media. A stressful event in adulthood may then infuse the brain with a massive dose of depressive memes. Thus, a brain that is already inhabited with a large number of depressive memes (most of which may be unconscious) may be overwhelmed by addition of new infection resulting in a depressive syndrome, a state of total control by the depressive memes (Fig. 3.2).

Ross postulated that a person becomes vulnerable to "psychosomatic memes" when in distress [13]. He writes, "the anguish of distress compels the sufferer to give it a name…a meaning…Like a virus that incorporates into a cell by fitting a forged protein into a cell receptor, a psychosomatic meme incorporates into a host by providing the "key" to the suffering."

Explanatory concepts of symptoms and disease are all memeplexes and undergo evolution within and across cultures. Somatic sensation may be amplified by memes ("I have a serious disease") to the point of hypochondriasis. Psychosomatic memes may be epidemic, as in the case of pseudohypoglycemia in the 1970s [14].

Posttraumatic stress disorder (PTSD) may be likened to a tumor of event-related memes. In massive traumatic stress, there may be an invasion of massive amounts of memes both representing the trauma (visual, auditory, tactile perceptions) as well as the meaning of the trauma (anxiety/fear memes, anger memes, regret memes, guilt memes). The massive infusion of memes results in massive stress hormone activation.

Hippocampus plays an important role in shutting off the HPA activation – any damage or atrophy of the hippocampus attenuates this resulting in a prolonged HPA activation to stress [15, 16]. Certain types of acute stress and many chronic stressors suppress neurogenesis or cell survival in the hippocampus. Glucocorticoids, excitatory amino acids acting on *N*-methyl-D-aspartic acid (NMDA) receptors, and endogenous opioids mediate the suppression [17]. Stress also affects the shape and abundance of dendrites in the hippocampus, amygdala, and prefrontal cortex. Generally, stress results in retraction and simplification of dendrites.

In sum, stress hormones tend to disconnect incoming memes from existing memes (memories), which in turn attenuates resident protective memes, allowing unchecked replication of newly introduced stress memes. These unchecked stress memes find every opportunity to reinforce themselves and replicate as in flashbacks and nightmares. Hypervigilance and avoidance in PTSD may be compensatory mechanisms to reduce the stress meme replication.

3.5 Treatment Approaches

Treatment of depression and stress-related disorders should be geared to (1) attenuating or reversing the brain state that is hospitable to pathologic memes, (2) attenuating or eradicating the strength of the pathologic memes that have taken control of the brain, and (3) regulating the memes in the environment, that is, reducing noxious memes and increasing beneficial memes.

Pharmacologic and surgical (e.g., deep brain stimulation) treatments are primarily geared to changing the brain state. Psychotherapies are essentially treatment modalities geared toward memes, but without the conceptualization of memes, they tend to be haphazard and imprecise and seem mutually exclusive or contradictory. Among extant psychotherapies, cognitive-behavioral therapy (CBT) comes closest to a more explicit understanding of the memes, particularly when the underlying "delusions," which are pathogenic memes, are identified.

As with antibiotics, meme-oriented therapies may be classified into broad-spectrum and specific therapies. Broad-spectrum anti-meme therapies suppress replication of all memes through activities such as meditation, mindfulness, relaxation training, autogenic training, music, dance, and exercise therapies. Specific anti-meme therapies include psychotherapies specifically geared to delusions, phobias, conflicts, etc. The concept of memes may lead to more specific and direct methods of identifying and neutralizing specific memes, for example, through introduction of counter-memes which may be in the form of images, melodies, or sounds.

Placebo is an excellent example of meme-oriented therapy that can result in robust physiologic and brain changes [18–20]. Non-deceptive placebo, in which patients are told that they will be taking a "sugar pill" that has been shown to help symptoms, has been shown to be effective in treating irritable bowel syndrome patients [21]. Virtual reality may be used to create conducive memetic environments, and avatars, images of oneself, may be used as memetic identification figures [22, 23].

In this gene × meme × environment interaction model of epigenetic development, prevention must play a key role. Prevention of epigenetic changes that cause vulnerability to illness, such as childhood abuse, as well as prevention through strengthening of the effective meme-filtering activity of critical thinking is essential in preventing mental, psychosomatic, and stress-related illnesses.

3.6 Conclusions

The brain evolved as a specialized organ for processing information. Information was stored in the brain as memory and died with the organism. With the acquisition of language in humans, memory became portable and spreadable – *memes*. Memes can be stored outside the brain in books and electronic media and spread widely. There are endemic memes we call culture that are introduced into the brains of children from early life. Such endemic memes may be protective or pathogenic. Memes associated with early stress and nurturance cause epigenetic changes and determine genetic vulnerability/resilience for later stress. In the course of development, memes that are stored in the brain as reinforced neural clusters undergo Darwinian natural selection, and some memes become dominant while others become attenuated or dormant. Later stress may result in hormonal changes leading to an attenuation of hippocampal function resulting in an attenuation of protective dominant memes, allowing a massive infusion of stress memes that in turn awaken dormant pathologic memes. This cascade may result in mental and stress-related psychosomatic illness. Treatment of psychosomatic illness should thus be geared to the suppression of pathologic memes as well as toward the prevention and treatment of pathogenic epigenetic changes. Broad-spectrum and specific memetic therapies should be considered. Childhood nurturance, prevention of abuse, and enhancement of meme processing through education are important factors in psychosomatic health.

References

1. Dawkins, R. (1976). *The selfish gene*. New York: Oxford University Press. 224pp.
2. Kandel, E. R. (2006). *In search of memory: The emergence of a new science of mind* (1st ed.). New York: WW Norton & Co. 510pp.
3. Yang, G., Tang, Z., Zhang, Z., et al. (2007). A flexible annealing chaotic neural network to maximum clique problem. *International Journal of Neural Systems, 17*, 183–192.
4. Lin, L., Osan, R., & Tsien, J. Z. (2006). Organizing principles of real-time memory encoding: Neural clique assemblies and universal neural codes. *Trends in Neurosciences, 29*, 48–57.
5. Edelman, G. M. (1987). *Neural Darwinism: The theory of neuronal group selection*. New York: Basic Books. 371pp.
6. Blackmore, S. J. (1999). *The meme machine*. Oxford/New York: Oxford University Press. 264pp.
7. Lotrich, F. E., & Pollock, B. G. (2004). Meta-analysis of serotonin transporter polymorphisms and affective disorders. *Psychiatric Genetics, 14*, 121–129.
8. Hu, S., Brody, C. L., Fisher, C., et al. (2000). Interaction between the serotonin transporter gene and neuroticism in cigarette smoking behavior. *Molecular Psychiatry, 5*, 181–188.
9. Lerman, C., Carporaso, N. E., Audrein, J., et al. (2000). Interacting effects of the serotonin transporter gene and neuroticism in smoking practices and nicotine dependence. *Molecular Psychiatry, 5*, 189–192.
10. Yeo, A., Boyd, P., Lumsden, S., et al. (2004). Association between a functional polymorphism in the serotonin transporter gene and diarrhoea predominant irritable bowel syndrome in women. *Gut, 53*, 1452–1458.
11. Caspi, A., Hariri, A. R., Holmes, A., et al. (2000). Genetic sensitivity to the environment: The case of the serotonin transporter gene and its implications for studying complex diseases and traits. *The American Journal of Psychiatry, 167*, 509–527.
12. Sugden, K., Arseneault, L., Harrington, H., et al. (2010). Serotonin transporter gene moderates the development of emotional problems among children following bullying victimization. *Journal of the American Academy of Child and Adolescent Psychiatry, 49*, 830–840.
13. Ross, S. E. (1999). "Memes" as infectious agents in psychosomatic illness. *Annals of Internal Medicine, 131*, 867–871.
14. Welch, M. (1971). Hypoglycemia. *Ladies Home Journal, 88*, 98–103.
15. McEwen, B. S. (2007). Physiology and neurobiology of stress and adaptation: Central role of the brain. *Physiological Reviews, 87*, 873–904.
16. McEwen, B. S., & Milner, T. A. (2007). Hippocampal formation: Shedding light on the influence of sex and stress on the brain. *Brain Research Reviews, 55*, 343–355.
17. Gould, E., McEwen, B. S., Tanapat, P., et al. (1997). Neurogenesis in the dentate gyrus of the adult tree shrew is regulated by psychosocial stress and NMDA receptor activation. *Journal of Neuroscience, 17*, 2492–2498.
18. Benedetti, F., Mayberg, H. S., Wager, T. J., et al. (2005). Neurobiological mechanisms of the placebo effect. *Journal of Neuroscience, 25*, 10390–10402.
19. Stein, D. J., & Mayberg, H. (2005). Placebo: The best pill of all. *CNS Spectrums, 10*, 440–442.
20. Mayberg, H. S., Silva, J. L., Brannan, S. K., et al. (2002). The functional neuroanatomy of the placebo effect. *The American Journal of Psychiatry, 159*, 728–737.
21. Kaptchuk, T. J., Friedlander, E., Kelley, J. M., et al. (2002). Placebos without deception: A randomized controlled trial in irritable bowel syndrome. *PLoS One, 5*, e15591.
22. Bailenson, J. N. (2006). Transformed social interaction in collaborative virtual environments. In P. Messaris & L. Humphreys (Eds.), *Digital media: Transformations in human communication* (pp. 255–264). New York: Peter Lang.
23. Bailenson, J. N., Yee, N., Blascovich, J., et al. (2008). The use of immersive virtual reality in the learning sciences: Digital transformations of teachers, students, and social context. *Journal of the Learning Sciences, 17*, 102–141.

Chapter 4
Alexithymia and Somatic Symptoms

Gen Komaki

4.1 Introduction

A person's limited ability to understand, process, or describe his/her feelings is referred to as alexithymia, literally "no words for feelings." This concept was first introduced by Sifneos [1] and was formulated from observations of psychosomatic patients who had deficits in their ability to identify, describe, and work with their own feelings as well as having difficulty in distinguishing between their feelings and their bodily sensations. In addition to these deficits, the concept of alexithymia also includes a very limited fantasy life and a cognitive style that is excessively focused on external details.

Although the term "alexithymia" was in the past mainly used for patients suffering from psychosomatic disorders, the concept of alexithymia is currently being used to refer to deficits in the emotional functioning of broader populations with common medical diseases and psychiatric disorders. Assessment of "alexithymia," as reported in the medical literature, is generally based on the Toronto Alexithymia Scale (TAS)-20 [2]. This self-reported alexithymia scale, however, reflects "subjective" difficulties in identifying and describing feelings that can differ from "objectively" identified difficulties. Consequently, it is possible that patients with neuroticism and/or somatization are being identified rather than those who are truly alexithymic. As Sifneos emphasized at every turn, what is really needed is for physicians to learn to recognize the difference between neurotic and alexithymic patients [3].

G. Komaki, M.D., Ph.D. (✉)
School of Health Sciences at Fukuoka, International University of Health and Welfare,
137-1 Enokizu, Ohkawa, Fukuoka 831-8501, Japan
e-mail: komaki@iuhw.ac.jp

K.B. Koh (ed.), *Somatization and Psychosomatic Symptoms*,
DOI 10.1007/978-1-4614-7119-6_4, © Springer Science+Business Media New York 2013

4.2 Alexithymia and Somatic Symptoms

Because of their inability to communicate their feelings, people with alexithymia are prone to communicate through their bodily sensations, seeking help from primary care physicians rather than getting the psychological treatment they need. A quantitative review of the literature showed a small to moderate association between the total score of TAS-20 and somatic symptoms [4]. In many studies, significant associations have been found between alexithymia and somatoform disorder symptoms or somatic symptoms in clinical [5–7] and nonclinical samples [7]. However, contradictory findings have also been reported [8, 9]. When trait anxiety and depression were controlled, no significant association between alexithymia and somatic complaints was found in a community sample [10]. Patients with a tendency to over-report physical symptoms scored significantly high on the TAS-20 "difficulty in identifying feelings" and "difficulty in describing feelings" subscales [7], whereas another subscale, "externally oriented thinking," was not related to somatic symptoms but rather to fewer medical outpatient visits [8]. Because the above studies were dependent on self-reported symptoms and "externally oriented thinking" may truly reflect a tendency toward alexithymia [11], it is difficult to draw concrete conclusions about the relationship between specific dimensions of alexithymia and somatic symptoms, regardless of whether or not the symptoms can be medically explained. As discussed later in 4–5, alexithymia may be associated with a "decoupling" of subjective emotional experience from physiological reactivity in emotionally arousing situations [12]. Neuroimaging studies may help to elucidate the relationship between alexithymia and somatic symptoms [13].

4.3 Alexithymia and Depression

The so-called dimensions associated with difficulties in communicating feelings have been positively related to negative affects such as depression and anxiety [11, 14]. Studies have shown that "difficulty in identifying and describing feelings" is associated with depression. Several studies showed a relationship between "measured alexithymia" and depression [15–18]. One study found that the "difficulty in identifying feelings" and "difficulty in describing feelings" subscale scores were significantly correlated with scores of the Beck Depression Inventory (BDI) [18]. In fact, depressed mood may potentiate alexithymia [19], but alexithymia differs from the cognitive distortions of depression as measured by the BDI. People who score high on the "difficulty in identifying feelings" and "difficulty in describing feelings" subscales may be viewed by others as emotionally aware, or they may use emotional language in relatively complex ways [20]. Clearly, people with high negative affect differ substantially from those with alexithymia who are much less interested in their own psychological and emotional lives.

4.4 Alexithymia and Personality

People with high neuroticism make fewer and less effective attempts at emotional regulation [21], and neuroticism itself is considered to be a stable dimension of normal personality [22]. Although the concept of neurosis has been excluded from the Diagnostic and Statistical Manual of Mental Disorders (DSM), it encompasses a variety of clinical manifestations: depression, anxiety (panic, phobia), hysterical symptoms, hypochondriasis, depersonalization, irritability, and abnormal eating behavior [23]. Neurotic people are aware of their predisposition to experience negative affect and are concerned about negative affect-eliciting situations, and they prefer to avoid them. Neuroticism is a trait that involves a predisposition to experience negative affect and that is considered to have a biological basis [24], whereas alexithymia is a personality trait that reflects a deficiency in emotional experience [20]. Similar to the findings for depression, as stated above, subjects with high TAS-20 scores are prone to show significantly more neurotic traits [25]. However, whether or not a patient's alexithymia scores are truly associated with this personality dimension should be carefully determined. Scores of the "difficulty in identifying feelings" and "difficulty in describing feelings" subscales of TAS-20 showed significant and positive correlations with the neuroticism scores of both the NEO-Five-Factor Inventory (FFI) [26] and the Eysenck Personality Questionnaire [2, 26, 27]. However, for the subscale that assessed "externally oriented thinking," no significant association with neuroticism was shown [2, 26]. In contrast with the "difficulty in identifying feelings" and "difficulty in describing feelings" of TAS-20, "externally oriented thinking" is the cognitive section of TAS-20 and is more accurately rated because the items related to this subscale ask people to rate themselves on a skill or habit that they are easily aware of [28]. Externally oriented thinking is also less influenced by depression or anxiety [29]. Although some researchers have questioned if it represents a salient feature of the alexithymia construct [24, 30], there is a significant and moderate negative correlation between "externally oriented thinking" of TAS-20 and "openness" of the NEO-FFI, which coincides with the results of a previous study [2]. People with low openness are deficient in imaginative ability, so it must be remembered that alexithymic patients have difficulty in finding the appropriate words to describe their feelings. Therefore, this impairment may be due to their impoverished fantasy life [3]. The negative association between "openness" and "externally oriented thinking" also supports the latter as corresponding to a passive and negative attitude toward observing, analyzing, and coping with unknown events and conflicts. Thus, the evidence indicates a strong overlap between the alexithymia construct and "openness to experience," which may be the key personality dimension [22].

4.5 Alexithymia and Interoceptive Awareness

As noted by Craig [31, 32], individual differences in emotional awareness are directly related to differences in the capacity for interoceptive feeling. Alexithymia is considered to be inversely associated with the processing and perception of interoceptive signals, because the characteristics of alexithymia are negatively associated with emotional awareness. However, there are contradictory findings on the interoceptive awareness of subjects with alexithymia.

Researchers have hypothesized that people with alexithymia may be excessively aware of or attuned to their bodies or the undifferentiated arousal that generates somatic sensations, which results in amplification of the sensations as symptoms of physical illness [33, 34]. Further, studies on the relationship between alexithymia and panic disorders have confirmed such tendencies [35–37]. Of the dimensions of TAS-20, however, "difficulty in identifying feelings" had a positive correlation with the severity of anxiety and panic symptoms, which suggests that "high" alexithymia may be associated with the amplification of panic symptoms in patients with panic disorder. In contrast, the experimental studies on alexithymia by Näring et al. [38] and Herbert et al. [39] found rather poorer or blunted perception of heart rate changes, which suggests a lack of interoceptive awareness (e.g., subjects with varying degrees of alexithymia and anxiety/depression). Because heart rate perception correlates with the ability to detect changes in other autonomically innervated organs, it can be said that this variable reflects a general sensitivity to visceral processes, i.e., interoceptive awareness. In fact, these findings showed that, in contrast with the findings for panic disorder patients [36, 37], there was no significant difference in the strength of association between interoceptive awareness, affective alexithymia component related to "difficulty in identifying and describing feelings," and cognitive alexithymia component related to "externally oriented thinking" [39]. Although the cognitive pathways, i.e., neural dysfunction of frontolimbic circuits, have been reported to possibly underlie the panic with "high" levels of alexithymia and hyperarousal toward emotionally related bodily stimuli [37], it remains unknown if and how alexithymia is associated with either physiological hyper- or hypoarousal in the different stages of emotional processing [39]. Further studies are necessary to examine the interaction between interoceptive awareness and the various aspects of alexithymia during physiological arousal with and without different emotional processing. In relation with this, it will be interesting to do neuroimaging studies to examine the relationship between alexithymia and interoceptive awareness [13].

Ikemi Y [40] first coined the term "alexisomia" to designate a condition wherein certain people have difficulty in expressing how their bodies feel. He noted that many people with alexithymia seemed to have reduced awareness of and difficulty in expressing their feelings about both normal and abnormal bodily sensations. This concept of impairment in the awareness of somatic feeling may overlap or be identical to alexithymia, i.e., a deficit in interoceptive awareness.

4.6 Validity Issues in the Assessment of Alexithymia

Recent studies on the relationship of TAS-20 scores with performance-based measurement of emotional ability and the developmental aspects of the emotional awareness in adolescents suggest that the assessment of "alexithymia" based on self-reported questionnaires should be reexamined [41, 42]. To prevent false-positive alexithymia, it would be better to use TAS-20 in combination with non-self-report measures of alexithymia. The non-self-report measures include the Modified Beth Israel Questionnaire, which is based on an interview [43]; Haviland's California Q-Set alexithymia Prototype [44] and his Observer Alexithymia Scale [45], which are rated by collateral informants; and Lane's Levels of Emotional Awareness Scale (LEAS). The LEAS is a tool for assessing the complexity of emotional responses to vignettes and contains performance subtests of various emotional abilities [46].

Igarashi et al. [41] investigated the relationship between the LEAS and TAS-20 scores among college students and found that only the "externally oriented thinking" subscale score of TAS-20 was significantly and negatively correlated with the LEAS scores. This is consistent with the findings of other studies for somatoform disorder patients [11, 47]. Furthermore, "externally oriented thinking" has been more closely associated with various objective measurements regarding emotional regulation, such as physiological indices (e.g., baseline heart rate) [47] and the Affect Consciousness Interview, than the two dimensions related to difficulties in communicating feelings [14, 48]. Therefore, the "externally oriented thinking" subscale may be more fit than the other subscales for the measurement of alexithymia in college students [41] because it is significantly associated with objective measures of emotional awareness (e.g., LEAS) and emotional regulation of bodily functions (e.g., baseline heart rate), as mentioned above.

One study [26] examined the relationship between the alexithymia subscales and age in a normative sample of more than 2,700 people and found that the TAS-20 total score and the "difficulty in identifying feelings" and "difficulty in describing feelings" subscale scores were highest in teenagers, thereafter declined with age, and from the 30s did not change significantly (Fig. 4.1). In contrast, "externally oriented thinking" subscale scores showed an almost linear, positive correlation with age. "Difficulty in identifying feelings" subscale scores were higher for women, while "externally oriented thinking" subscale scores were higher for men, without any interaction between gender and age differences. Such age-related differences in TAS-20 subscale scores indicate developmental aspects of emotional regulation; alexithymia has two components with different developmental paths: "difficulty in identifying feelings/difficulty in describing feelings" and "externally oriented thinking." In particular, this age-related difference in "difficulty in identifying feelings" and "difficulty in describing feelings" might reflect age-related alteration (linear decline with age) of self-consciousness, an aspect of neuroticism that is related to the discrete-emotion construct of shame [49].

Another study [42] indicated that alexithymia in early adolescence is not adequately assessed by self-report questionnaires such as the TAS-20, particularly the "difficulty in identifying feelings" and "difficulty in describing feelings" subscales. More than half of the items of TAS-20 had to be eliminated after exploratory factor analysis due to low factor loading, which indicates the necessity of modifying the content of these subscales or perhaps the need to create a new item pool. As described above, even when teenagers score significantly high on the "difficulty in identifying feelings" and "difficulty in describing feelings" subscales, the scores still might not

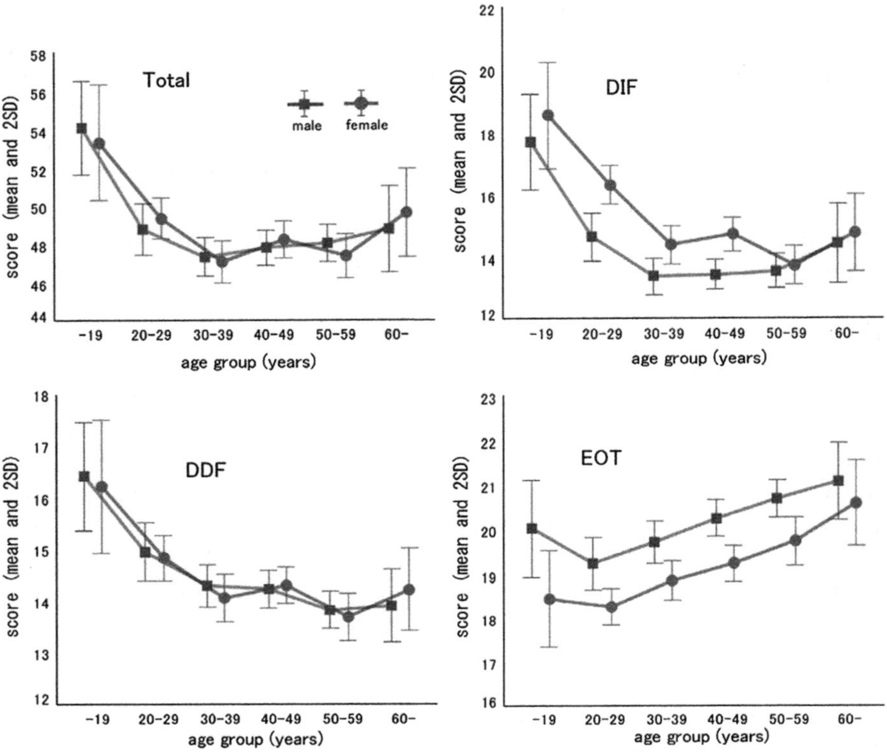

Fig. 4.1 Age-related comparison of TAS-20 total score and subscales scores (mean ± SE) in men and women. *DIF* difficulty in identifying feelings, *DDF* difficulty in describing feelings, *EOT* externally oriented thinking. TAS-20 total score and the DIF and DDF subscale scores were highest for teenagers, thereafter declined with age, and from the 30s did not change significantly. In contrast, EOT subscale scores showed a positive correlation with age ($p<0.05$). DIF subscale scores were higher in women, while EOT subscale scores were higher in men ($p<0.05$) (From Moriguchi et al. [26])

represent a tendency toward alexithymia. Therefore, self-reported questionnaires for alexithymia need to be carefully constructed and examined, for both adolescents and adults.

4.7 Conclusions

Whether or not somatic symptoms can be medically explained, many studies have indicated that somatoform disorders, depression, panic symptoms, and neuroticism are associated with alexithymia. However, critical analysis of the current methods of assessment shows weaknesses in that alexithymia has been defined only by its affective aspects, such as difficulty in identifying and/or describing feelings, and that assessment has been based on self-reported measurements, such as TAS-20. Because affect and cognition are not ontologically separate, but perhaps phenomenologically distinctive, future studies need to examine how the affective and cognitive aspects of alexithymia are associated with difficulty in distinguishing between feelings and emotional arousal-related bodily sensations.

To determine the relationship between alexithymia and somatic symptoms, it is necessary to use a package that can cover all the aspects of the alexithymia construct: self-reported questionnaires (e.g., TAS-20), performance-based measurements, expert judgments, and the ratings of collateral informants. In addition, neuroimaging studies may help to elucidate the relationship between alexithymia and somatic symptoms.

References

1. Sifneos, P. E. (1973). The prevalence of 'alexithymic' characteristics in psychosomatic patients. *Psychotherapy and Psychosomatics, 22*, 255–262.
2. Bagby, R. M., Taylor, G. J., & Parker, J. D. (1994). The twenty-item Toronto Alexithymia Scale-II. Convergent, discriminant, and concurrent validity. *Journal of Psychosomatic Research, 38*, 33–40.
3. Sifneos, P. E. (1975). Problems of psychotherapy of patients with alexithymic characteristics and physical disease. *Psychotherapy and Psychosomatics, 26*, 65–70.
4. De Gucht, V., & Heiser, W. (2003). Alexithymia and somatisation. A quantitative review of the literature. *Journal of Psychosomatic Research, 54*, 425–434.
5. Bach, M., & Bach, D. (1996). Alexithymia in somatoform disorder and somatic disease: A comparative study. *Psychotherapy and Psychosomatics, 65*, 150–152.
6. Rief, W., Heuser, J., & Fichter, M. M. (1996). What does the Toronto Alexithymia Scale TAS-R measure? *Journal of Clinical Psychology, 52*, 423–429.
7. Mattila, A. K., Kronholm, E., Jula, A., et al. (2008). Alexithymia and somatization in general population. *Psychosomatic Medicine, 70*, 716–722.
8. Bach, M., Bach, D., Böhmer, F., et al. (1994). Alexithymia and somatization: Relationship to DSM-III-R diagnoses. *Journal of Psychosomatic Research, 38*, 529–538.
9. Rasmussen, N. H., Agerter, D. C., Colligan, R. C., et al. (2008). Somatisation and alexithymia in patients with high use of medical care and medically unexplained symptoms. *Mental Health in Family Medicine, 5*, 139–148.
10. Lundh, L. G., & Simonsson-Sarnecki, M. (2001). Alexithymia, emotion, and somatic complaints. *Journal of Personality, 69*, 483–510.
11. Cohen, K., Auld, F., & Brooker, H. (1994). Is alexithymia related to psychosomatic disorder and somatizing? *Journal of Psychosomatic Research, 38*, 119–127.
12. Nemiah, J. C., Sifneos, P. E., & Apfel-Savitz, R. (1977). A comparison of the oxygen consumption of normal and alexithymic subjects in response to affect-provoking thoughts. *Psychotherapy and Psychosomatics, 28*, 167–171.
13. Moriguchi, Y., & Komaki, G. (2013). Neuroimaging studies of alexithymia: physical, affective, and social perspectives. *Biopsychosocial Medicine, 7*, 8 (online).
14. Waller, E., & Scheidt, C. E. (2004). Somatoform disorders as disorders of affect regulation: A study comparing the TAS-20 with non-self-report measures of alexithymia. *Journal of Psychosomatic Research, 57*, 239–247.
15. Haviland, M. G., Hendryx, M. S., Cummings, M. A., et al. (1991). Multidimensionality and state dependency of alexithymia in recently sober alcoholics. *The Journal of Nervous and Mental Disease, 179*, 284–290.

16. Haviland, M. G., Shaw, D. G., Cummings, M. A., et al. (1988). Alexithymia: Subscales and relationship to depression. *Psychotherapy and Psychosomatics, 50*, 164–170.
17. Hendryx, M. S., Haviland, M. G., & Shaw, D. G. (1991). Dimensions of alexithymia and their relationships to anxiety and depression. *Journal of Personality Assessment, 56*, 227–237.
18. Wise, T. N., Jani, N. N., Kass, E., et al. (1988). Alexithymia: Relationship to severity of medical illness and depression. *Psychotherapy and Psychosomatics, 50*, 68–71.
19. Parker, J. D., Bagby, R. M., & Taylor, G. J. (1991). Alexithymia and depression: Distinct or overlapping constructs? *Comprehensive Psychiatry, 32*, 387–394.
20. Lumley, M. A. (2000). Alexithymia and negative emotional conditions. *Journal of Psychosomatic Research, 49*, 51–54.
21. John, O. P., & Gross, J. J. (2007). Individual differences in emotion regulation. In J. J. Gross (Ed.), *Handbook of emotion regulation*. New York: Guilford Press.
22. Taylor, G. J., Bagby, R. M., & Parker, J. D. (1993). Is alexithymia a non-neurotic personality dimension? A response to Rubino, Grasso, Sonnino & Pezzarossa. *The British Journal of Medical Psychology, 66*(part 3), 281–287. Discussion 289–294.
23. Van Praag, H. M. (1992). About the centrality of mood lowering in mood disorders. Plenary Lecture ECNP Congress, Monte Carlo, October 1991. *European Neuropsychopharmacology, 2*, 393–404.
24. Costa, P. T., & McCrae, R. R. (1992). *NEO PI-R professional manual*. Odessa, FL: Psychological Assessment Resouces.
25. Mann, L. S., Wise, T. N., Trinidad, A., et al. (1994). Alexithymia, affect recognition, and the five-factor model of personality in normal subjects. *Psychological Reports, 74*, 563–567.
26. Moriguchi, Y., Maeda, M., Igarashi, T., et al. (2007). Age and gender effect on alexithymia in large, Japanese community and clinical samples: A cross-validation study of the Toronto Alexithymia Scale (TAS-20). *Biopsychosocial Medicine*, 1, 7 (online).
27. Parker, J. D., Bagby, R. M., & Taylor, G. J. (1989). Toronto Alexithymia Scale, EPQ, and self-report measures of somatic complaints. *Personality and Individual Differences, 10*, 599–604.
28. Lane, R. D., Sechrest, L., Reidel, R., et al. (1996). Impaired verbal and nonverbal emotion recognition in alexithymia. *Psychosomatic Medicine, 58*, 203–210.
29. Henry, J. D., Phillips, L. H., Crawford, J. R., et al. (2006). Cognitive and psychosocial correlates of alexithymia following traumatic brain injury. *Neuropsychologia, 44*, 62–72.
30. Bach, M., de Zwaan, M., Ackard, D., et al. (1994). Alexithymia: Relationship to personality disorders. *Comprehensive Psychiatry, 35*, 239–243.
31. Craig, A. D. (2004). Human feelings: Why are some more aware than others? *Trends in Cognitive Sciences, 8*, 239–241.
32. Craig, A. D. (2009). How do you feel-now? The anterior insula and human awareness. *Nature Reviews Neuroscience, 10*, 59–70.
33. Lumley, M. A., Stettner, L., & Wehmer, F. (1996). How are alexithymia and physical illness linked? A review and critique of pathways. *Journal of Psychosomatic Research, 41*, 505–518.
34. Wise, T. N., & Mann, L. S. (1994). The relationship between somatosensory amplification, alexithymia, and neuroticism. *Journal of Psychosomatic Research, 38*, 515–521.
35. Parker, J. D., Taylor, G. J., Bagby, R. M., et al. (1993). Alexithymia in panic disorder and simple phobia: A comparative study. *The American Journal of Psychiatry, 150*, 1105–1107.
36. Marchesi, C., Fontò, S., Balista, C., et al. (2005). Relationship between alexithymia and panic disorder: A longitudinal study to answer an open question. *Psychotherapy and Psychosomatics, 74*, 56–60.
37. Galderisi, S., Mancuso, F., Mucci, A., et al. (2008). Alexithymia and cognitive dysfunctions in patients with panic disorder. *Psychotherapy and Psychosomatics, 77*, 182–188.
38. Näring, G. W., & van der Staak, C. P. (1995). Perception of heart rate and blood pressure: The role of alexithymia and anxiety. *Psychotherapy and Psychosomatics, 63*, 193–200.
39. Herbert, B. M., Herbert, C., & Pollatos, O. (2011). On the relationship between interoceptive awareness and alexithymia: Is interoceptive awareness related to emotional awareness? *Journal of Personality, 79*, 1149–1175.

40. Ikemi, Y., & Ikemi, A. (1986). An oriental point of view in psychosomatic medicine. *Psychotherapy and Psychosomatics, 45*, 118–126.
41. Igarashi, T., Komaki, G., Lane, R. D., et al. (2011). The reliability and validity of the Japanese version of the Levels of Emotional Awareness Scale (LEAS-J). *Biopsychosocial Medicine*, 5, 243 (online).
42. Nishimura, H., Komaki, G., Igarashi, T., et al. (2009). Validity issues in the assessment of alexithymia related to the developmental stages of emotional cognition and language. *Biopsychosocial Medicine*, 3, 1244 (online).
43. Komaki, G., Moriguchi, Y., Gondo, M., et al. (2009). The development of a precise inventory for the evaluation of alexithymia in Japan: A structured interview using a modified Japanese version of the Beth Israel Hospital Psychosomatic Questionnaire (SIBIQ). In S. Fassino, G. A. Fava, G. A. Daga, et al. (Eds.), *Panminerva medica* (Vol. 51(suppl. 13)). Turin: Edizioni Minerva Medica. pp62.
44. Haviland, M. G. (1998). The validity of the California Q-set alexithymia prototype. *Psychosomatics, 39*, 536–539.
45. Haviland, M. G., Warren, W. L., & Riggs, M. L. (2000). An observer scale to measure alexithymia. *Psychosomatics, 41*, 385–392.
46. Lane, R. D., Quinlan, D. M., Schwartz, G. E., et al. (1990). The Levels of Emotional Awareness Scale: A cognitive-developmental measure of emotion. *Journal of Personality Assessment, 55*, 124–134.
47. Wehmer, F., Brejnak, C., Lumley, M., et al. (1995). Alexithymia and physiological reactivity to emotion-provoking visual scenes. *The Journal of Nervous and Mental Disease, 183*, 351–357.
48. Monsen, J. T., Eilersten, D. E., Melgard, T., et al. (1996). Affects and affect consciousness: Initial experience with the assessment of affect integration. *Journal of Psychotherapy Practice and Research, 5*, 238–249.
49. Magai, C. (2008). Long-lived emotions. A life course perspective on emotional development. In M. Lewis, J. M. Haviland-Jones, & L. F. Barrett (Eds.), *Hand book of emotions* (3rd ed.). New York: The Guilford Press.

Chapter 5
Culture and Somatic Symptoms: *Hwa-byung*, a Culture-Related Anger Syndrome

Sung Kil Min

5.1 Introduction

Many psychiatric illnesses or symptoms are known to evolve in a sociocultural context. Culture may not only affect the labeling of certain illnesses or symptoms but also affect people's belief in the occurrence of a certain illness or symptom according to their reaction pattern via modulation of sensitivity to a particular stressor as well as susceptibility to a particular organ [1]. Culture is closely related to the clinical history or the precipitants of a certain health problem. Accordingly, understanding the influence of culture on psychiatric disorders is critical to the biopsychosocial formulation and treatment planning for patients with such disorders.

Particularly, somatic symptoms are probably the most typical symptoms that reflect the influences of culture on psychiatric symptoms. For example, somatic symptoms are frequently described in different names according to different cultures, as if they are really different illnesses, although they are substantially identical. The opposite is possible, too: the same label of symptoms or illnesses for a substantially different pathology. However, there have been limited studies on how a particular culture affects the development of symptoms along with their labeling.

In Korea as well, a few studies have been reported to date regarding the influences of culture on the occurrence of somatic symptoms, on the labeling of somatic symptoms, and on the explanation of etiology. In the study of such culture influences, a culture-related psychiatric syndrome may be the most suitable subject. In Korea, *hwa-byung* is the case.

In this chapter, several studies will be reviewed on how somatic symptoms are differently manifested, described, and explained according to the traditional and contemporary cultures of Korea in general; a case of *hwa-byung*, a culture-related syndrome will also be analyzed.

S.K. Min, M.D., Ph.D. (✉)
Professor Emeritus, Yonsei University College of Medicine, Seoul Metropolitan Eunpyeong Hospital, 90 Baengnyeonsan-ro, Eunpyeong-gu, Seoul 122-913, Korea
e-mail: skmin518@yuhs.ac

K.B. Koh (ed.), *Somatization and Psychosomatic Symptoms*,
DOI 10.1007/978-1-4614-7119-6_5, © Springer Science+Business Media New York 2013

5.2 Somatization in Koreans

5.2.1 Somatizing Tendency of Koreans

It has been argued that Koreans have a high tendency to express their psychological or emotional problems in somatic terms, not only in psychiatric illnesses, but also in an ordinary conversation. Kim [2] related such high somatization tendency to old primitive concepts based on shamanism and Asian ancient medicine. In an ordinary conversation, Koreans frequently use somatic, especially visceral, terms in order to express their psychological or emotional matters. For example, there is a frequently stated Korean proverb which says, "when one's cousin buys a piece of land, they get sick to their stomach." In this proverb, the major characteristics of the traditional Korean culture are reflected, including traditional agrarian culture, historical poverty, emotional reaction to unfairness, and people's utmost concern for eating (gastrointestinal function) [3]. In Korea, the greeting "Good morning" used to be "Did you eat breakfast?" Min and Kim [4] reported that Korean depressives tended to somatize their depression, especially in visceral symptoms including indigestion, abdominal discomfort, heart pounding, and respiratory stuffiness.

5.2.2 Biology and Culture

Based on the biopsychosocial model of human behavior, research has suggested the complex interactions between the body, mind, and sociocultural environments. This complexity has been attributed to a marked increase in the number of neurons in the human brain. Additionally, the increase of interconnections among neurons, which are shaped by an environmental input of long-term evolutionary changes as well as by development after birth, also affects the complexity. Certain somatic symptoms may be localized in the brain where culture may exert influence. An example illustrating the influences of culture on brain localization is handedness. Handedness may be developed differently according not only to the genetic predisposition but to the cultural pressure on handedness. Min and Lee [5] reported the differences of the lateralized pattern of somatic symptoms in Korean patients with depression, anxiety disorders, and somatization disorders in relation to handedness.

5.2.3 International Comparative Studies

In an epidemiological study in Korea [6], using the original American version of DIS-III, the lifetime prevalence of somatization disorders was reported to be 0.06 % of the general population. However, when the Korean version of DIS-III was used, including the Korean culture-related somatic symptoms (i.e., heat sensation, respiratory stuffiness, and a feeling of something pushing up in the chest) in the diagnostic criteria of somatization disorders, the prevalence rate increased to 5.45 %. This result suggested not only a high tendency of somatization in Koreans along with the influence of Korean culture on naming of certain symptoms or a selection of symptomatic organs but a necessity for modification of the diagnostic criteria according to different cultures since the occurrence of somatization symptoms and naming of symptoms are strongly influenced by culture.

An international comparative study on the differences in the prevalence rate of symptoms of depression in three Asian countries, Japan, China, and Korea [7], reported that Korean depressives were more likely to show a depressive mood, psychic anxiety, somatic anxiety, and gastrointestinal and genital symptoms in comparison with the Japanese and Chinese depressives. In addition, Koreans had relatively more frequently complained of palpitation, indigestion, general weakness, and loss of libido.

However, Kim et al. [8] reported a different finding. They compared depressive symptoms among the three groups of depressed patients: Koreans residing in Seoul, Korea; Korean Chinese in Yanbian, China; and Chinese in Yanbian, China, using the rating scales for depression. The results revealed that Korean depressives in Korea complained of more psychological symptoms, Chinese depressives of more somatic symptoms, and Korean Chinese depressives of symptoms that lie between the other two groups on a somatic–psychological continuum. The differences between the two studies may be explained by time differences of the studies. During the 1991–1999 period, the Korean society had been significantly changed in its cultural context.

5.2.4 Comparative Studies Within Korea

Within the same ethnic group, somatic symptoms can transform in quantity and quality in relation to a cultural change over time. For example, Min and Suh [9] reported that, during a period of 15 years between the 1950s and 1970s, the number of admitted patients with hysterical disorder had decreased. Moreover, the classical symptoms such as convulsion, fainting, or other motor–sensory symptoms had decreased in patients with this disorder, whereas pain or visceral symptoms had increased. These changes were considered related to the cultural changes in the Korean society, from a simple agrarian undeveloped culture to a more industrialized, educated, and sophisticated culture.

5.3 Korean Culture-Related Syndrome, *Hwa-byung*

5.3.1 Clinical Correlates of Hwa-byung

Symptoms of *hwa-byung*, especially its somatic symptoms, reveal how the Korean culture is related not only to the concept and naming of a certain disorder and its symptoms but to the explanation of the cause and development of the disorder and to its treatment [10]. The name *hwa-byung* itself is cultural: *Hwa* (火) in *hwa-byung* means anger and fire in Korean, and *byung* (病) means disease or illness; accordingly, *hwa-byung* literally means "anger disorder" or "fire disease."

Self-labeled *hwa-byung* was reported in 4.2 % of the general population in Korea; it was most frequently reported in middle-aged or older women of lower socioeconomic status, who seem to have kept the Korean traditional culture [11].

When diagnoses were made according to the criteria of the DSM-III-R or DSM-IV in patients with self-labeled *hwa-byung*, many of them were diagnosed with a major depressive disorder, generalized anxiety disorder, an atypical somatization disorder, or their comorbid state [11]. However, in a study using the research diagnostic criteria for *hwa-byung* [12], only about 16.8 % of the patients with the so-called "neurotic" disorders were found to have only *hwa-byung* [13], suggesting the existence of a new category of "anger" disorder [14].

Regarding the biology of *hwa-byung*, Lee et al. [15] reported that in a study using functional magnetic resonance imaging (fMRI) on neural responses to neutral, sad, and angry facial stimuli, the effect of anger suppression resulted in an aberrant function of the brain regions related to the visual pathways. Moreover, this functional impairment in the anterior cingulate cortex may contribute to the pathophysiology of *hwa-byung*.

The precipitating factors of *hwa-byung* were reported to be traumatic experiences to one's self-esteem. The most common typical factor was domestic violence: husbands and/or mothers-in-law committing violent acts toward wives/daughters-in-law [10]. According to the patients' explanation, anger reactive to the unfairness should be "suppressed" in order not to jeopardize harmonious familial and/or social relationships [16]. However, if the anger-provoking situation is repeated, then the suppressed anger accumulates and becomes dense(鬱), which patients usually describe as *wool-hwa* (鬱火), meaning dense *hwa* (anger or fire), and finally resulting in *hwa-byung*.

Hwa-byung has been argued to be the result of incomplete suppression and somatization of anger [10]. Defense style or coping strategies include oral consumption, avoidance of stimulus, externalization (projection), help-seeking behavior, impulsiveness (acting out), pseudo-altruism, omnipotence, fatalism, self-pity, and fantasy [17]. Roberts et al. [18] suggested that *hwa-byung* is characterized by anger, hopelessness, general health problems, and gastrointestinal symptoms. Lee et al. [19] examined the temperament of patients with *hwa-byung* and suggested that *hwa-byung* was positively correlated with impulsiveness, harm avoidance, and self-transcendence; *hwa-byung* was negatively related with self-directedness, self-acceptance, and acceptance. Moreover, global severity of *hwa-byung* showed positive association with self-transcendence, its subscale being self-forgetfulness, and anticipatory worry, but negative association with attachment and compassion.

Hwa-byung was reported to be a chronic illness [20]. Supportive psychotherapy, family therapy, and selective serotonin reuptake inhibitors (SSRIs) are suggested as effective treatments for h*wa-byung* [20, 21].

A Case Vignette

A 49-year-old housewife visited the outpatient clinic with the chief complaint of pent-up anger, "*hwa*," which was intermittently accompanied by a hot sensation, which had to be cooled with a fan, along with a feeling of something pushing up in her chest. The other symptoms were "many things accumulated" in the epigastrium and respiratory stuffiness that used to be relieved by frequent sighs. At times, she felt so angry and so "*uk-wool*" (a feeling of unfairness) that she almost felt like losing control or losing her mind. Her self-diagnosis was *hwa-byung*. The reason for her anger was her family situation with her husband and her mother-in-law. Her anger began 15 years ago just after her marriage, when she realized that she had been deceived by her husband regarding his past history. He had never been in college and was in a much worse economic condition than what he had claimed before marriage. Since then, she lived with an angry feeling, with a frustration related to her hard life. Moreover, her mother-in-law had lived together with her family only because her husband was the first son. Her mother-in-law began to treat her unfairly and, furthermore, she interfered in her everyday private and marital life. To keep peace in the family, the patient had to suppress her anger and hide her hatred toward her husband and mother-in-law; she obeyed her husband and his mother. While living with her husband, she found her husband to be a truly good man, and that is why she kept their marriage intact until now. Nevertheless, she gradually became irritable and nervous. She recently became more irritable and began to beat her husband and even throw things at her children to the point that she abused them. She said the children never understood why she was so angry. When she recently stood up against her mother-in-law for the first time in her life, she felt "cool" (relieved) at the moment.

During the interview, she talked extensively, with sighs and tears, about how she had suffered from a life of "*uk-wool* and anger" and with "much *haan*." However, she said she did not feel depressed and had never thought about suicide. Rather, she has tried to live enthusiastically and actively; she regularly worked as an employee (cleaning buildings). She attempted to avoid being isolated from her fellow workers since she believed they might think of her as a "good" person. She revealed her painful past memory of how she had been discriminated by her mother for being a daughter. Finally, her mother's favoritism to sons and her gender discrimination did not allow the patient to complete her middle school education.

5.3.2 Symptoms of Hwa-byung

Symptoms of *hwa-byung* have been studied in patients who self-labeled themselves with *hwa-byung* [10, 22] and in *hwa-byung* patients diagnosed with the Research Diagnostic Criteria for *hwa-byung* [12, 23]. The typical psychological symptoms of *hwa-byung* include subjective pent-up anger (*hwa*), a feeling of unfairness, *uk-wool* (抑鬱) and *boon* (憤), and hate/hostility and revengeful mind toward someone who caused the anger. Patients also typically complain of *haan*, which means grudge, embitterment, or distress (*haan* will be described in detail later). Other psychological symptoms are many thoughts (雜念, rumination), irritability, being easily frightened, sad and pessimistic mood, nihilistic ideas, and guilt feeling. *Hwa-byung* patients sometimes report "cannot find what to do" or "absentmindedness," which seems to be a feeling of losing control. Typical *hwa-byung* patients work hard, eat well, sleep well, and associate well with others as seen in the case history. They usually express a strong will to live and do not have any thoughts about suicide.

The most typical factor is somatic symptoms including a heat/hot sensation in or on the body, appearing mainly in the upper trunk. Heat may appear as a hot flush on the head, a feeling of boiling inside, or by sweating. Sometimes, a hot sensation in the trunk is accompanied by a cold sensation with cold sweat on the limbs. Other typical somatic symptoms include palpitations, the feeling of something pushing up in the chest, and dry mouth. The "something" used to be a mass of fire/anger. The "pushing up" usually extends up to "the end of the head" and causes the head to become hot, resulting in a headache. These symptoms seem to reflect the symbolical relation between anger and physical nature of fire/smoke. Patients with *hwa-byung* sometimes complain of respiratory stuffiness (chest oppression or chest tightness), which is relieved by letting out a deep sigh. This action of sighing seems to symbolize the release of suppressed anger/fire as well as the choking smoke. Less frequent but typical factor is epigastric mass or a feeling of mass formation in the neck, chest, or abdomen. This mass is referred to as *dung-u-ri*, like a piece of stone, which seems to symbolize suppression, accumulation, and increased density of anger/fire; it is also attributed to respiratory stuffiness.

Behaviorally, *hwa-byung* patients are generally polite and docile, but at times, they show irritability, ill temper, aggressive words, violent gestures, or, rarely, aggressive action such as throwing things or quarreling. They are generally reluctant to talk about their inner and familial life, suggesting a suppression of anger. But once the talk is ignited, their talk on their life distress and *haan* is extended for a long period of time accompanied by frequent tears and sighs (*hasoyeon*); it becomes hard for them to stop the conversation. Talking, tears, and sighing seem to be symbolic measures of releasing suppressed anger and feeling of unfairness (*uk-wool*). Patients with *hwa-byung* are intolerant to a warm and closed space. To cool down the heat, they use fans and ice cubes, ventilate the air, or go out to feel the cool air. At times, they walk around without a destination, or they get on a bus, go to the last stop, and come back. These behaviors seem to symbolize their intention to avoid or release anger/fire/smoke.

Other less frequent symptoms include insomnia, anorexia, headache, and general aches, all of which seem to symbolize a general psychological distress.

5.4 The Relationship Between Somatic Symptoms and Korean Culture

Traditional shamanism and Asian traditional medicine has provided Koreans with concrete and physical explanation for nature, emotion, and human suffering (disease), whereas the traditional philosophy like Confucianism has taught a way of life in which people suppress emotional reaction not to jeopardize harmonious interpersonal relationships. In this culture, Koreans have learned to express their suppressed emotion in somatized form while saving their face.

5.4.1 Shamanism

Shamanism has provided people with an explanation of the world, life, and disease. Traditionally in Korea, shamanism used to relate suffering or symptoms of any diseases with physical harming of spirits who died from unfairness (*"uk-wool"*), and thus, they became evil spirits because of their unresolved anger and revengefulness [24].

5.4.2 Traditional Asian Medicine

Somatization tendency of Koreans, particularly the frequentness of visceral or gastrointestinal symptoms, can be related to the traditional medicine. In traditional medicine, based on traditional philosophies, the human body can be explained in physical terms of five cosmic elements including fire, water, wood, metal, and earth. The body is also operated with cosmic positive or negative energy (*qi*), *yin* and *yang,* of five elements. In this medicine, emotions were also understood as energy, which is related to five major body organs including the liver, heart, stomach, spleen, and kidney. According to this theory, Koreans' body image has been formed, with which they believe that health can be kept in harmonious balance between those *kis* in these visceral organs; unbalanced impact of emotion may disturb the function of the autonomic nervous visceral organs. In particular, the impact of anger has been identified with the energy of fire (*hwa-qi*), and such emotion is supposed to affect the visceral organs, mostly the heart and liver, resulting in a disease such as *hwa-byung*, fire disease.

5.4.3 Traditional Social System

Traditional philosophies including Confucianism and the traditional patriarchal authoritative culture have supported the development of unique familial collectivism in Korea. In this culture, fathers, teachers, and kings are identified to be in the same authority. People have been taught to suppress anger and not to jeopardize social or familial harmony with those authority figures, engendering a suppression of anger. These traditional cultures have also been supportive in the development of gender discrimination and social class-related oppression, which has contributed to the social unfairness for women and lower-class people in their sociopolitical life. Under the influence of such traditional cultures, the socially weak, especially women, have adopted somatization or *hwa-byung* presentation as a way for a nonverbal communication of their suffering and also as a help-seeking method in order for the people around them to understand their feeling or suffering, while saving their faces, in the Korean cultural context.

5.4.4 Traditional Affect of Haan

Haan (恨) has been defined as a chronic mixed mood of missing, sadness, and "everlasting woe," [25] beyond its literal meaning [26], and is known to be a unique traditional collective sentiment or pathos for Koreans. Similar to *hwa-byung*, *haan* has been said to be resulting from the accumulation of suppressed anger, feeling of unfairness (*uk-wool*), and/or even revengeful mind.

Haan has been argued to have developed in the psyche of Koreans, who have endured repeated traumas from international violence (invasion of China, Mongolia, Japan and, recently, communist North Korea) and domestic violence throughout not only their nation's history but also from their personal lives. Their *haan* includes *haan* of poverty, *haan* of the weak, *haan* of not being educated, and women's *haan* [18, 27, 28]. Accordingly, the Korean history of 5,000 years used to be referred to as a history of *haan*. Accordingly, *hwa-byung* and *haan* are frequently found in the socially weak group of people, especially among women. *Haan* has been suggested as a within normal range of emotion providing positive energy for survival or creativity, while *hwa-byung* seems to be a personal illness, a negative or illness form of *haan* [29, 30].

Naturally, *haan* and *hwa-byung* have many common factors in clinical correlates including etiological emotion of anger and feeling of unfairness, precipitating factors in sociocultural context, and defense styles including suppression and somatization [17, 30], and clinical signs such as sighing, tears, respiratory stuffiness, *hasoyeon,* and lamenting with frequent deep sighs and tears and *eung-u-ri*, a feeling of a mass in the chest (a bit vague concept compared to the more concrete *dung-u-ri* in *hwa-byung*).

Metaphorically, *hwa-byung* is like an inactive volcano, from which fire, smoke, and lava leak. In this metaphor, an anger attack or intermittent explosive disorder is like an active volcano with an explosive eruption of the flame and lava. *Haan* is like an extinct volcano; the crater became a lake which is surrounded by a forest. The volcano may look peaceful and beautiful; yet the flame under it is ready to erupt at any time [14].

It is natural that Koreans have developed social devices for solving *haan,* generally referred to as "*haan-puri*." Collectively, historical *haan* of poverty has been solved by working hard and educating children. *Haan* of the socially weak was solved by protesting against the oppression of rulers, by sublimation through satirizing them, through artistic activities including humorous paintings by unknown people, or elegant ceramics making by unknown masters. Therefore, the Korean traditional culture is called as a culture of *haan*.

Personal *haan-puri* includes wish fulfillment, revenge, shaman ritual, or achieving final success after longtime effort and endurance of the hardship. For example, a mother's *haan-puri* can be achieved by a divorce or more desirably by the success of her son whom she has nurtured with long-term sacrifices of herself despite unfair treatment from her husband and/or mother-in-law. Productive and creative *haan-puri* may provide a theoretical frame for the treatment of *hwa-byung*.

Koreans' passion to overcome their historical *haan*, especially the *haan* of poverty, has stimulated modern Koreans to educate their children enthusiastically (education fever) and work very hard, resulting in the recent rapid economic growth. However, their children, who had been educated on democracy and human rights, began to protest against the military dictators in order to solve *haan* of the politically suppressed. At the same time, such economic growth and high competitiveness in the society had produced many losers and stimulated a new anger or unfairness reaction, or a new *haan* among them and a new form of acute *hwa-byung*, contrasting to traditional chronic *hwa-byung*.

5.5 Conclusions

The review of research on somatization in Koreans and unique somatic symptoms of *hwa-byung*, a culture-related anger syndrome of Korea, suggests the significant influence of culture on somatic symptoms. Further, the review on the specific historical and cultural experiences as national and personal traumas may contribute to understanding specific emotional reaction patterns as well as specific somatization symptom patterns in Koreans to evolve. Also, the symbolic meaning of names of such somatic symptoms as well as the dynamic analysis of such symptom development could be explained by a traditional view on nature, body, and, most importantly, the emotions of the Korean, which still continues up to the present time. Further research is needed in order to develop the culture-relevant treatment methods for Koreans with health problems.

References

1. Tseng, W. S. (2001). *Handbook of cultural psychiatry*. San Diego: Academic Press.
2. Kim, K.-L. (1977). A study on somatization tendency of Koreans. *New Medicine, 15*, 1440–1443.
3. Min, S. K. (1981). Psychodynamic in somatization. In Kang, S. H., et al. (Eds.), *Tao and Human Science* (pp. 413–428). Seoul, Korea: Samil-dang.
4. Min, S. K., & Kim, K. H. (1988). Somatic symptoms in depression. *Journal of Korean Neuropsychiatric Association, 17*, 149–154.
5. Min, S. K., & Lee, B. W. (1997). Laterality in somatization. *Psychosomatic Medicine, 59*, 236–240.

6. Lee, H. Y., Namgoong, K., Lee, M. H., et al. (1989). The psychiatric epidemiological study of Kanghwa Island (III). The prevalence of major psychiatric disorders. *Journal of Korean Neuropsychiatric Association, 28*, 984–999.
7. Nakane, Y., Ohta, Y., Radford, M., et al. (1991). Comparative study of affective disorders in three Asian Countries. II. Differences in prevalence rate and symptom presentation. *Acta Psychiatrica Scandinavica, 84*, 313–319.
8. Kim, K.-I., Li, D., & Kim, D.-H. (1999). Depressive symptoms in Koreans, Korean-Chinese and Chinese: A transcultural study. *Transcultural Psychiatry, 36*, 303–316.
9. Min, S. K., & Suh, S. Y. (1979). A clinical study on hysterical neurosis and change of its symptom pattern for last 16 years in Korea. *Journal of Korean Neuropsychiatric Association, 18*, 75–81.
10. Min, S. K., Lee, M. H., Kang, H. C., et al. (1987). A clinical study of hwa-byung. *Journal of the Korean Medical Association, 30*, 187–197.
11. Min, S. K., Namkoong, K., & Lee, H. Y. (1990). An epidemiological study of hwa-byung. *Journal of Korean Neuropsychiatric Association, 29*, 867–874.
12. Min, S. K., Suh, S. Y., Hur, J. S., et al. (2009). Development of the hwa-byung scale and the research criteria of hwa-byung. *Journal of Korean Neuropsychiatric Association, 48*, 77–85.
13. Min, S. K., & Suh, S.Y. (2010). Anger syndrome, hwa-byung and its comorbidity. *Journal of Affective Disorders, 124*, 211–214.
14. Min, S. K. (2008). Clinical correlates of hwa-byung and a proposal of a new anger disorder. *Psychiatry Investigation, 5*, 125–141.
15. Lee, B. T., Paik, J. W., Kang, R. H., et al. (2008). The neural substrates of affective face recognition in patients with hwa-byung and healthy individuals in Korea. *The World Journal of Biological Psychiatry, 10*, 552–559.
16. Min, S. K. (1989). A study on the concept of hwa-byung. *Journal of Korean Neuropsychiatric Association, 28*, 604–615.
17. Min, S. K., Park, C. S., & Hahn, J. O. (1993). Defense mechanisms and coping strategies in hwa-byung. *Journal of Korean Neuropsychiatric Association, 32*, 506–516.
18. Roberts, M. E., Han, K. H., & Weed, N. C. (2006). Development of a scale to assess hwa-byung, a Korean culture bound syndrome, using the Korean MMPI-2. *Transcultural Psychiatry, 43*, 383–400.
19. Lee, J., Min, S. K., Kim, K. H., et al. (2012). Differences in temperament and character dimensions of personality between patients with hwa-byung, an anger syndrome, and patients with major depressive disorder. *Journal of Affective Disorders, 138*, 110–116.
20. Min, S. K. (2004). Treatment and prognosis of hwa-byung. *Psychiatry Investigation, 1*, 29–36.
21. Min, S. K., Suh, S. Y., Jeon, D. I., et al. (2009). Effects of paroxetine on symptoms of hwa-byung. *Korean Journal of Psychopharmacology, 20*, 90–97.
22. Min, S. K., & Kim, K. H. (1998). Symptoms of hwa-byung. *Korean Journal of Psychopharmacology, 37*, 1138–1145.
23. Min, S. K., Suh, S.Y., & Song, K. J. (2009). Symptoms to use for the diagnostic criteria of hwa-byung. *Psychiatry Investigation, 6*, 7–12.
24. Rhi, B. Y. (1970). The legend of won-ryung and psychology of haan. In H. K. Kim (Ed.), *Traditional society and people's art* (pp. 95–107). Seoul, Korea: Min-um Sa.
25. Kim, L (1997, May). *Haan and hwabyung*. Presented at the 150th Annual Meeting of the American psychiatric Association, San Diego, pp. 14–17.
26. Han, W. S., & Kim, S. K. (1980). *An essay on haan in popular sociological concept*. Seoul, Korea: Hankil-sa.
27. Lee, H. J. (1978). *Haan of Korean women*. Seoul, Korea: Chungwoo-sa.
28. Chung, H. K. (1991). *Struggle to be the sun again*. Maryknoll, NY: Orbis Books.
29. Min, S. K. (1991). Hwa-byung and the psychology of haan. *Journal of Korean Medical Association, 34*, 1189–1198.
30. Min, S. K., Lee, J. S., & Hahn, J. O. (1997). A psychiatric study on haan. *Journal of Korean Neuropsychiatric Association, 36*, 603–611.

Chapter 6
Molecular Mechanism of Sleep–Wake Regulation: From Basic to Translational Research

Yoshihiro Urade

6.1 Introduction

Sleep gives our body its needed rest, which prepares us for the next day's activities. In our modern society, people suffer from sleep deprivation, which leads to an inability to concentrate, to a loss of judgment, and to an increased risk of accidents. It is reported that 1 in 4–5 Japanese has a sleep problem and that 1 in 9 Japanese uses sleeping pills regularly. Hypnotic drugs are prescribed for insomnia patients. The current sleeping pills developed from tranquilizers are much safer than the ones used in the past, as the latter were developed from anesthetic agents, which brought death in case too many pills were taken. However, the current type of sleeping pills causes a coma in case of an overdose. Such pills are sometimes used in crimes such as coma robbery cases.

What people demand now is some methods to adjust the sleep–wake rhythm based on our innate sleep–wake regulatory system and sleeping pills that induce natural sleep without any side effects. To develop such sleep aids, it is necessary that we understand the mechanism of sleep–wake regulation. However, there is still much mystery regarding sleep and questions to be answered, such as why we sleep and how to gain comfortable sleep. Sleep research has only a 90-year history and is currently being advanced due to highly interdisciplinary input based on recent findings from brain science, genetic engineering, and computer and information–communication technology.

Y. Urade, Ph.D. (✉)
Department of Molecular Behavioral Biology, Osaka Bioscience Institute,
6-2-4, Furuedai, Suita-shi, Osaka 565-0874, Japan
e-mail: uradey@obi.or.jp

K.B. Koh (ed.), *Somatization and Psychosomatic Symptoms*,
DOI 10.1007/978-1-4614-7119-6_6, © Springer Science+Business Media New York 2013

6.2 Sleep–Wake Regulation by Endogenous Sleep Substances: Prostaglandin (PG) D_2 and Adenosine

6.2.1 Prostaglandin (PG) D_2 as an Endogenous Sleep Substance

Many endogenous molecules have been isolated and proposed to act as sleep-promoting substances. Among them, PGD_2 is the most potent endogenous sleep-promoting substance, and its sleep-induction mechanism is best characterized in terms of production and action sites, and signal transduction system, whose characterization has been made by the use of various pharmacological tools and gene-knockout mice for the synthases or receptors.

In the 1980s, PGD_2 was found to be the most abundant PG in the brains of rats [1] and other mammals including humans [2], thus suggesting that it has an important function in the central nervous system. The sleep-promoting effect of PGD_2 was then discovered after the microinjection of nano-molar quantities of PGD_2 into the rat brain, which causes profound enhancement of both non-rapid eye movement (non-REM, NREM) and REM sleep [3]. Based on electrophysiological and behavioral criteria, PGD_2-induced sleep is indistinguishable from physiological sleep. During the infusion of PGD_2, for instance, rats are easily aroused by a clap sound, and their sleep is episodic, indicating that PGD_2 does not interfere with the basal wakefulness crucial to the survival of the animal. The somnogenic effect of PGD_2 was later confirmed in a nonhuman primate, when PGD_2 was infused via the intracerebroventricular (i.c.v.) route into a rhesus monkey (*Macaca mulatta*) [4]. The electroencephalogram (EEG) power spectrum of NREM sleep during the PGD_2 infusion into monkeys was the same as that of their natural sleep at night, but clearly different from benzodiazepine-induced sleep, which is characterized by a decrease in the theta range and the appearance of a rapid wave with a peak at around 20 Hz. In addition, PGD_2 was reported to be involved in the pathogenesis of mastocytosis, a disorder characterized by episodic production of endogenous PGD_2, which accompanies deep-sleep episodes [5]. Also, the PGD_2 concentration, but not that of PGE_2 or IL-1ß, is elevated time-dependently in the CSF of patients with African sleeping sickness, which is a disease caused by an infection with *Trypanosoma* [6]. These findings suggest that PGD_2 induces sleep in humans as well as in rodents and monkeys.

To study the molecular mechanism of PGD_2-induced sleep, we established a sleep bioassay system using the EEG to monitor brain waves, and the electromyogram to monitor the muscle tension, of freely moving mice during the continuous i.c.v. infusion of drugs (Fig. 6.1). We also developed SLEEPSIGN software (Kissei Comtec Co., Ltd., Nagano, Japan) for automatic scoring of the vigilance states of rats and mice, based on the fast Fourier transform (FFT) analysis of the EEG [7].

When PGD_2 is infused into the lateral ventricle of wild-type mice at a rate of 50 pmol/min during a wake period at night, it induces potent NREM sleep (about 35 min/h) almost equal to the maximum level of NREM sleep during a sleep period in the morning, but induces only a small amount of REM sleep (about 5 min/h, Fig. 6.2). In contrast, DP_1-knockout mice do not respond to the PGD_2 infusion at all,

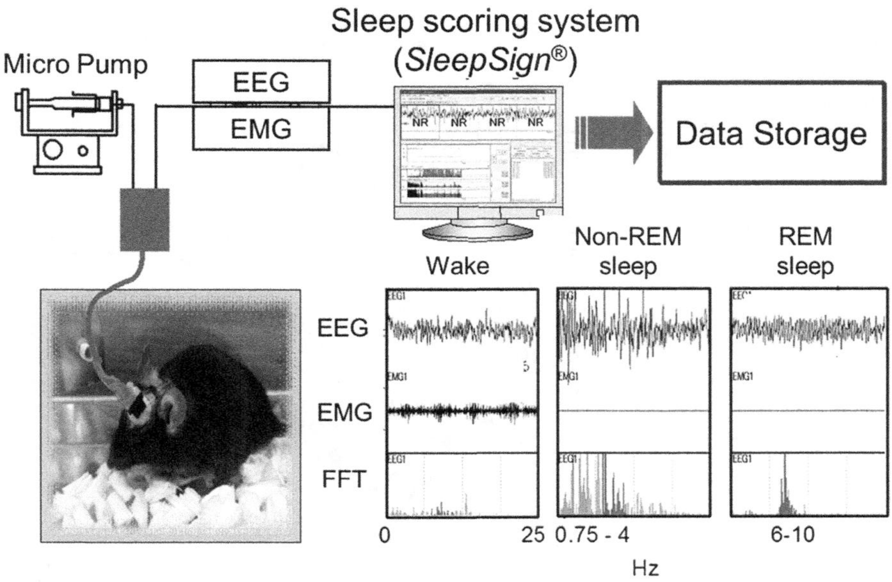

Fig. 6.1 Sleep bioassay system EMG, electromyogram

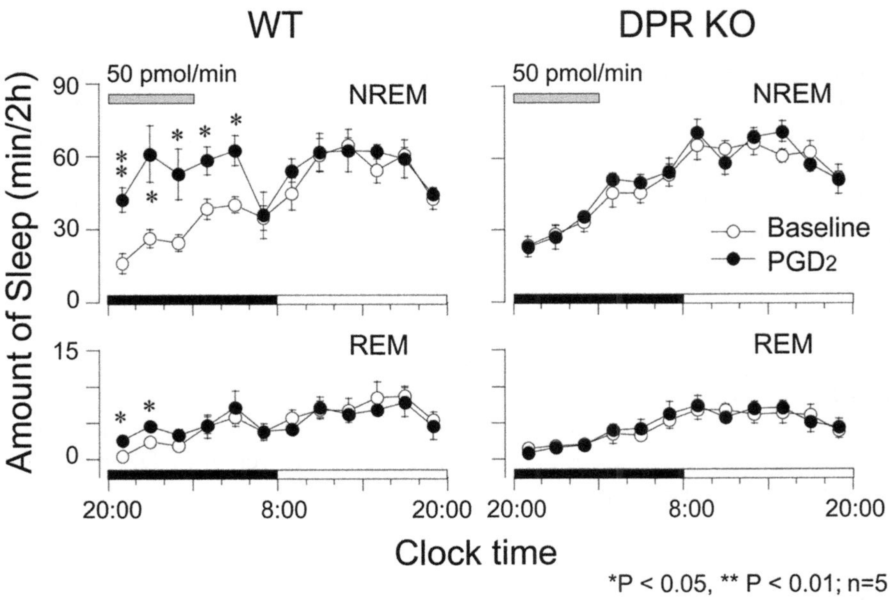

Fig. 6.2 Sleep induction by i.c.v. infusion of PGD_2 in wild-type (*WT*) and DP_1 receptor-knockout (*DPR KO*) mice (From Mizoguchi et al. [8], reprinted by permission of *Proceedings of the National Academy of Sciences*)

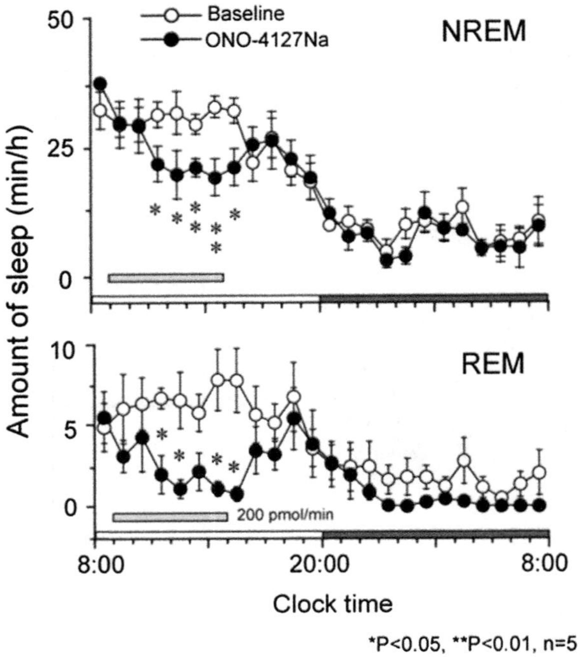

Fig. 6.3 DP_1 antagonist inhibits sleep in rats. ONO-4127Na was given between 09:00 and 15:00 for 6 h, as indicated by the *horizontal bars* (From Qu et al. [9], reprinted by permission of *Proceedings of the National Academy of Sciences*)

indicating that the remarkable NREM sleep induction by PGD_2 is completely dependent on DP_1 receptors [8].

Ono Pharmaceutical Co., Ltd. (Osaka, Japan) developed a novel DP_1 antagonist, ONO-4127Na, which exhibits a highly specific binding affinity ($Ki=2.5$ nM) for and excellent antagonistic effects ($pA_2=9.73$) on DP_1 receptors. We examined the effect of ONO-4127Na on sleep in rats by infusing it into the subarachnoid space under the rostral basal forebrain, where DP_1 receptors are the most abundant [9]. The antagonist infusion reduces NREM sleep by 23 % and 28 % and REM sleep by 49 % and 63 % at 100 and 200 pmol/min, respectively, during perfusion for 6 h and post-infusion for 1 h. ONO-4127Na infusion at 200 pmol/min decreases NREM sleep by 30–40 % per hour and REM sleep by 60–90 % 2 h after the start of ONO-4127Na infusion, as compared with the baseline (Fig. 6.3). Due to the low solubility of ONO-4127Na, the antagonist cannot be used at doses higher than 200 pmol/min. These results clearly show that the DP_1 antagonist dose-dependently attenuates NREM and REM sleep, suggesting that endogenous PGD_2 acting via DP_1 receptors is essential for the maintenance of physiological sleep.

6.2.2 Adenosine as a Paracrine Sleep-Promoting Molecule

The infusion of PGD_2 into the subarachnoid space of wild-type mice increases the extracellular adenosine concentration in a dose-dependent manner. This PGD_2-induced increase in extracellular adenosine is absent in DP_1 receptor-knockout mice,

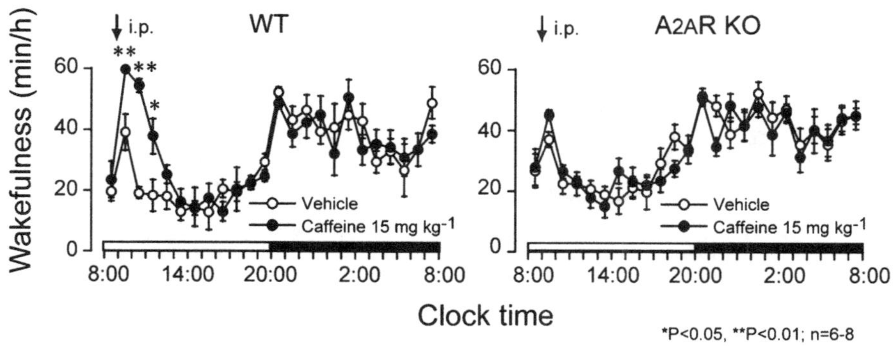

Fig. 6.4 Caffeine-induced arousal in adenosine receptor gene-manipulated mice. Caffeine (15 mg/kg, i.p.)-induced arousal in wild-type (*WT*) and A_1 receptor-knockout mice, but not in A_{2A} receptor-knockout (*$A_{2A}R$ KO*) mice (From Huang et al. [10], reprinted by permission of Nature Publishing Group)

indicating that DP_1 receptors are required for this increase [8]. Adenosine has also been proposed to be an endogenous sleep substance, because a number of stable adenosine analogues induce sleep when administered to rats and other animal species. For example, when CGS21680, an A_{2A} receptor agonist, is infused into the lateral ventricle of wild-type mice, NREM sleep is induced dose-dependently. Comparatively, CGS21680 is tenfold or more potent than PGD_2, the unstable natural ligand, in terms of the potency to induce NREM sleep. The infusion of CGS21680 at a dose of 5 pmol/h increases NREM sleep to 35 min/h. In contrast, N6-cyclopentyladenosine, an A_1 receptor-selective agonist, is totally inactive even when infused at 5 nmol/h, indicating that A_{2A}, but not A_1, receptors play a major role in NREM sleep regulation.

Caffeine is a nonselective antagonist of adenosine A_1 and A_{2A} receptors. Caffeine induces complete insomnia in wild-type mice (Fig. 6.4) for 2–3 h after an intraperitoneal (i.p.) injection at a dose of 15 mg/kg, a dose corresponding to an intake of approximately three cups of coffee in humans. Earlier we used knockout mice for A_1 or A_{2A} receptors and their respective wild-type littermates of the inbred C57BL/6 strain to test which subtype of the adenosine receptor is involved in the caffeine-induced wakefulness [10]. The caffeine-induced arousal in A_1 receptor-knockout mice was observed to have the same intensity and duration as that in the wild-type mice. In contrast, A_{2A} receptor-knockout mice did not show any change in time spent in wakefulness after the caffeine administration, indicating that A_{2A} receptors are crucial for the caffeine-induced wakefulness and that these receptors play an important role in the regulation of the sleep–wake cycle.

The DP_1 antagonist ONO-4127Na inhibits sleep in rats and caffeine, a nonselective antagonist of adenosine A_1 and A_{2A} receptors, induces complete insomnia in wild-type mice, suggesting that the PGD_2/adenosine system is important for the maintenance of physiological sleep, as described above. However, knockout mice for DP_1, A_1, and A_{2A} receptors show essentially the same circadian profiles and daily amounts of sleep as wild-type mice. These results suggest that a deficiency of one system in a complicated sleep–wake regulatory network is effectively compensated by collateral systems formed during embryonic development. Therefore,

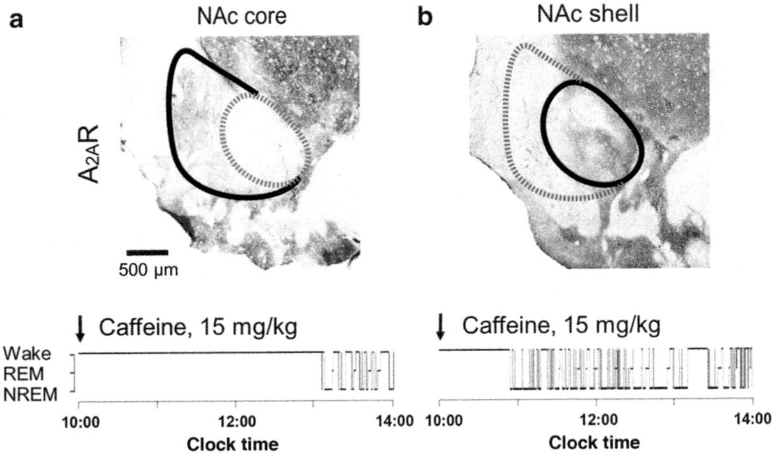

Fig. 6.5 Effects on caffeine-induced arousal of focal deletion of adenosine A_{2A} receptors in the core (**a**) or shell (**b**) of the NAc of rats. Caffeine (15 mg/kg, i.p.)-induced arousal in rats with A_{2A} receptors in the NAc shell (**a**), but not after removal of A_{2A} receptors in the NAc shell (**b**) (From Lazarus et al. [11], reprinted by permission of *Journal of Neuroscience*)

pharmacological approaches, such as receptor antagonists, and conditional gene suppression based on the Cre/loxP system or the focal RNA interference strategy are useful to minimize functional compensation in sleep–wake regulation.

Adenosine A_{2A} receptors are densely expressed in the basal ganglia of the brain, which contains the caudate putamen, which is involved in locomotion; the nucleus accumbens (NAc), which is important for motivation and addiction; and the olfactory tubercle, a structure involved in olfaction. To identify the active center of the caffeine-induced insomnia, we used focal knockdown of A_{2A} receptors by microinjecting adeno-associated virus-carrying short-hairpin RNA into the A_{2A} receptor-expressing brain regions of rats [11]. As shown in Fig. 6.5, caffeine-induced wakefulness in rats is not affected by the focal removal of A_{2A} receptors from the NAc core or other A_{2A} receptor-positive areas of the basal ganglia, but is remarkably decreased by their removal from the NAc shell. These results indicate that caffeine promotes arousal by activating pathways that traditionally have been associated with motivational and motor responses in the brain.

6.3 Translational Sleep Research for Sleepless Modern Society

6.3.1 Sleep Condition of Modern Society

Figure 6.6 summarizes the sleep length in the Asia-Pacific region, surveyed by The Nielsen Company, New York, USA, in 2004. As clearly seen, Japanese and Korean people are increasingly suffering from sleep deprivation which has pronounced

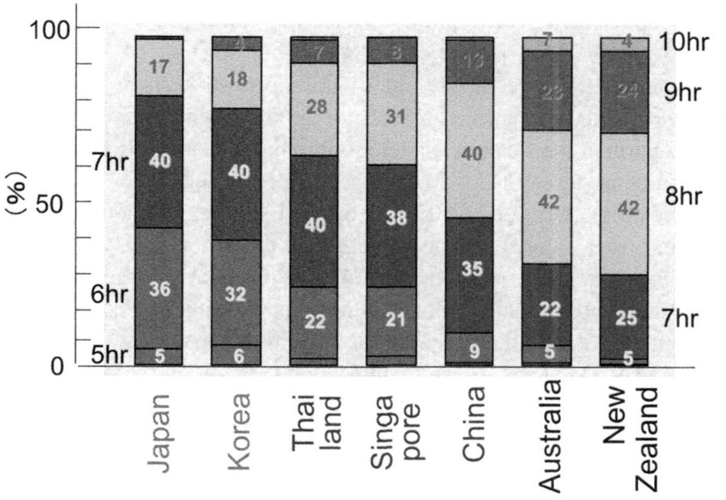

Fig. 6.6 Sleep length in Asia-Pacific regions (The Nielsen Company 2004) (Depicted from data of the Nielsen Company 2004). The number in the rectangle indicates the percentage of hours of sleep

negative effects on performance and increases the risk of accidents as well as negatively affects the health outcome in the case of cardiovascular disease and certain forms of cancer. However, there seems at present to be no way to eliminate most of the negative effects of insomnia on human physiology and cognition. Therefore, the development of products that are safe and effective for the treatment of insomnia is demanded. Toward this end we have used our sleep-scoring system to identify sleep-promoting components in various foods and herbal raw materials.

6.3.2 Identification of Natural Sleep-Promoting Components

6.3.2.1 Hastatoside and Verbenalin from Herbal Tea *Verbena officinalis*

Herbal tea made from *Verbena officinalis* has traditionally been used for the treatment of insomnia and other nervous conditions. Oral administration of hastatoside or verbenalin (0.25 and 0.5 g/kg of body weight, respectively), two major iridoid compounds of *V. officinalis*, increases NREM sleep in rats during a 9-h period in the dark time (when rats are active) 1.8- and 1.4-fold, respectively, with a lag time of about 3–5 h after the administration at the lights-off time. Both compounds also increase the delta activity during NREM sleep. However, verbascoside, a major polyphenol of *V. officinalis*, has no effect on the amount of sleep, indicating that hastatoside and verbenalin are major sleep-promoting components of this herb [12].

6.3.2.2 L-Stepholidine from Chinese Herb *Stephonia*

L-Stepholidine is an active ingredient of the Chinese herb *Stephonia*, the first compound with mixed dopamine D_1 receptor agonist/D_2 antagonist properties, and is used as a treatment medication for schizophrenia. When stepholidine is administered i.p. to mice at doses of 20–80 mg/kg, it shortens the sleep latency to NREM sleep, increases the amount of NREM sleep, and prolongs the duration of NREM sleep episodes, with a concomitant reduction in the amount of wakefulness [13]. Stepholidine also increases the number of state transitions from wakefulness to NREM sleep and subsequently from NREM sleep to wakefulness. However, stepholidine has no effect on either the amount of REM sleep or EEG power density of either NREM or REM sleep. These results suggest the potential application of this herb for the treatment of insomnia.

6.3.2.3 Ornithine

Ornithine supplementation has recently been used for attenuation of physical fatigue in healthy people. When we examined the effects of this molecule on the sleep–wake cycle of freely moving mice after oral administration at lights-off time, we found that ornithine (1.0 and 3.0 g/kg of body weight) increases the amount of NREM sleep 1.6- and 2.0-fold, respectively, for 2 h after its administration, with a peak at 1 h post administration compared with that of the vehicle-administered mice, without changing the amount of REM sleep [14]. Ornithine may also be considered to improve human sleep.

6.3.2.4 Crocin, Crocetin, and Safranal from *Crocus sativus L.* (Saffron)

Crocus sativus L. (saffron) has been traditionally used for the treatment of insomnia and other diseases of the nervous systems. Two carotenoid pigments, crocin and crocetin, are the major components responsible for the various pharmacological activities of *C. sativus L.* When crocin (30 and 100 mg/kg, i.p.) is administered to mice, it increases the total time of NREM sleep 1.6- and 2.7-fold, respectively, during a 4-h period after administration at a lights-off time [15]. When crocin is given to histamine H1 receptor-knockout mice, its sleep-promoting effects are attenuated, suggesting that the histaminergic system is involved in crocin-induced sleep. Crocetin (100 mg/kg, i.p.) also increases 1.5-fold the total time of NREM sleep after its administration. These compounds do not change the amount of REM sleep or show any adverse effects, such as rebound insomnia, after the induction of sleep. In hypnotic-model mice treated with a low dose (20 mg/kg) of pentobarbital, oral administration of safranal (100–300 mg/kg), another component of *C. sativus L.*, increases the duration of NREM sleep, shortens NREM sleep latency, increases the number of stage transitions between episodes of NREM sleep and wakefulness, and enhances the delta power activity of NREM sleep [16]. These findings indicate that crocin, crocetin, and safranal may be useful for the promotion of sleep in humans.

6.3.2.5 Honokiol and Magnolol from Chinese Herb Houpu (*Magnolia officinalis*)

Decoctions of the Chinese herb houpu (*Magnolia officinalis*) contain honokiol and magnolol and are used to treat a variety of mental disorders including depression. Honokiol (10 and 20 mg/kg, i.p.) significantly shortens the sleep latency to NREM sleep in mice and increases the amount of NREM sleep [17] and the number of state transitions from wakefulness to NREM sleep and subsequently from NREM sleep to wakefulness. However, honokiol has no effect on either the amount of REM sleep or EEG power density of either NREM or REM sleep. Magnolol (5 and 25 mg/kg, i.p.) also increases NREM sleep in mice [18]. Pretreatment with flumazenil (1 mg/kg, i.p.), an antagonist of the benzodiazepine-binding site of $GABA_A$ receptors, completely abolishes the somnogenic effects of honokiol and magnolol, indicating that these compounds promote NREM sleep through the $GABA_A$/benzodiazepine receptor complex. Therefore, these compounds may be used for the treatment of insomnia, especially for patients with difficulty in falling asleep, as well as for sleep maintenance.

6.3.3 Development of Portable 1-Channel EEG Device and a Simple Scoring System for Human Sleep

To measure sleep stages in hospitals, a polysomnographic test is normally used, in which data are analyzed with major devices and many electrodes to measure brain waves, eye movement, electromyogram, breathing, and snoring. However, we have established a simple sleep-scoring system for animals by using an EEG system with only two electrodes. Based on this unique technology, we developed a portable 1-channel EEG device and a simple sleep-scoring system for measuring the human EEG at home or while traveling. This device is the smallest in size in the world, weighing only 60 g, and it is easy to wear and does not bring about any uncomfortable feeling (Fig. 6.7a).

This portable EEG device is used daily to evaluate the quality of a person's sleep easily, so that the wearer can detect intrinsic sleep problems as soon as they occur in the early stages of mental disorders such as depression. We have started a collaborative research project with the National Institute of Polar Research of Japan and Japan Aerospace Exploration Agency (JAXA). Our device was used by members of the 50th and 51st Antarctic observation teams to evaluate an effect of a long stay in the polar regions on their psychological implication and their biological rhythm. Our device was also used by a Japanese astronaut, during his long stay in the International Space Station (Fig. 6.7b).

This device and sleep-scoring system will make it possible to improve the quality of sleep, thus providing a safer environment, as well as prevent traffic accidents and, eventually, improve the mental health of the wearer. It is hoped that people's quality of life will also be improved. Importantly, this portable EEG device allows a person to evaluate quite easily the quality of his or her daily sleep.

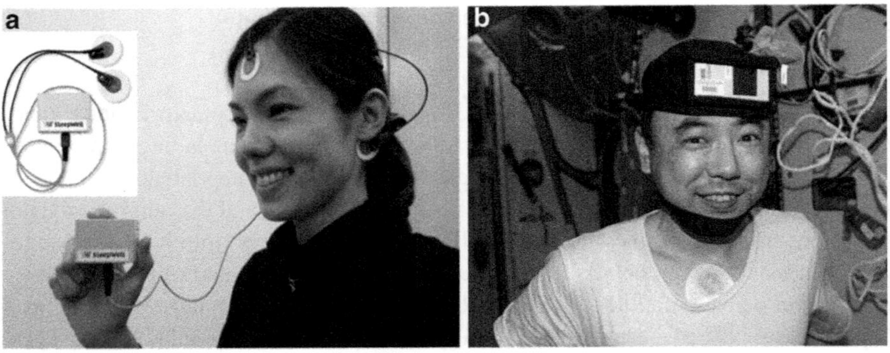

Fig. 6.7 Portable 1-channel EEG device used for evaluation of sleep-promoting health foods (**a**) and daily sleep of Japanese astronaut, Mr. Furukawa, while staying in the International Space Station (**b**) (Reprinted by permission of Sleep Well Co., Ltd., and Mr. Satoshi Furukawa, JAXA)

6.4 Conclusions

PGD_2 is the most potent endogenous sleep-promoting substance, and its action mechanism is the best characterized at a molecular level among various endogenous sleep-promoting substances. PGD_2 stimulates DP_1 receptors, which increases the local concentration of extracellular adenosine. Adenosine acts as a paracrine sleep-promoting molecule to activate adenosine A_{2A} receptor-expressing sleep-promoting neurons in the brain. The administration of a DP_1 antagonist (ONO-4127Na) or an adenosine $A_{1/2A}$ receptor antagonist (caffeine) suppresses sleep, indicating that the PGD_2-adenosine system is crucial for the maintenance of physiological sleep.

Earlier we established a sleep-scoring system to measure the EEG of various gene-manipulated mice. This system is used to identify sleep-promoting components in various food and herbal raw materials, such as hastatoside and verbenalin from *Verbena officinalis*; L-stepholidine, an active ingredient of the Chinese herb *Stephonia*; ornithine, a noncoding amino acid in the urea cycle; crocin, crocetin, and safranal from *Crocus sativus* L. (saffron); and honokiol and magnolol from the Chinese herb houpu (*Magnolia officinalis*). These findings will contribute to the production of health foods and pharmaceuticals that improve the quality of sleep.

By using sleep-scoring technology for animals, we also developed a small portable device for measuring human EEG activity at home or while traveling. This EEG device is useful to allow an individual to self-evaluate easily his or her quality of daily sleep. This "self-diagnostic system" as well as "supplements for good sleep" will make it possible for one to improve his or her quality of sleep in addition to proper exercise, an appropriate bathing practice, and selection of the best kinds of food.

Acknowledgments We thank Drs. Michael Lazarus and Zhi-Li Huang for helpful comments on this manuscript. This work was supported by grants from the Japan Society for the Promotion of Science, Japan Science and Technology Agency, Takeda Science Foundation, Sankyo Foundation, the Program of Basic and Applied Researches for Innovations in Bio-oriented Industry of Japan, Takeda Pharmaceutical Co., Ltd., Ono Pharmaceutical Co., Ltd, and Osaka City.

References

1. Narumiya, S., Ogorochi, T., Nakao, K., et al. (1982). Prostaglandin D_2 in rat brain, spinal cord and pituitary: Basal level and regional distribution. *Life Sciences, 31*, 2093–2103.
2. Ogorochi, T., Narumiya, S., Mizuno, N., et al. (1984). Regional distribution of prostaglandins D_2, E_2, and $F_{2\ alpha}$ and related enzymes in postmortem human brain. *Journal of Neurochemistry, 43*, 71–82.
3. Ueno, R., Ishikawa, Y., Nakayama, T., et al. (1982). Prostaglandin D_2 induces sleep when microinjected into the preoptic area of conscious rats. *Biochemical and Biophysical Research Communications, 109*, 576–582.
4. Onoe, H., Ueno, R., Fujita, I., et al. (1988). Prostaglandin D_2, a cerebral sleep-inducing substance in monkeys. *Proceedings of the National Academy of Sciences of the United States of America, 85*, 4082–4086.
5. Roberts, L. J., Sweetman, B. J., Lewis, R. A., et al. (1980). Increased production of prostaglandin D2 in patients with systemic mastocytosis. *The New England Journal of Medicine, 303*, 1400–1404.
6. Pentreath, V. W., Rees, K., Owolabi, O. A., et al. (1990). The somnogenic T lymphocyte suppressor prostaglandin D_2 is selectively elevated in cerebrospinal fluid of advanced sleeping sickness patients. *Transactions of the Royal Society of Tropical Medicine and Hygiene, 84*, 795–799.
7. Kohtoh, S., Taguchi, Y., Matsumoto, N., et al. (2008). Algorithm for sleep scoring in experimental animals based on fast Fourier transform power spectrum analysis of the electroencephalogram. *Sleep and Biological Rhythms, 6*, 163–171.
8. Mizoguchi, A., Eguchi, N., Kimura, K., et al. (2001). Dominant localization of prostaglandin D receptors on arachnoid trabecular cells in mouse basal forebrain and their involvement in the regulation of non-rapid eye movement sleep. *Proceedings of the National Academy of Sciences of the United States of America, 98*, 11674–11679.
9. Qu, W. M., Huang, Z. L., Xu, X. H., et al. (2006). Lipocalin-type prostaglandin D synthase produces prostaglandin D_2 involved in regulation of physiological sleep. *Proceedings of the National Academy of Sciences of the United States of America, 103*, 17949–17954.
10. Huang, Z. L., Qu, W. M., Eguchi, N., et al. (2005). Adenosine A_{2A}, but not A_1, receptors mediate the arousal effect of caffeine. *Nature Neuroscience, 8*, 858–859.
11. Lazarus, M., Shen, H. Y., Cherasse, Y., et al. (2011). Arousal effect of caffeine depends on adenosine A_{2A} receptors in the shell of the nucleus accumbens. *Journal of Neuroscience, 31*, 10067–10075.
12. Makino, Y., Kondo, S., Nishimura, Y., et al. (2009). Hastatoside and verbenalin are sleep-promoting components in *Verbena officinalis*. *Sleep and Biological Rhythms, 7*, 211–217.
13. Qiu, M. H., Qu, W. M., Xu, X. H., et al. (2009). D1/D2 receptor-targeting L-stepholidine, an active ingredient of the Chinese herb *Stephonia*, induces non-rapid eye movement sleep in mice. *Pharmacology, Biochemistry and Behavior, 94*, 16–23.
14. Omori, K., Kagami, Y., Yokoyama, C., et al. (2012). Promotion of non-rapid eye movement sleep in mice after oral administration of ornithine. *Sleep and Biological Rhythms, 10*, 38–45.
15. Masaki, M., Aritake, K., Tanaka, H., et al. (2012). Crocin promotes non-rapid eye movement sleep in mice. *Molecular Nutrition & Food Research, 56*, 304–308.
16. Liu, Z., Xu, X. H., Liu, T. Y., et al. (2012). Safranal enhances non-rapid eye movement sleep in pentobarbital-treated mice. *CNS Neuroscience & Therapeutics. 18*, 623–630.
17. Qu, W. M., Yue, X. F., Sun, Y., et al. (2012). Honokiol promotes non-rapid eye movement sleep via the benzodiazepine site of the $GABA_A$ receptor in mice. *British Journal of Pharmacology. 167*, 587–598.
18. Chen, C., Zhou, X., Luo, Y., et al. (2012). Magnolol, a major bioactive constituent of the bark of *Magnolia officinalis*, induces sleep via the benzodiazepine site of $GABA_A$ receptor in mice. *Neuropharmacology. 63*, 1191–1199.

Part IV
Practical Approaches to Patients and Family

Chapter 7
Psychosomatic Approach to Clinical Practice

Eliana Tossani and Giovanni Andrea Fava

7.1 Introduction

Stemming from Lipowski's original definition [1] and subsequent developments [2–4], psychosomatic medicine may be defined as a comprehensive and interdisciplinary framework for:

(a) Assessment of psychosocial factors affecting individual vulnerability, course, and outcome of any type of disease
(b) Holistic consideration of patient care in clinical practice
(c) Integration of psychological therapies in the prevention, treatment, and rehabilitation of medical diseases (psychological medicine)

The psychosomatic approach has resulted in important clinical developments, which have been outlined in a recent monograph [5]. We will summarize here the most important implications.

E. Tossani, Ph.D.
Department of Psychology, University of Bologna, Viale Berti Pichat 5, Bologna 40127, Italy
e-mail: eliana.tossani2@unibo.it

G.A. Fava, M.D. (✉)
Laboratory of Psychosomatics and Clinimetrics, Department of Psychology, University of Bologna, Viale Berti Pichat 5, Bologna 40127, Italy

Department of Psychiatry, State University of New York at Buffalo, Buffalo, NY, USA
e-mail: giovanniandrea.fava@unibo.it

K.B. Koh (ed.), *Somatization and Psychosomatic Symptoms*,
DOI 10.1007/978-1-4614-7119-6_7, © Springer Science+Business Media New York 2013

7.2 Assessing Psychosocial Factors Affecting Individual Susceptibility to Illness

It is becoming increasingly clear that we can improve medical care by paying more attention to psychological aspects of medical assessment [6], with particular reference to the role of stress [2–4, 7–9]. A number of factors have been implicated to modulate individual vulnerability to disease; for example, healthy habits and psychological well-being positively promote health rather than merely reduce disease.

7.2.1 *Early Life Events*

The role of early developmental factors in susceptibility to disease has been a frequent object of psychosomatic investigation [7,8]. Using animal models, events such as premature separation from the mother have consistently induced pathophysiological modifications, such as increased hypothalamic–pituitary–adrenal (HPA) axis activation. They may render the human individual more vulnerable to the effects of stress later in life. There has been also considerable interest in the association of childhood physical and sexual abuse with medical diseases, such as chronic pain and irritable bowel syndrome [10]. A history of childhood maltreatment was significantly associated with several adverse health outcomes, for example, functional disability and greater number of health risk behaviors, yet the evidence currently available does not allow any firm conclusions [11].

7.2.2 *Recent Life Events*

The notion that events and situations in a person's life, which are meaningful to him/her, may be followed by ill health has been a common clinical observation. The introduction of structured methods of data collection and control groups has allowed to substantiate the link between life events and a number of medical diseases, encompassing endocrine, cardiovascular, respiratory, gastrointestinal, autoimmune, skin, and neoplastic diseases [8, 9, 12–16].

7.2.3 *Stress and Allostatic Load*

The role of life change and stress has evolved from a simplistic linear model to a more complex multivariant conception embodied in the "allostatic" construct. McEwen and Stellar [12] proposed a formulation of the relationship between stress and the processes leading to disease based on the concept of allostasis, the ability of the organism to achieve stability through change. The concept of allostatic load refers to the wear and tear that results from either too much stress or insufficient coping, such as not turning off the stress responses when it is no longer needed. Biological parameters of allostatic load, such as glycosylated proteins, coagulation/fibrinolysis, and hormonal markers, have been linked to cognitive and physical functioning and mortality [8]. Recently, clinical criteria for determining the presence of allostatic load have been determined [9]. Thus, life changes are not the only source of psychological stress and subtle and long-standing life situations should not too readily be dismissed as minor and negligible, since chronic, daily life stressors may be experienced by the individual as taxing or exceeding his/her coping skills.

7.2.4 Health Attitudes and Behavior

Unhealthy lifestyle is a major risk factor for many of the most prevalent diseases, such as diabetes, obesity, and cardiovascular illnesses [17].

7.2.5 Social Support

Prospective population studies have found associations of measures of social support with mortality, psychiatric and physical morbidity, and adjustment to and recovery from chronic diseases [2]. An area that is now called "social neuroscience" is beginning to address the effects of the social environment on the brain and the physiology it regulates [8].

7.2.6 Psychological Well-Being

Positive health is often regarded as the absence of illness, despite the fact that, half a century ago, the World Health Organization defined health as a "state of complete physical, mental and social well-being and not merely the absence of disease or infirmity" [18]. Research on psychological well-being has indicated that it derives from the interaction of several related dimensions [19,20]. Several studies have suggested that psychological well-being plays a buffering role in coping with stress and has a favorable impact on disease course [21,22].

7.2.7 Personality Factors

The notion that personality variables can affect vulnerability to specific diseases was prevalent in the first phase of development of psychosomatic medicine (1930–1960) and was particularly influenced by psychoanalytic investigators, who believed that specific personality profiles underlie specific "psychosomatic disorders." This hypothesis was not supported by subsequent research [1,2]. Two personality constructs that can potentially affect general vulnerability to diseases, type A behavior and alexithymia (the inability to express emotion), have attracted considerable attention, but their relationship with health is still controversial [23,24].

7.2.8 *Psychiatric Disorders*

Psychiatric disorders, depression and anxiety in particular, are strongly associated with medical diseases. Mental disorders increase the risk for communicable and noncommunicable diseases; at the same time, many health conditions increase the risk for mental disorders, and comorbidity complicates recognition and treatment of medical diseases [25,26]. The potential relationship between medical diseases and psychiatric symptoms ranges from a purely coincidental occurrence to a direct causal role of organic factors – either medical diseases or drug treatment – in the development of psychiatric symptoms. The latter is often subsumed under the rubric of organic mental disorder whose key feature is the resolution of psychiatric symptoms by specific treatment of the organic condition, such as depression in Cushing's syndrome [27]. Not surprisingly, a correct diagnosis of depression in primary care is a difficult task. A recent meta-analysis [28,29] indicated that there are more false positives than either missed or identified cases.

Major depression has emerged as an extremely important source of comorbidity in medical diseases [30]. It was found to affect quality of life and social functioning and lead to increased health-care utilization, to be associated with higher mortality (particularly in the elderly), to have an impact on compliance, and to increase susceptibility to medical diseases [30–36]. The relationship between anxiety disorders and comorbid medical diseases has also been found to entail important clinical implications [37–39].

7.2.9 *Psychological Symptoms*

Current emphasis in psychiatry is about assessment of symptoms resulting in syndromes identified by diagnostic criteria of the Diagnostic and Statistical Manual of Mental Disorders (DSM). However, emerging awareness that also psychological symptoms which do not reach the threshold of a psychiatric disorder may affect quality of life and entail pathophysiological and therapeutic implications led to the development of the Diagnostic Criteria for Psychosomatic Research (DCPR) [40] together with a specific interview to assess patients [41]. The DCPR were introduced in 1995 and tested in various clinical settings [40–43]. They do provide also a classification for illness behavior, as the ways in which individuals experience, perceive, evaluate, and respond to their own health status. The DCPR allow a far more sophisticated qualitative assessment of patients than the one-dimensional DSM checklist of psychological symptoms.

Fava and Wise [44] have suggested to modify the DSM-IV category concerned with psychological factors affecting medical conditions that is a poorly defined diagnosis with virtually no impact on clinical practice (Table 7.1). They suggested a new

Table 7.1 Proposed classification for psychological factors affecting either identified or feared medical conditions

Hypochondriasis (DSM)
Disease phobia (DCPR)
Persistent somatization (DCPR)
Conversion symptoms (DCPR)
Illness denial (DCPR)
Demoralization (DCPR)
Irritable mood (DCPR)

DSM Diagnostic and Statistical Manual of Mental Disorders, *DCPR* Diagnostic Criteria for Psychosomatic Research

section which consists of the six most frequent DCPR syndromes [41]. The clinical specifiers include the DSM diagnosis of hypochondriasis and its prevalent variant, disease phobia. Both the DSM somatization disorder and undifferentiated somatoform disorder are replaced by the DCPR persistent somatization, conceptualized as a cluster of functional symptoms involving different organ systems [45]. Conversion may be redefined according to Engel's stringent criteria [46], involving features such as ambivalence, histrionic personality, and precipitation of symptoms by psychological stress of which the patients is unaware. DCPR illness denial, demoralization, and irritable mood offer further specifiers. Persistent denial of having a medical disease and needing treatment (e.g., lack of compliance, delay in seeking medical attention) frequently occurs in the medical setting [47]. Demoralization connotes the patient's consciousness of having failed to meet his or her own expectations (or others' expectations) with feelings of helplessness, hopelessness, or giving up [48,49]. It can be found in almost a third of medical patients and can be differentiated from depressive disorders. Furthermore, demoralization predicted a decline of both physical and psychological quality of life in consultation–liaison psychiatry patients [43,50].

Irritable mood, which may be experienced as brief episodes or be prolonged and generalized, has also been associated with the course of several medical diseases, carrying important clinical implications [51].

The advantage of this classification is that it departs from the organic/functional dichotomy and from the misleading and dangerous assumption that if organic factors cannot be identified, there should be psychiatric reasons which may be able to fully explain the somatic symptomatology. The presence of a nonfunctional medical disease does not exclude but indeed increases the likelihood of psychological distress and abnormal illness behavior [50,52].

In 2004, Tinetti and Fried [53] suggested that time has come to abandon diseases as the primary focus of medical care and suggest that the goal of treatment should be the attainment of individual goals, with identification and treatment of all modifiable biological and nonbiological factors, according to Engel's biopsychosocial model [54].

How should we assess these nonbiological variables? In clinical medicine there is the tendency to rely exclusively on "hard data," preferably expressed in the dimensional numbers of laboratory measurements, excluding "soft information" such as impairments and well-being. This soft information can now, however, be reliably assessed by clinical rating scales and indices which have been validated and used in psychosomatic research and practice [55,56].

7.3 The Clinimetric Approach in Clinical Research and Practice

In 1967, Alvan Feinstein dedicated a monograph to an analysis of clinical reasoning that underlies medical evaluations, such as the appraisal of symptoms, signs, and the timing of individual manifestations [57]. In 1982, he introduced the term "clinimetrics" [58] to indicate a domain concerned with the measurement of clinical issues that do not find room in customary clinical taxonomy. Such issues include types, severity, and sequence of symptoms; rate of illness progression (staging); severity and types of comorbidity; problems of functional capacity; reasons for medical decisions (e.g., treatment choices); and many other aspects of daily life, such as well-being and distress [59].

Clinimetrics has a set of rules that govern the structure of indices, the choice of component variables, and the evaluation of consistency, validity, and responsiveness. It may help in expanding the narrow range of information that is currently used in clinical science. The clinimetric perspective provides an intellectual home for clinical judgment, whose implementation is likely to improve outcomes in both clinical research and practice [60,61].

Feinstein, when he introduced the concept of comorbidity, referred to any "additional coexisting ailment" separated from the primary disease, even in the case this secondary phenomenon does not qualify as a disease per se [62]. Indeed, in clinical medicine, the many methods that are available for measuring comorbidity are not limited to disease entities [63].

A new method has been developed for organizing clinical data as variables in clinical reasoning. Emmelkamp et al. [64,65] have introduced the concept of macroanalysis (a relationship between co-occurring syndromes and problems is established on the basis of where treatment should commence in the first place). Fava and Sonino [55] have applied macroanalysis to assessing the relationship between medical and psychological variables. Macroanalysis starts from the assumption that in most cases there are functional relationships with different more or less clearly defined problem areas [64] and that the targets of treatment may vary during the course of disturbances [55].

The hierarchical organization that is chosen may depend on a variety of contingent factors (urgency, availability of treatment tools, etc.), which also include the patient's preferences and priorities. Indeed, macroanalysis is not only a tool for the therapist but can also be used to inform the patient of the relationship between different problem areas and motivate the patient to change [64,65]. The concept of shared decision is getting increasing attention in clinical medicine [66], but it is still seldom practiced in psychiatry [67]. Macroanalysis also requires reference to the staging method, whereby a disorder is characterized according to seriousness, extension, and longitudinal development [68].

Macroanalysis should be supplemented by microanalysis, a detailed analysis of specific symptoms (onset and course of the complaints, circumstances that worsen symptoms and consequences) [64,65]. For instance, when anxiety characterizes the clinical picture, it is necessary to know under which circumstances the anxiety becomes manifest, what the patient does when he/she becomes anxious, whether an avoidant behavior occurs, and what the long-term consequences of the avoidance behavior are.

Feinstein [69] remarks that, when making a diagnosis, thoughtful clinicians seldom leap from a clinical manifestation to a diagnostic end point. The clinical reasoning goes through a series of "transfer stations," where potential connections between presenting symptoms and pathophysiological process are drawn. These stations are a pause for verification, or change to another direction. In psychiatric assessment, however, disturbances are generally translated into diagnostic end points, where the clinical process stops. This does not necessarily explain the mechanisms by which the symptom is produced [69]. Not surprisingly, psychological factors are often advocated as an exclusion resource when symptoms cannot be explained by standard medical procedures, which is a diagnostic oversimplification which both Engel [70] and Lipowski [57] refused. Macroanalysis may allow to identify modifiable factors and their interactions. One case example is included to illustrate how clinical assessment and management follow similar patterns in case the disorder is either functional or organic.

The case which is illustrated in Box 7.1, Figs. 7.1 and 7.2 exemplifies the use of macroanalysis in the setting of nonulcer dyspepsia.

Box 7.1 A 24-Year-Old Woman with Nonulcer Dyspepsia

Ms. X is a 45-year-old woman who was diagnosed with **nonulcer dyspepsia**, on the basis of her symptomatology, after extensive negative medical work-up. He had taken gastroprotector therapy as prescribed without relief. She was convinced that she had stomach cancer. She also suffered from recurrent back pain. She was referred for psychosomatic consultation. Interviewing did not identify a specific psychiatric disorder, but disclosed the presence of a considerable ***allostatic load*** (she felt overwhelmed by her job demands as a lawyer's assistant and marital problem), ***agoraphobia*** (fear of public spaces and going out alone) without history of panic disorder and also ***high reactivity to social environment*** (both at work and within her family), and ***hypochondriasis***. No psychotropic drugs were prescribed. She was referred to a clinical psychologist who first introduced some lifestyle modifications as to her allostatic load. It was explained to her that agoraphobia is a psychological disorder and that there is a correlation between psychological stressors and physiological symptoms. The psychologist then addressed abnormal illness behavior with explanatory therapy for correcting hypochondriacal fears and beliefs, emotional instability with cognitive restructuring, and lack of assertiveness with well-being therapy. A brief course of individual cognitive treatment by a psychologist (five treatment sessions, one 50-min session per week), which included emotion regulation techniques and relationship skills training, did improve her relationship problems, emotional regulation, and agoraphobia. After a few months, there was a significant general improvement, which was maintained at a 2-year follow-up.

The various elements of macroanalysis are highlighted (underlined bold letters) and shown in Figs. 7.1 and 7.2.

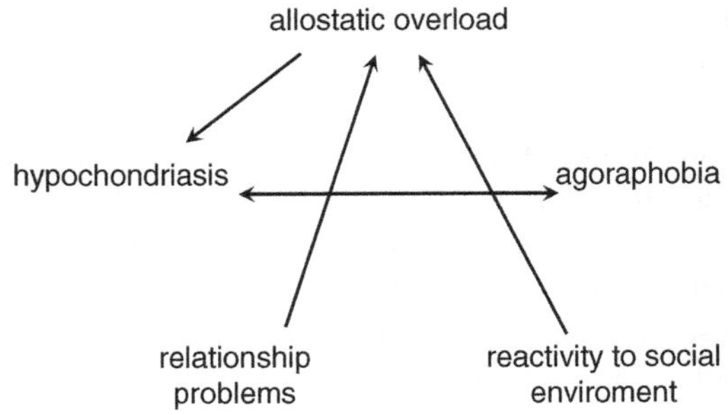

Fig. 7.1 Assessment by macroanalysis

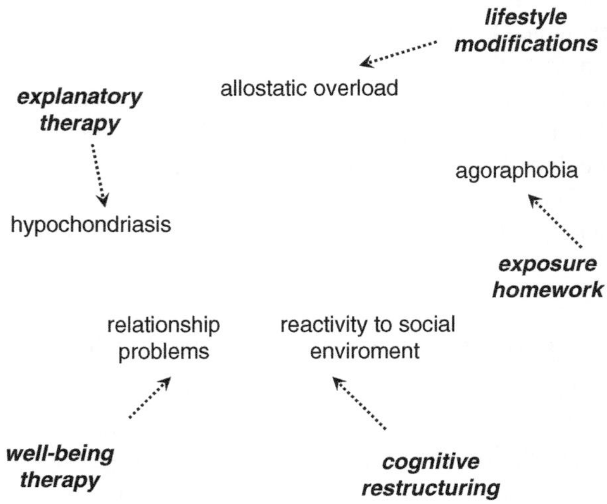

Fig. 7.2 Therapeutic approaches according to macroanalysis

The fear or idea of having a serious disease (cancer) based on misinterpretation of bodily symptoms, for more than 6 months, occurs without adequate organic pathology to account for preoccupation with the disease and despite medical reassurance, which indicates a syndrome of hypochondriasis [41]. This category identifies patients in whom psychophysiological symptoms tend to cluster [45], as is frequently the case in patients with hypochondriasis [71]. The clinical psychologist approached the psychological problems according to a sequential approach [72], starting from lifestyle modification proceeding to explanatory therapy [73] and then to exposure, cognitive restructuring, and well-being therapy [74]. The treatment team was multidisciplinary and involved the collaboration of a primary care physician who referred the patient to a psychiatrist, a gastroenterologist, and a clinical psychologist.

The issue is to take full advantage of clinimetric tools within the clinical process. It is not that certain disorders lack an organic explanation; it is that our assessment is inadequate in most clinical encounters and this particularly strikes when "hard data" are missing. It is noteworthy that Feinstein said, "even when the morphologic evidence shows the actual lesion that produces the symptoms of a functional disorder, a mere citation of the lesion does not explain the functional process by which the symptom is produced. (...) Thus, the clinician may make an accurate diagnosis of gallstones, but if the diagnosed gallstones do not account for the abdominal pain, a cholecystectomy will not solve the patient's problem" [75].

7.4 Mechanisms and Pathophysiological Implications

Alvan Feinstein was also the one who warned against the destruction of the pathophysiological bridges from bench to bedside [76]. Indeed, the lack of a psychosocial perspective, as is generally the case in current medicine, deprives the clinical process of a number of important links:

(a) The biological correlates of allostatic load [8,9], such as glycosylated proteins, coagulation/fibrinolysis, and hormonal markers, carry important clinical implications in terms of vulnerability risk.
(b) Recent advances in psychoneuroimmunology offer links between endogenous danger signals and the brain cytokine system that organizes the sickness response in its subjective, behavioral, and metabolic components [77]. The neurobiology of illness behavior, including the placebo effect [78], is beginning to unravel a number of clinical phenomena [78,79].
(c) The autonomic system has been a traditional target for exploration of psychosomatic research. Autonomic imbalance, such as a state of low heart rate variability, may be associated with a wide range of psychological and medical dysfunctions [80,81] and may affect responses to medical treatments [82].
(d) Mood and anxiety disorders have been associated with a variety of medical conditions [30,83]. The neurotransmitter imbalances associated with reinforcement–reward dysregulation, central pain, and psychomotor functioning may provide pathophysiological bridges for a number of clinical phenomena [84]. Similar considerations apply to the neurobiology of anger and irritability [85,86].
(e) Research on the neurobiologic correlates of resilience and well-being [87] has disclosed how different circuits may involve the same brain structures, particularly the amygdala, the nucleus accumbens, and the medial prefrontal cortex.
(f) The neurobiology of personality features, such as reward dependence and novelty seeking [88], alexithymia [24], and type A behavior [41,89], provides other valuable pathophysiological insights into the tendency to develop symptoms and abnormal illness behavior in the setting of medical diseases.

7.5 Clinical Implications

A satisfactory psychosomatic assessment yields a number of implications for management of medical diseases:

7.5.1 Subtyping According to Psychological Variables

There is now increasing evidence on the fact that the presence of psychological variables such as depressed mood in the medically ill is associated with a worse prognosis and deserves specific consideration [25,27,30–36,90]. Interestingly, the need for subtyping has recently emerged within the psychiatric definition of depression [91–93]. Several recent studies have attempted to characterize depression in the medically ill applying cluster analysis [94,95]. Guidi et al. [94] identified two distinct trajectory clusters: depressed somatizers and irritable/anxious depression. The first cluster accounted for about 60 % of total cases and was characterized by DCPR somatization syndromes (persistent somatization, functional somatic symptoms secondary to a psychiatric disorder, conversion symptoms, and anniversary reactions) and alexithymia. The second cluster encompassed about 40 % of cases and was characterized by DCPR irritability (irritable mood and type A behavior) and DSM-IV anxiety disorders. Subtyping major depressive disorders in the setting of medical diseases may yield improved targets for psychosomatic research and treatment trials [94]. These findings suggest that the mood and anxiety disorders are intertwined with somatization processes [95].

7.5.2 Lifestyle Modification

An increasing body of evidence links the progression of severe medical diseases to specific lifestyle behaviors [96]. The benefits of modifying lifestyle have been particularly demonstrated in coronary heart disease [13] and type 2 diabetes [97]. Further, a number of psychological treatments have been found to be effective in health-damaging behaviors, such as smoking [98]. A basic psychosomatic assumption is the consideration of patients as partners in managing a disease. The partnership paradigm includes collaborative care (a patient–physician relationship in which physicians and patients make health decisions together) [66,67] and self-management (a plan that provides patients with problem-solving skills to enhance their self-efficacy) [99].

7.5.3 Treatment of Psychiatric Comorbidity

Psychiatric disorders, particularly major depression, are frequently unrecognized and untreated in medical settings, with widespread harmful consequences for the individual and the society. Treatment of psychiatric comorbidity such as depression, with either pharmacological or psychotherapeutic interventions, markedly improves depressive symptoms, health-related functioning, and the patient's quality of life, even though an effect on medical outcome has not been demonstrated [100,101].

7.5.4 *Psychosocial Interventions*

Use of psychotherapeutic strategies (cognitive-behavioral therapy, stress management procedures, brief dynamic therapy) in controlled investigations has yielded a substantial improvement in a number of medical diseases [102–104]. Examples are interventions that increase social support, improve mood and enhance health-related behavior in patients with cancer [105–108], foster self-control and self-management in chronic pain [109] and asthma [110], and improve emotional disclosure [111,112].

7.5.5 *Treatment of Abnormal Illness Behavior*

For many years, abnormal illness behavior has been viewed mainly as an expression of personality predisposition and considered to be refractory to treatment by psychotherapeutic methods. There is now evidence to challenge such pessimistic stance [41]. For instance, several controlled studies on psychotherapy indicate that hypochondriasis is a treatable condition by the use of simple cognitive strategies [73]. The correlation between abnormal illness behavior and health habits may have implications in preventive efforts; individuals with excessive health anxiety were found to take worse care of themselves than control subjects in several studies [113]. Indeed, they may be so distressed by their belief of having an undiagnosed or neglected disease that choices yielding benefits in the distant future appear to be irrelevant to them.

7.6 Conclusions

There have been major transformations in health-care needs in the past decades. Chronic disease is now the principal cause of disability, and the use of health services for patients with chronic diseases consumes almost 80 % of health expenditures.

The exponential spending on preventive medication justified by the potential long-term benefits to a small segment of the population is now being challenged, whereas the benefits of modifying lifestyle by population-based measures are increasingly demonstrated and are in keeping with the biopsychosocial model.

Medically unexplained symptoms occur in up to 30–40 % of medical patients and increase medical utilization and costs. The traditional medical specialties, based mostly on organ systems (e.g., cardiology, gastroenterology), appear to be more and more inadequate in dealing with symptoms and problems which cut across organ system subdivisions. The need for a holistic approach is underscored by the implementation of interdisciplinary services.

The need to include consideration of functioning in daily life, productivity, performance of social roles, intellectual capacity, emotional stability, and well-being, has emerged as a crucial part of clinical investigation and patient care. These aspects have become particularly important in chronic diseases where cure cannot take place and also extend over family caregivers of chronically ill patients and health providers.

References

1. Lipowski, Z. J. (1986). Psychosomatic medicine: Past and present. Part II. Current state. *Canadian Journal of Psychiatry, 31*, 8–13.
2. Fava, G. A., & Sonino, N. (2010). Psychosomatic medicine. *International Journal of Clinical Practice, 64*, 1155–1161.
3. Wise, T. N. (2010). Psychosomatic medicine: An approach needed now more than ever. *International Journal of Clinical Practice, 64*, 999–1001.
4. Fava, G. A., & Sonino, N. (2010). Psychosomatic medicine: A name to keep. *Psychotherapy and Psychosomatics, 79*, 1–3.
5. Fava, G. A., Sonino, N., & Wise, T. N. (Eds.). (2012). *The psychosomatic assessment. Strategies to improve clinical practice* (Advances in psychosomatic medicine, Vol. 32). Basel, Switzerland: Karger.
6. Kroenke, K. (2002). Psychological medicine. *BMJ, 324*, 1536–1537.
7. Novack, D. H., Cameron, O., Epel, E., et al. (2007). Psychosomatic medicine: The scientific foundation of the biopsychosocial model. *Academic Psychiatry, 31*, 388–401.
8. McEwen, B. S. (2007). Physiology and neurobiology of stress and adaptation: Central role of the brain. *Physiological Reviews, 87*, 873–904.
9. Fava, G. A., Guidi, J., Semprini, F., et al. (2010). Clinical assessment of allostatic load and clinimetric criteria. *Psychotherapy and Psychosomatics, 79*, 280–284.
10. McCauley, J., Kern, D. E., Kolodner, K., et al. (1997). Clinical characteristics of women with a history of childhood abuse. *JAMA: The Journal of the American Medical Association, 277*, 1362–1368.
11. Romans, S., & Cohen, M. (2008). Unexplained and underpowered: The relationship between psychosomatic disorders and interpersonal abuse. *Harvard Review of Psychiatry, 16*, 35–44.
12. McEwen, B. S., & Stellar, E. (1993). Stress and the individual. Mechanisms leading to disease. *Archives of Internal Medicine, 153*, 2093–2101.
13. Rozanski, A., Blumenthal, J. A., & Kaplan, J. (1999). Impact of psychological factors on the pathogenesis of cardiovascular disease and implications for therapy. *Circulation, 99*, 2192–2217.
14. Sonino, N., Tomba, E., & Fava, G. A. (2007). Psychosocial approach to endocrine disease. *Advances in Psychosomatic Medicine, 28*, 21–33.
15. Wright, R. J., Rodriguez, M., & Cohen, S. (1998). Review of psychosocial stress and asthma. *Thorax, 53*, 1066–1074.
16. Picardi, A., & Abeni, D. (2001). Stressful life events and skin disease. *Psychotherapy and Psychosomatics, 70*, 118–136.
17. Mokdad, A. H., Marks, J. S., Stroup, D. F., et al. (2004). Actual causes of death in the United States, 2000. *JAMA: The Journal of the American Medical Association, 291*, 1238–1245.
18. World Health Organization. (1948). *Constitution of the World Health Organization basic document*. Geneva, Switzerland: Author.
19. Ryff, C. D., & Singer, B. (1996). Psychological well-being. *Psychotherapy and Psychosomatics, 65*, 14–23.
20. Caprara, G. V., Alessandri, G., & Barbaranelli, C. (2010). Optimal functioning. *Psychotherapy and Psychosomatics, 79*, 328–330.

21. Pressman, S. D., & Cohen, S. (2005). Does positive affect influence health? *Psychological Bulletin, 131*, 925–971.
22. Chida, Y., & Steptoe, A. (2008). Positive psychological well-being and mortality. *Psychosomatic Medicine, 70*, 741–756.
23. Shah, S. U., White, A., White, S., et al. (2004). Heart and mind: (1) Relationship between cardiovascular and psychiatric conditions. *Postgraduate Medical Journal, 80*, 683–689.
24. Taylor, G. J. (2010). Affects, trauma, and mechanisms of symptom formation. A tribute to John C. Nemiah, MD (1918–2009). *Psychotherapy and Psychosomatics, 79*, 339–349.
25. Prince, M., Patel, V., Saxena, S., et al. (2007). No health without mental health. *Lancet, 370*, 859–877.
26. Pohle, K., Domscheke, K., Roehrs, T., et al. (2009). Medical comorbidity affects antidepressant treatment response in patients with melancholic depression. *Psychotherapy and Psychosomatics, 78*, 359–363.
27. Sonino, N., Fava, G. A., & Fallo, F. (2010). Psychosomatic aspects of Cushing's syndrome. *Reviews in Endocrine & Metabolic Disorders, 11*, 95–104.
28. Aj, M., Vaze, A., & Rao, S. (2009). Clinical diagnosis of depression in primary care: A meta-analysis. *Lancet, 374*, 609–619.
29. Mitchell, A. J., Rao, S., & Vaze, A. (2010). Do primary care physicians have particular difficulty identifying late-life depression? A meta-analysis stratified by age. *Psychotherapy and Psychosomatics, 79*, 285–294.
30. Katon, W. J. (2003). Clinical and health services relationships between major depression, depressive symptoms, and general medical illness. *Biological Psychiatry, 54*, 216–226.
31. Schulz, R., Drayer, R. A., & Rollman, B. L. (2002). Depression as a risk factor for non-suicide mortality in the elderly. *Biological Psychiatry, 52*, 205–225.
32. di Matteo, M. R., Lepper, H. S., & Croghan, T. W. (2000). Depression is a risk factor for noncompliance with medical treatment. *Archives of Internal Medicine, 160*, 2101–2107.
33. Frasure-Smith, N., & Lesperance, F. (2003). Depression and other psychological risks following myocardial infarction. *Archives of General Psychiatry, 60*, 627–636.
34. Lemogne, C., Nabi, H., Zins, M., et al. (2010). Hostility may explain the association between depressive mood and mortality: Evidence from the French GAZEL cohort study. *Psychotherapy and Psychosomatics, 79*, 164–171.
35. Dirmaier, J., Watzke, B., Koch, U., et al. (2010). Diabetes in primary care: Prospective associations between depression, nonadherence and glycemic control. *Psychotherapy and Psychosomatics, 79*, 172–178.
36. Kojima, M., Hayano, J., Suzuki, S., et al. (2010). Depression, alexithymia and long-term mortality in chronic hemodialysis patients. *Psychotherapy and Psychosomatics, 79*, 303–311.
37. Roy-Byrne, P. P., Davidson, K. W., Kessler, R. C., et al. (2008). Anxiety disorders and comorbid medical illness. *General Hospital Psychiatry, 30*, 208–225.
38. Fava, G. A., Porcelli, P., Rafanelli, C., et al. (2010). The spectrum of anxiety disorders in the medically ill. *The Journal of Clinical Psychiatry, 71*, 910–914.
39. Beutel, M. E., Bleichner, F., von Heymann, F., et al. (2010). Anxiety disorders and comorbidity in psychosomatic inpatients. *Psychotherapy and Psychosomatics, 79*, 58.
40. Fava, G. A., Fabbri, S., Sirri, L., et al. (2007). Psychological factors affecting medical condition: A new proposal for DSM-V. *Psychosomatics, 48*, 103–111.
41. Porcelli, P., & Sonino, N. (Eds.). (2007). *Psychological factors affecting medical conditions. A new classification for DSM-V*. Basel, Switzerland: Karger.
42. Wise, T. N. (2009). Diagnostic criteria for psychosomatic research are necessary for DSM-V. Psychotherapy *and Psychosomatics, 78*, 330–332.
43. Porcelli, P., Bellomo, A., Quartesan, R., et al. (2009). Psychosocial functioning in consultation-liaison psychiatry patients. *Psychotherapy and Psychosomatics, 78*, 352–358.
44. Fava, G. A., & Wise, T. N. (2007). Psychological factors affecting either identified or feared medical conditions: A solution for somatoform disorders. *The American Journal of Psychiatry, 164*, 1002–1003.

45. Kellner, R. (1994). Psychosomatic syndromes, somatization and somatoform disorders. *Psychotherapy and Psychosomatics, 61*, 4–24.
46. Engel, G. L. (1970). Conversion symptoms. In C. M. Mac Bryde & R. S. Blacklow (Eds.), *Signs and symptoms* (pp. 650–699). Philadelphia: Lippincott.
47. Goldbeck, R. (1997). Denial in physical illness. *Journal of Psychosomatic Research, 43*, 575–593.
48. Cockram, C. A., Doros, G., & de Figueiredo, J. M. (2009). Diagnosis and measurement of subjective incompetence: The clinical hallmark of demoralization. *Psychotherapy and Psychosomatics, 78*, 342–345.
49. Mangelli, L., Fava, G. A., Grandi, S., et al. (2005). Assessing demoralization and depression in the setting of medical disease. *The Journal of Clinical Psychiatry, 66*, 391–394.
50. Sirri, L., Fava, G. A., & Wise, T. N. (2011). Psychiatric classification in the setting of medical disease: Comparing the clinical value of different proposals. *Journal of Psychosomatic Research, 70*, 493–495.
51. Mangelli, L., Fava, G. A., Grassi, L., et al. (2006). Irritable mood in Italian patients with medical disease. *The Journal of Nervous and Mental Disease, 194*, 226–228.
52. Härter, M., Baumeister, H., Reuter, K., et al. (2007). Increased 12-month prevalence rates of mental disorders in patients with chronic somatic diseases. *Psychotherapy and Psychosomatics, 76*, 354–360.
53. Tinetti, M. E., & Fried, T. (2004). The end of the disease era. *American Journal of Medicine, 116*, 179–185.
54. Engel, G. L. (1977). The need for a new medical model: A challenge for biomedicine. *Science, 196*, 129–136.
55. Fava, G. A., & Sonino, N. (2009). Psychosomatic assessment. *Psychotherapy and Psychosomatics, 78*, 333–341.
56. Sonino, N., & Peruzzi, P. (2009). A psychoneuroendocrinology service. *Psychotherapy and Psychosomatics, 78*, 346–351.
57. Lipowski, Z. J. (1974). Physical illness and psychopathology. *International Journal of Psychiatry in Medicine, 5*, 483–497.
58. Feinstein, A. R. (1982). The Jones criteria and the challenge of clinimetrics. *Circulation, 66*, 1–5.
59. Feinstein, A. R. (1987). *Clinimetrics*. New Haven, CT: Yale University Press.
60. Fava, G. A., Tomba, E., & Sonino, N. (2012). Clinimetrics: The science of clinical measurements. *International Journal of Clinical Practice, 66*, 11–15.
61. Fava, G. A., Rafanelli, C., & Tomba, E. (2012). The clinical process in psychiatry: A clinimetric approach. *The Journal of Clinical Psychiatry, 73*, 177–184.
62. Feinstein, A. R. (1970). The pre-therapeutic classification of comorbidity in chronic disease. *Journal of Chronic Diseases, 23*, 455–468.
63. deGroot, V., Beckerman, H., Lankhorst, G. J., et al. (2003). How to measure comorbidity: A critical review of available methods. *Journal of Clinical Epidemiology, 56*, 221–229.
64. Emmelkamp, P. M. G., Bouman, T. K., & Scholing, A. (1993). *Anxiety disorders* (pp. 55–67). Chichester, England: Wiley.
65. Emmelkamp, P. M. G. (2004). The additional value of clinimetrics needs to be established rather than assumed. *Psychotherapy and Psychosomatics, 73*, 142–144.
66. Joosten, E. A. G., De Fuentes-Merillas, L., de Weert, G. H., et al. (2008). Systematic review of the effects of shared-decision making on patient satisfaction, treatment adherence and health status. *Psychotherapy and Psychosomatics, 77*, 219–226.
67. Joosten, E. A. G., de Jong, C. A. J., de Weert-van Oene, G. H., et al. (2009). Shared decision making reduces drug use and psychiatry severity in substance-dependent patients. *Psychotherapy and Psychosomatics, 78*, 245–253.
68. Fava, G. A., & Kellner, R. (1993). Staging: A neglected dimension in psychiatric classification. *Acta Psychiatrica Scandinavica, 87*, 225–230.
69. Feinstein, A. R. (1973). An analysis of diagnostic reasoning. I The domains and disorders of clinical macrobiology. *The Yale Journal of Biology and Medicine, 46*, 212–232.

70. Engel, G. L. (1967). The concept of psychosomatic disorder. *Journal of Psychosomatic Research, 11*, 3–9.
71. Aaron, L. A., & Buchwald, D. (2001). A review of the evidence for overlap among unexplained clinical conditions. *Annals of Internal Medicine, 134*, 868–881.
72. Fava, G. A., Tomba, E., & Grandi, S. (2007). The road to recovery from depression. *Psychotherapy and Psychosomatics, 76*, 260–265.
73. Fava, G. A., Grandi, S., Rafanelli, C., et al. (2000). Explanatory therapy of hypochondriasis. *The Journal of Clinical Psychiatry, 61*, 317–322.
74. Fava, G. A., & Tomba, E. (2009). Increasing psychological well-being and resilience by psychotherapeutic methods. *Journal of Personality, 77*, 1903–1934.
75. Feinstein, A. R. (1973). An analysis of diagnostic reasoning. II. The strategy of intermediate decisions. *The Yale Journal of Biology and Medicine, 46*, 264–283.
76. Feinstein, A. R. (1999). Basic biomedical science and the destruction of the pathophysiological bridge from bench to bedside. *American Journal of Medicine, 107*, 461–467.
77. Dantzer, R. (2005). Somatization: A psychoneuroimmune perspective. *Psychoneuroendocrinology, 30*, 947–952.
78. Price, D. D., Finniss, D. G., & Benedetti, F. (2008). A comprehensive review of the placebo effect. *Annual Review of Psychology, 59*, 565–590.
79. Walach, H., Bosch, H., Lewith, G., et al. (2008). Effectiveness of distant healing for patients with chronic fatigue syndrome. *Psychotherapy and Psychosomatics, 77*, 158–166.
80. Thayer, J. F., & Brosschot, J. F. (2005). Psychosomatics and psychopathology. *Psychoneuroendocrinology, 30*, 1050–1058.
81. Tak, L. M., Janssens, K. A., Dietrich, A., et al. (2010). Age-specific associations between cardiac vagal activity and functional somatic symptoms: A population-based study. *Psychotherapy and Psychosomatics, 79*, 179–187.
82. Zachariae, R., Paulsen, K., Mehlsen, M., et al. (2007). Chemotherapy-induced nausea, vomiting and fatigue. *Psychotherapy and Psychosomatics, 76*, 376–384.
83. Bech, P. (2009). Fifty years with the Hamilton Scales for anxiety and depression. *Psychotherapy and Psychosomatics, 78*, 202–211.
84. Carroll, B. J. (1994). Brain mechanisms in manic depression. *Clinical Chemistry, 40*, 303–308.
85. Fava, G. A. (1987). Irritable mood and physical illness. *Stress Medicine, 3*, 293–299.
86. Kamarck, T. W., Haskett, R. F., Muldoon, M., et al. (2009). Citalopram intervention for hostility. *Journal of Consulting and Clinical Psychology, 77*, 174–188.
87. Charney, D. S. (2004). Psychobiological mechanisms of resilience and vulnerability. *The American Journal of Psychiatry, 161*, 195–216.
88. Cloninger, C. R. (1987). Systematic method for clinical description and classification of personality. *Archives of General Psychiatry, 44*, 573–588.
89. Fava, M., Littman, A., & Halperin, P. (1987). Neuroendocrine correlates of the type A behavior pattern. *International Journal of Psychiatry in Medicine, 17*, 289–307.
90. Rapp, M. A., Rieckmann, N., Lessman, D. A., et al. (2010). Persistent depressive symptoms after acute coronary syndrome are associated with compromised white matter integrity in the anterior cingulate: A pilot study. *Psychotherapy and Psychosomatics, 79*, 149–155.
91. Lichtenberg, P., & Belmaker, R. H. (2010). Subtyping major depressive disorder. *Psychotherapy and Psychosomatics, 79*, 131–135.
92. Bech, P. (2010). The struggle for subtypes in primary and secondary depression and their mode-specific treatment or healing. *Psychotherapy and Psychosomatics, 79*, 331–338.
93. Baumeister, H., & Parker, G. (2010). A second thought on subtyping major depression. *Psychotherapy and Psychosomatics, 79*, 388–389.
94. Guidi, J., Fava, G. A., Picardi, A., et al. (2011). Subtyping depression in the medically ill by cluster analysis. *Journal of Affective Disorders, 132*, 383–388.
95. Fava, G. A., Guidi, J., Porcelli, P., et al. (2012). A cluster analysis-derived classification of psychological distress and illness behavior in the medically ill. *Psychological Medicine, 42*, 401–407.

96. Tomba, E. (2012). Assessment of lifestyle in relation to health. *Advances in Psychosomatic Medicine, 32*, 72–96.
97. Narayan, K. M. V., Kanaya, A. M., & Gregg, E. W. (2003). Lifestyle intervention for the prevention of type 2 diabetes mellitus. *Treatments in Endocrinology, 2*, 315–320.
98. Compas, B. E., Haagon, D. A., Keefe, F. J., et al. (1998). Sampling of empirically supported psychological treatments from health psychology: Smoking, chronic pain, cancer, and bulimia nervosa. *Journal of Consulting and Clinical Psychology, 66*, 89–112.
99. Bodenheimer, T., Lorig, K., Holman, H., et al. (2002). Patient self-management of chronic disease in primary care. *JAMA: The Journal of the American Medical Association, 288*, 2469–2475.
100. Jackson, J. L., de Zee, K., & Berbano, E. (2004). Can treating depression improve disease outcomes? *Annals of Internal Medicine, 140*, 1054–1056.
101. Pigott, H. E., Leventhal, A. M., Alter, G. S., et al. (2010). Efficacy and effectiveness of antidepressants. *Psychotherapy and Psychosomatics, 79*, 267–279.
102. Balon, R. (2009). Cognitive-behavioral therapy, psychotherapy and psychosocial interventions in the medically ill. *Psychotherapy and Psychosomatics, 78*, 261–264.
103. Kaupp, J. W., Rapaport-Hubschman, N., & Spiegel, D. (2005). Psychosocial treatments. In J. L. Levenson (Ed.), *Textbook of psychosomatic medicine* (pp. 923–956). Washington, DC: American Psychiatric Press.
104. Abbass, A., Kisely, S., & Kroenke, K. (2009). Short-term psychodynamic psychotherapy for somatic disorders. *Psychotherapy and Psychosomatics, 78*, 265–274.
105. Andersen, B. L., Yang, H. C., Farrar, W. B., et al. (2008). Psychologic intervention improves survival for breast cancer patients. *Cancer, 113*, 3450–3458.
106. Herschbach, P., Berg, P., Waadt, S., et al. (2010). Group psychotherapy of dysfunctional fear of progression in patients with chronic arthritis or cancer. *Psychotherapy and Psychosomatics, 79*, 31–38.
107. Grassi, L., Sabato, S., Rossi, E., et al. (2010). Effects of supportive-expressive group therapy in breast cancer patients with affective disorders: A pilot study. *Psychotherapy and Psychosomatics, 79*, 39–47.
108. Tulipani, C., Morelli, F., Spedicato, M. R., et al. (2010). Alexithymia and cancer pain: The effect of psychological intervention. *Psychotherapy and Psychosomatics, 79*, 156–163.
109. Turk, D. C., Swanson, K. S., & Tunks, E. R. (2008). Psychological approaches in the treatment of chronic pain patients. *Canadian Journal of Psychiatry, 53*, 213–223.
110. Lahmann, C., Nickel, M., Schuster, T., et al. (2009). Functional relaxation and guided imagery as complementary therapy in asthma: A randomized controlled clinical trial. *Psychotherapy and Psychosomatics, 78*, 233–239.
111. Frisina, P. G., Borod, J. C., & Lepore, S. J. (2004). A meta-analysis of the effects of written emotional disclosure on the health outcomes of clinical populations. *The Journal of Nervous and Mental Disease, 192*, 629–634.
112. van Middendorp, H., Geenen, R., Sorbi, M. J., et al. (2009). Health and physiological effects of an emotional disclosure intervention adapted for application at home: A randomized clinical trial in rheumatoid arthritis. *Psychotherapy and Psychosomatics, 78*, 145–151.
113. Sirri, L., Grandi, S., & Fava, G. A. (2008). The illness attitude scales. *Psychotherapy and Psychosomatics, 77*, 337–350.

Chapter 8
Emotional Intelligence, Alexithymia, and the Doctor-Patient Relationship

Arnstein Finset

8.1 Introduction

8.1.1 Emotions in Doctor-Patient Encounters

Emotional topics are common in medical consultations as well as in psychotherapy. Patients often present to the doctors and therapists their hopes, uncertainties, feelings, and worries. However, patients often will refrain from conveying their emotions explicitly in the consultation. Rather, emotions may be expressed as an indirect hint about underlying worries or concerns, often referred to as cues [1–3] or clues [4]. However, studies indicate that most consultations contain few cues to underlying emotions. Feelings may also be expressed more unambiguously, labeled in the literature, for instance, as concerns [1] or empathic opportunities [5].

Studies show large variations in how health professionals respond to patients' emotion. Most studies have assessed physicians' responses. For instance, Mjaaland [6] found in a study of medical interviews in a general hospital across specialties that physicians provided room for further disclosure in response to about half of all emotional cues and concerns, but more often with reference to the medical than the affective content of the cue or concern. Similarly, Butow et al. [7] reported that oncologists effectively identified and responded to the majority of informational cues; however, they were less effective in addressing cues for emotional support. In another study on cancer care, Pollak et al. [8] found that oncologists reacted with empathy to 29 % of patients' expression of negative emotion. A number of studies report similar results, indicating that the emotional aspect of patients' messages is often overlooked and not responded to by physicians [6, 9–11]. Rather than follow

A. Finset, Ph.D. (✉)
Department of Behavioural Sciences in Medicine, Institute of Basic Medical Sciences, Faculty of Medicine, University of Oslo, P.O.Box 1111, Blindern N-0317 Oslo, Norway
e-mail: arnstein.finset@medisin.uio.no

K.B. Koh (ed.), *Somatization and Psychosomatic Symptoms*,
DOI 10.1007/978-1-4614-7119-6_8,

up on emotional cues, physicians often, but not always, respond with biomedical questioning and information giving or rather nonspecific acknowledgment or premature reassurance [9–12].

The responses of nurses to cues and concerns have also been investigated and the results vary. In a study from a surgical oncology clinic, Uitterhoeve et al. [13] found that nurses explored or acknowledged 45 % of patients' emotional expressions, but more than half of the expressions were met with distancing behaviors. Eide et al. [14], on the other hand, found that 75 % of all emotional expressions were met with implicit recognition, whereas another 13 % were explicitly recognized in a study of admittance interviews at a pain clinic [14]. The differences between findings may be due to both methodological differences and different clinical tasks and settings.

In a recent study, Del Piccolo et al. [15] investigated cues and concerns in psychiatric consultations. They found that psychiatrists quite often provided space for further disclosure of the emotional cue, but most often without an explicit reference to the cue or concern. Psychiatrists made a specific mention of the patient's cue or concern only when the emotional expression had been initiated by them, but empathic responses were infrequent.

Many patients welcome the opportunity to talk about their feelings, but other patients are rather reluctant. However, in any case, awareness toward patients' emotions is an important element in the clinician's repertoire of clinical skills, both in conventional medical consultations and psychotherapy. In a conventional consultation, the main purpose of the consultation is most often to set a diagnosis or somehow monitor an already known disease as well as provide information and treatment to the patient. Psychotherapy, "the talking cure," aims to reduce distress and modify behavior, most often within a series of encounters, ranging from a few hours of short-term therapy to treatment lasting for several years. In both cases, the clinician may be faced with patients' emotion and will be challenged to find ways to respond. Expression and non-expression of emotion are important elements in the ongoing relationship between doctors and patients.

8.1.2 Individual Differences in How to Handle Emotions

Emotional expressions vary in terms of valence and intensity of the emotion expressed, from fervent rage to calm delight, from deep sadness to animated joy. But there are individual differences, not only in what patients feel but in the way patients handle their emotions as well as how clinicians respond. These differences may relate to what we call regulatory aspects of emotion. Emotion regulation is defined by Gross [16] as the processes by which emotions are influenced, when one has them, and how one experiences and expresses them. Studies on emotion regulation attempt to find answers to a number of different questions: To which extent are the emotional qualities of the stimuli perceived? How is the emotion identified (and with what degree of clarity), tolerated, labeled, and expressed, verbally and nonverbally? How attentive is the person to his or her emotions, and how well are emotions monitored and controlled?

A number of different terms have been suggested to cover these aspects of emotional behavior, with different emphases, operationalizations, and theoretical foundations, such as affect regulation, mood awareness, levels of emotional awareness, affect consciousness, and emotional approach coping.

Some of the research on emotion regulation seeks to find general elements in the process of emotion regulation. Other research seeks to identify stable individual profiles of emotion regulation. The two most frequently studied concepts in the latter tradition are alexithymia and emotional intelligence.

Thirty-five years ago, Peter Sifneos and his colleagues [17] observed that patients with psychosomatic disorders often had difficulties to express emotions in medical consultations. He coined the term alexithymia, which literally means lack of words for feelings (a-lexi-thymia), which he considered a stable personality trait in some individuals. Alexithymia has been defined and operationalized in different ways. Currently, the most commonly used method to measure alexithymia is the Toronto Alexithymia Scale, developed by Taylor et al. [18]. In the 20-item version, TAS-20, alexithymia is defined as a cognitive-affective style or trait involving (1) difficulty identifying feelings and distinguishing between feelings and bodily sensations, (2) difficulties expressing and communicating subjective feelings verbally, and (3) a certain concrete, externally oriented, bluntly reality-based style of thinking.

Around 1990 Peter Salovey et al. [19] developed the concept of emotional intelligence. Emotional intelligence is described as an individual characteristic that reflects the "ability to monitor one's own and other's emotions, to discriminate among them and to use this information to guide one's thinking and actions [20]." The concept has gained popularity in psychological research over the last 10 years. The term has also become a household word in popular psychology, not the least through the best-selling book on emotional intelligence by Daniel Goleman [21].

In spite of the increasing number of research papers, few researchers have investigated the impact of alexithymia and emotional intelligence on the doctor-patient relationship. Interestingly, a few studies have been done on either clinicians' emotional intelligence or patients' alexithymia. However, there have been no studies on the relationship of clinicians' alexithymia or of patients' emotional intelligence with the doctor-patient relationship. Nor has there to our knowledge been any study which simultaneously investigates emotion regulation or affective awareness components in both patients' and clinicians' behavior.

8.2 Clinicians' Emotional Intelligence and the Doctor-Patient Relationship

Arora et al. [22] have recently reviewed the research literature on the relationship of emotional intelligence with clinical competence and skills in medicine. Their expectation was to find positive association between measures of emotional intelligence and variables relevant to the doctor-patient relationship.

The findings in the empirical literature give partial support to this expectation. Weng [23] studied the association between emotional intelligence and variables related to the doctor-patient relationship in a sample of 983 patients and 39 physicians representing 11 different specialties. The measure of physicians' emotional intelligence was based on ratings by nurses who had collaborated closely with the physicians. The strongest association was found between physicians' emotional intelligence and patients' trust in physicians. Patients' trust in physicians was strongly related to their satisfaction, but there was no direct link between physicians' emotional intelligence and patients' satisfaction [23].

In a subsequent study, Weng et al. [24] investigated the associations of emotional intelligence of surgeons with patients' ratings of the quality of the doctor-patient relationship, surgeons' empathy, and patients' satisfaction. The surgeons' emotional intelligence predicted the quality of the doctor-patient relationship, but again no direct association was found between physicians' emotional intelligence and patients' satisfaction.

Recently Kaplowitz et al. [25] studied the impact of therapists' emotional intelligence on psychotherapy in a small pilot study of 23 therapist-patient dyads [25]. The researchers found, to use their own words, "… modest preliminary evidence for the hypothesis that therapists' emotional skills positively influence therapeutic efficacy." Higher emotional intelligence of therapist predicted better improvement of patients' interpersonal problems, as assessed by the therapists. Moreover, higher therapists' emotion management abilities (a component of the emotional intelligence measure applied) were significantly associated with greater improvement in patient-rated symptomatology. However, no significant relationship was found between therapists' emotional intelligence and working alliance.

8.3 Patients' Alexithymia and the Doctor-Patient Relationship

The concept of alexithymia was based on the observations of Peter Sifneos in psychotherapy with patients with psychosomatic complaints. Still there is surprisingly little research on the potential impact of alexithymia on the process and outcome of psychotherapy. Krystal [26] suggested 30 years ago that psychotherapists often assume that patients generally have "the affective functions necessary for the utilization of psychotherapy." However, this is not always the case. Ogrodniczuk and his colleagues [27] have recently elaborated on Krystal's observation in a series of studies on the effects of alexithymia on the process and outcome of psychotherapy.

Ogrodniczuk et al. [27] point to a number of myths regarding alexithymia and psychotherapy. One myth is that patients with alexithymia not only are reluctant to talk about emotions in therapy sessions but also are reluctant to even take part in psychotherapy. However, in a study of 145 new patients from two different psychiatric outpatient clinics, they found that alexithymia scores (as measured with the TAS-20) did not significantly differ between groups of patients who chose medication treatment, psychotherapy, or no treatment at all [27]. Another myth is the notion that alexithymia is resistant to change even in those patients who engage in psychotherapy. However, a number of studies have reported that alexithymia scores may decline during psychotherapy and that such changes are correlated with improvements in therapy.

However, consistent with earlier studies, what Ogrodniczuk et al. [27] confirmed was the widely held idea that alexithymia is associated with poor outcome in psychotherapy. Interestingly, the researchers found that the therapists' reactions to the patients partially mediated the effect of alexithymia on the outcome of psychotherapy. The negative effects of patients' difficulties in communicating feelings and of externally oriented thinking were mediated by therapists' negative attitudes and reactions toward these patients.

There are few studies on the effect of emotion regulation and affect awareness on the doctor-patient relationship outside of psychotherapy. A series of studies on arranged consultations in a laboratory setting have investigated how individual differences in terms of trait anxiety and alexithymia influence how patients respond to emotional talk in medical consultation.

In our first study, students with high and low trait anxiety volunteered to take part in arranged consultations with a physician [28]. They were instructed to bring up any medical complaint that they had at the present or had suffered in the past or a medical concern about their parents or other close relatives. The interviews were performed in two different experimental conditions. In one condition, labeled as patient-centered, the physician attended to psychosocial topics and responded explicitly to emotional concerns. In the other condition, labeled as physician-centered, the physician concentrated strictly on the medical complaints and largely ignored psychosocial issues and emotional concerns. Dependent variables were affective responses as measured with the Profiles of Mood States (POMS) and cortisol responses. We expected stronger emotional responses to the consultation in patients with high state anxiety. Moreover, we expected that patients with high state anxiety would respond with attenuated emotional activation in the patient-centered condition. However, contrary to our expectation, this study found a significant interaction effect between trait anxiety and experimental conditions, with higher arousal among high-anxiety patients in the patient-centered than in the physician-centered condition, while the opposite among low-anxiety patients [28].

Our subsequent study found physician-patient interaction in arranged consultations with fibromyalgia patients with and without alexithymia. Similar to the study of high- and low-anxiety students, fibromyalgia patients with alexithymia reported more confusion, less vigor, and higher heart rate activation in arranged consultations with a "patient-centered" psychosocially focused communication style as compared to a "physician-centered" symptom-focused communication style [29]. Yet, it was found that these patients were more satisfied with many empathic statements from the doctor [30]. When the patients later viewed the videos of the consultations, patients with alexithymia displayed more confusion, less vigor, increased electrodermal activation, and a feeling of less control in consultations with a psychosocial emphasis. In contrast, for patients without alexithymia, the "patient-centered" psychosocially focused communication style was associated with fewer phasic electrodermal responses (as measured by the number of spikes) and a feeling of more control in the consultation than was the physician-centered condition with a focus on symptoms [31].

8.4 Conclusions

There is some evidence that clinicians' emotional intelligence and patients' alexithymia may have some impact on the process and outcome of consultations. The following tentative conclusions can be drawn from some studies. First, clinicians' emotional intelligence seems to be associated with patients' experiences of trust in their physicians. Some findings indicate its positive impact on outcome in psychotherapy, but not on the therapeutic alliance. Second, alexithymia is negatively associated with outcome in psychotherapy. This effect is partially mediated by negative therapist's attitude toward patients with alexithymia. Third, some studies indicate a consistent interaction effect between alexithymia and communication style in patients' responses to emotional content in medical consultations. An emphasis on emotional themes in the consultation was associated with higher arousal, less feeling of control, and less satisfaction in patients with alexithymia, while it was associated with a more accepting reaction in patients without alexithymia. Applying measures of alexithymia as well as emotional intelligence both to clinicians and to patients could provide valuable information on the potential relationship between patients' and clinicians' emotion regulation and how such potential associations are related to qualities of the doctor-patient relationship.

References

1. Zimmermann, C., Del Piccolo, L., & Finset, A. (2007). Cues and concerns by patients in medical consultations: A literature review. *Psychological Bulletin, 133*, 438–463.
2. Maguire, P., Booth, K., Elliott, C., et al. (1996). Helping health professionals involved in cancer care acquire key interviewing skills -the impact of workshops. *European Journal of Cancer, 32A*, 1486–1489.
3. Lussier, M. T., & Richard, C. (2009). Handling cues from patients. *Canadian Family Physician, 55*, 1213–1214.
4. Levinson, W., Gorawara-Bhat, R., & Lamb, J. (2000). A study of patient clues and physician responses in primary care and surgical settings. *The Journal of the American Medical Association, 284*, 1021–1027.
5. Suchman, A. L., Markakis, K., Beckman, H. B., et al. (1997). A model of empathic communication in the medical interview. *The Journal of the American Medical Association, 277*, 678–682.
6. Mjaaland, T. A., Finset, A., Jensen, B. F., et al. (2011). Physicians' responses to patients' expressions of negative emotions in hospital consultations: A video-based observational study. *Patient Education and Counseling, 84*, 332–337.
7. Butow, P. N., Brown, R. F., Cogar, S., et al. (2002). Oncologists' reactions to cancer patients' verbal cues. *Psycho-Oncology, 11*, 47–58.
8. Pollak, K. I., Arnold, R., Alexander, S. C., et al. (2010). Do patient attributes predict oncologist empathic responses and patient perceptions of empathy? *Supportive Care in Cancer, 18*, 1405–1411.
9. Bell, R. A., Kravitz, R. L., Thom, D., et al. (2002). Unmet expectations for care and the patient-physician relationship. *Journal of General Internal Medicine, 17*, 817–824.

10. Pollak, K. I., Arnold, R. M., Jeffreys, A. S., et al. (2007). Oncologist communication about emotion during visits with patients with advanced cancer. *Journal of Clinical Oncology, 25*, 5748–5752.
11. Ryan, H., Schofield, P., Cockburn, J., et al. (2005). How to recognize and manage psychological distress in cancer patients. *European Journal of Cancer Care, 14*, 7–15.
12. Epstein, R. M., Hadee, T., Carroll, J., et al. (2007). "Could this be something serious?" Reassurance, uncertainty, and empathy in response to patients' expressions of worry. *Journal of General Internal Medicine, 22*, 1731–1739.
13. Uitterhoeve, R., Bensing, J., Dilven, E., et al. (2009). Nurse-patient communication in cancer care: Does responding to patient's cues predict patient satisfaction with communication. *Psycho-Oncology, 18*, 1060–1068.
14. Eide, H., Sibbern, T., Egeland, T., et al. (2001). Fibromyalgia patients' communication of cues and concerns: Interaction analysis of pain clinic consultations. *The Clinical Journal of Pain, 27*, 602–610.
15. Del Piccolo, L., Mazzi, M.A., Goss, C., et al. (2012). How emotions emerge and are dealt with in first diagnostic consultations in psychiatry. *Patient Education and Counseling*. doi:10.1016/j.pec. 2012.01.010, 88, 29–35.
16. Gross, J. J. (1998). The emerging field of emotion regulation: An integrative review. *Review of General Psychology, 2*, 271–299.
17. Sifneos, P. E., Apfel-Savitz, R., & Frankel, F. H. (1977). The phenomenon of 'alexithymia': Observations in neurotic psychosomatic patients. *Psychotherapy and Psychosomatics, 28*, 47–57.
18. Bagby, R. M., Parker, J. D. A., & Taylor, G. T. (1994). The twenty-item Toronto Alexithymia Scale – I: Item selection and cross-validation of the factor structure. *Journal of Psychosomatic Research, 38*, 23–32.
19. Mayer, J. D., DiPaolo, M., & Salovey, P. (1990). Perceiving affective content in ambiguous visual stimuli: A component of emotional intelligence. *Journal of Personality Assessment, 54*, 772–781.
20. Mayer, J. D., & Salovey, P. (1997). What is emotional intelligence? In P. Salovey & D. J. Suyter (Eds.), *Emotional development and emotional intelligence: Educational implications*. New York: Basic Books.
21. Goleman, D. (1995). *Emotional intelligence: Why it matters more than IQ*. London: Bloomsbury.
22. Arora, S., Ashrafian, H., Davis, R., et al. (2010). Emotional intelligence in medicine: A systematic review through the context of the ACGME competencies. *Medical Education, 44*, 749–764.
23. Weng, H.-C. (2008). Does the physician's emotional intelligence matter?: Impacts of the physician's emotional intelligence on the trust, patient-physician relationship, and satisfaction. *Health Care Management Review, 33*, 280–288.
24. Weng, H.-C., Steed, J. F., Yu, S.-W., et al. (2011). The effect of surgeon empathy and emotional intelligence on patient satisfaction. *Advances in Health Sciences Education, 16*, 591–600.
25. Kaplowitz, M. J., Safran, J. D., & Muran, C. J. (2011). Impact of therapist emotional intelligence on psychotherapy. *The Journal of Nervous and Mental Disease, 199*, 74–84.
26. Krystal, H. (1982–83). Alexithymia and the effectiveness of psychoanalytic treatment. *International Journal of Psychoanalytic Psychotherapy, 13*, 76–85.
27. Ogrodniczuk, J. S., Piper, W. E., & Joyce, A. S. (2011). Effect of alexithymia on the process and outcome of psychotherapy: A programmatic review. *Psychiatry Research, 190*, 43–48.
28. Graugaard, P. K., & Finset, A. (2000). Trait anxiety and reactions to patient-centered and doctor-centered styles of communication: An experimental study. *Psychosomatic Medicine, 62*, 33–39.
29. Finset, A., Graugaard, P., & Holt, E. (2006). *Communication induced stress responses in medical interviews with fibromyalgia patients: The role of alexithymia*. Presented at European Research Conference on Psychosomatic Medicine, Dubrovnik.

30. Graugaard, P. K., Holgersen, K., & Finset, A. (2004). Communicating with alexithymic and non-alexithymic patients: An experimental study of the effect of psychosocial communication and empathy on patient satisfaction. *Psychotherapy and Psychosomatics, 73*, 92–100.
31. Finset, A., Graugaard, P., & Holt, E. (2006). *Electrodermal responses to viewing a medical interview: The effect of affect regulation*. Presented at European Association of Communication in Health Care Conference, Basel.

Chapter 9
An Effective Approach to Somatization Assessment and Management

Kyung Bong Koh

9.1 Introduction

Somatization is a process in which there is inappropriate focus on physical symptoms and psychosocial problems are denied [1]. Somatization is highly prevalent in primary care where 20–30 % of patients fulfill criteria for somatoform disorders [2–4] and even more patients may present with medically unexplained symptoms of shorter duration [5]. In a general medical clinic in the USA, 84 % of presentations of common physical symptoms had no identified organic cause [5], and over half of new referrals to a Dutch medical outpatient clinic had symptoms that remained medically unexplained [6]. Despite its high prevalence, somatization often goes unrecognized [3, 7]. Somatizing patients suffer distress for a long time and seek treatment that results in disappointment because a correct diagnosis is not made by physicians. They doctor shop but cannot find a willing physician so they are called "medical orphans" [8]. They often make the complaint that "My symptoms are genuine, but everything is coming back negative" [9].

Somatic symptoms persist despite treatment [5] and patients are dissatisfied with aspects of their management. This may be because clinicians do not effectively address patients' needs other than the management of pathology [10]. Thus, treatment of somatoform disorder is challenging, and physicians are often frustrated because it cannot be treated according to the existing biomedical model [11].

Sophisticated technologies may facilitate diagnosis, but they also serve to reinforce the boundary between medically explained and medically unexplained symptoms [12]. The default use of biomedical approaches may cause iatrogenic harm and disable somatizing patients [13, 14].

K.B. Koh, M.D., Ph.D. (✉)
Department of Psychiatry, Yonsei University College of Medicine,
50 Yonsei-ro, Seodaemun-gu, Seoul 120-752, Korea
e-mail: kbkoh@yuhs.ac

K.B. Koh (ed.), *Somatization and Psychosomatic Symptoms*,
DOI 10.1007/978-1-4614-7119-6_9, © Springer Science+Business Media New York 2013

Such patients often express concern that practitioners and others presume their symptoms are "all in the mind." They might be seen to be "faking" their symptoms and so are not accepted by others as being "legitimately ill." Such concerns further amplify their marginalization from medical care and other forms of social support [9]. Therefore, normal test results present major problems for patients, physicians, and health services. Patients may be angry and dissatisfied, feeling that they are not being taken seriously or that the implication is that their problem is all in their minds [10]. Physicians are more likely to find the doctor-patient relationship difficult if symptoms are unexplained [15], and they often find it difficult to help patients with such symptoms [16].

Physicians may be less skilled in providing support and ongoing care against a background of diagnostic uncertainty [12]. Patients may be reluctant to accept the relevance of psychological factors, and negotiation to achieve this acceptance requires skill and care [10]. Therefore, this chapter reviews methods of educating medical students and physicians in the assessment and management of patients with somatization.

9.2 Comorbidity with Depressive Disorders and Anxiety Disorders

Depression, anxiety, and somatization are the most common mental disorders encountered in primary care [2]. General practitioners (GPs) are usually the first contact person for patients suffering from psychological and physical problems and therefore play a central role in the detection, prevention, and management of mental disorders. Adequate detection and management of these disorders pose a challenge to the health-care system [17–20].

Moreover, some somatoform disorders (somatization disorder and pain disorder) are highly comorbid with depressive disorders and anxiety disorders [21]. About 5 % of somatoform disorder patients have comorbid depressive and anxiety disorders [22]. Several possibilities may explain such comorbidity [23, 24]. First, it may be that the association is spurious because of methodological problems (e.g., recall bias may explain the observed comorbidity). Second, somatoform disorders may lead to the onset of depressive disorders and anxiety disorders. Third, depressive disorders and/or anxiety disorders may lead, in a causal way, to the onset of somatoform disorders. Fourth, there are common causes that lead to the onset of all three types of disorders (e.g., genetic or environmental factors). Finally, there may be more complex associations (e.g., somatoform disorders may influence remission or treatment responses of other disorders or vice versa).

Previous studies have reported that there is no empirical evidence to determine whether primary somatoform disorders predict subsequent depressive disorders/anxiety disorders or vice versa [21]. Furthermore, mental comorbidity is often associated with a more difficult doctor-patient relationship [22]. For GPs to have conversations with these patients, better continuing medical education in communication skills is needed [22].

9.3 Is "Somatization" a Defense Against the Acknowledgement of a Psychiatric Disorder?

Somatizing patients often show resistance to psychological explanations [9]. However, there is no evidence that experiencing multiple physical symptoms helps the individual deny the presence of psychiatric disorders [25]. Research on primary and secondary care in the United Kingdom has shown that patients' main expectations are for explanations and understanding, which are more important than expectations for support, testing, and diagnosis [26, 27]. Therefore, special skills and strategies are required by nonpsychiatric physicians to manage chronic somatizing patients for whom the acceptance of psychiatric treatment is essential [1].

9.4 When Should Psychological Skills Be Taught and by Whom?

Somatizing patients are good candidates for medical students and primary care physicians to learn about the biopsychosocial approach for patient-centered care because the symptoms of somatizing patients cannot be biomedically explained. Primary care physicians also feel that effective management strategies are lacking [28, 29]. Therefore, education for medical students and primary physicians is essential. Psychological skills should be taught to medical students during their clinical rotations and to GPs during their GP training period [1]. During these training periods, psychiatrists have an important role to play in helping other physicians develop the skills necessary to identify and manage patients with somatization [1].

9.5 Educational Programs

Educational programs should include a review of diagnostic criteria for somatization [30]; discussion of the role of stress, anger, and mood in the disorder [1, 31]; skills training in biopsychosocial history taking; a general treatment model for somatization; and advice on the management of chronic cases [30].

9.6 How Can Psychiatrists Educate Other Practitioners?

Several teaching techniques, particularly modeling, role-playing (Fig. 9.1), and video feedback, are known to be effective in teaching psychological skills both to psychiatrists [32] and to GPs [33, 34]. A few studies [35, 36] have stressed the

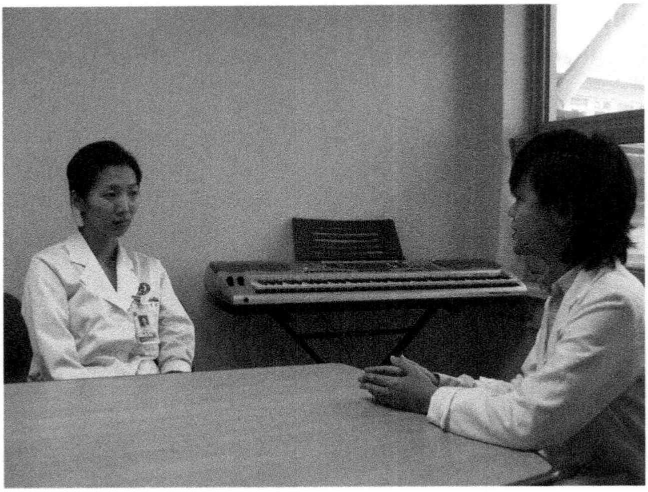

Fig. 9.1 A medical student is role-playing for preparation of a somatizing patient for psychiatric referral

importance of interview techniques in identifying somatizing patients. These techniques are often employed in teaching "reattribution" skills to GP trainees [35]. Most GPs recognize that helping a patient with a psychiatric illness to reattribute his or her somatic symptoms to a psychological rather than a physical etiology is an important, but difficult, task [37].

9.7 Approach to Patients: Attitude and Communication Skills

9.7.1 Empathic Listening and Patience

Empathic listening to patients' narratives is critical to effective patient-centered care. Practitioners can help by listening to patients' accounts of their symptoms and their attempts to overcome them [9]. Management of somatizing patients often requires patience from physicians because patients may be angry and dissatisfied, feeling that they are not being taken seriously [10]. At the same time, some physicians cannot tolerate patients' frequent complaints and demands, showing anger toward such patients not only because their illness behavior is different from other patients' but also their symptoms are not medically explained. This countertransference can be frequently observed during the management of somatizing patients [38, 39], which leads to the breaking down of the doctor-patient relationship.

9.7.2 *Accept Patient's Suffering*

People who suffer from an undiagnosed illness want their symptoms to be acknowledged as "genuine," and they also want to feel that practitioners will work with them to suggest and negotiate strategies that may help alleviate them and better "manage" their situation. Therefore, their suffering should be accepted by physicians as legitimate. Explanations of symptoms are more likely to be helpful if physicians avoid a strict mind/body dualism. However, attempts to integrate the mind and body may be challenging because such separation remains so culturally ingrained [9].

9.7.3 *Biopsychosocial Assessment*

There is no dichotomy between physical and psychological disorders. Rather, the proportion of physical or psychological etiology varies across a continuum [40]. Psychological factors such as health anxiety and symptom attributions may influence the genesis and presentation of physical symptoms, even in the absence of psychiatric disorders. Therefore, from the beginning of assessment, equal attention should be devoted to understanding biopsychosocial factors, such as somatic, psychological, dietary, environmental, and physiotherapeutic aspects in somatizing patients [10]. When taking the patient's history, physicians should be aware of psychosocial cues and then should be consistent and unambiguous in their management of the patients [1]. In particular, physicians should assess patients' anger because anger—especially anger suppression—may play an important role in somatization as seen in cases of hwabyung, or somatoform disorders [31].

A Case of hwabyung

A 49-year-old woman had to suppress her expression of emotion toward her husband since her marriage because he drank alcohol nearly every day and she reported that he beat her. Recently, she separated from him and stayed at her parents' home. She could not tolerate her somatic symptoms, which she described as feeling as if something heavy and hot in her chest was moving up, febrile sensations, and headaches.

9.7.3.1 Understand Patient's Illness Experience

Physicians need to understand the problems faced by people with undiagnosed illness. One way of helping people with an undiagnosed illness might be for practitioners to adopt more patient-centered styles of care. Physicians trained in biomedical models of care may be able to satisfactorily identify and treat disease but may be less at ease with providing care and support. Patient-centered care, with an emphasis not just on the disease but also the illness experience, may provide a framework for practitioners to provide enhanced care and support [41].

Patient-centered care also stresses the importance of finding common ground with the patient. In relation to an undiagnosed illness, it may be particularly helpful for physicians and patients to reach a mutual understanding and agreement of the problems. If a full biomedical explanation is not possible, then partial explanations that are consistent with the patient's point of view and make sense in their world-view may be very valuable to patients' outcomes [42].

9.7.3.2 Integrating Cognitive Therapy into the Assessment

Cognitive factors may contribute to the genesis of all physical symptoms and to associated distress, disability, and health-care use. A physical symptom has two essential components: first, the awareness of a bodily sensation and, second, the attribution of abnormality to that sensation. Attributions influence the sufferer's response to the sensation. Therefore, cognitions such as symptom attributions clearly have a role in the presentation of physical symptoms to medical care [10].

Cognitive therapy is a psychological treatment that, in the treatment of persistent and troubling physical symptoms, aims to change symptom attributions and thereby improve outcomes. This therapy is usually conducted individually in ten or more weekly sessions of about 1 h each. Patients are actively involved in testing out and modifying their dysfunctional beliefs about their physical symptoms. Cognitive therapy is time-consuming and expensive [10].

The twin obstacles of availability and acceptability of cognitive therapy can be overcome by integrating aspects of cognitive therapy into medical care [10]. Cognitive therapy of medically unexplained physical symptoms and hypochondriasis includes the identification and challenging of patients' evidence for their misinterpretations of bodily sensations [43, 44]. In a general hospital clinic, the clinician may act as a cognitive therapist and can do this by eliciting the patient's beliefs, explaining his or her view of the cause of the symptoms, and presenting evidence from the assessment to support his or her view and, if appropriate, challenge the patient's view. Therefore, the clinical assessment itself may modify cognitive factors such as symptom attribution and consequently improve outcomes [10].

An approach to the management of symptoms that acknowledges their basis in both pathophysiology and cognition opens up an additional therapeutic avenue. With the cognitive approach, the assessment—diagnosis and explanation—is potentially a powerful form of treatment. The therapeutic effect of the assessment is likely to be mediated cognitively by changing the sufferer's understanding of the meaning of the symptoms [10]. Assessment itself, without formal psychological therapy, may be used as a treatment regardless of whether relevant pathology is present. Although the potential treatment effect of the assessment will exist principally where tests are normal, it may also exist when relevant physical pathology is present. The relevant factor here is the direction of change in the patient's beliefs about the symptom. Therefore, an investigation does not need to be normal to be good news. Patients with abdominal pain, for example, may fear that their pain is due to cancer. The discovery of gastritis rather than cancer at gastroscopy may therefore be reassuring and thereby reduce symptom severity. Conversely, a normal test result in the presence of continuing symptoms may be considered bad news as the cause remains unexplained and untreatable. This dimensional approach to test results and health anxiety implies that the assessment may function as a treatment for physical symptoms whether the findings are normal or not [10].

A cognitive-educational intervention suffices without performing an investigation. There is some randomized evidence to support the therapeutic effect of explanation supported only by history taking and consultation. Perhaps clinicians can evoke similar therapeutic effects by using history taking and clinical examinations as well [45]. In sum, assessment is a vital and powerful part of treatment rather than being merely its subordinate and prelude [10]. Observational studies in patients with headache and bowel symptoms suggest that the consultation itself may improve outcomes [46, 47]. Thus, discussion of the problem and its cause appears to be therapeutic. Changes in symptom attributions are probably the mediator of the therapeutic effects arising from such discussions [10].

The potential power of this cognitive approach in the treatment of physical symptoms is evidenced in trials of cognitive therapy for a range of disorders that present to a general hospital. It is not possible to offer formal cognitive therapy to every patient presenting with physical symptoms, and such an approach would not be acceptable to many patients. However, simple cognitive approaches may be able to reframe cognitions and result in meaningful improvements in outcomes. The patient's understanding of the cause and prognosis of his/her symptoms may be elicited. History taking, a physical examination, and testing may contribute to evidence that can be used to confirm or refute patients' beliefs. If symptoms remain medically unexplained, a positive explanation of possible causes, combined with an optimistic prognosis, may be effective [10]. For example, in hypochondriasis, normal advice and reassurance is clearly ineffective. However, the ability of cognitive therapy to change cognitions and thereby improve other outcomes in this disorder demonstrates that this approach is powerful [10].

9.7.4 Learn Communication Skills

Once somatizing patients have been identified by physicians, these physicians need to develop the following skills:

1. Let the patient know his/her potential diagnosis and its prognosis by explaining test results and the nature of the illness.
2. Use general terms such as "tension" and "stress" and avoid using professional (or psychological) terms to minimize patients' resistance [11].
3. Explain the mechanisms of somatization by giving an example of common somatic symptoms, such as palpitation, headache, and backache [1, 48].
4. Make sure patients will improve when they receive treatment from specialists, such as psychiatrists.
5. Administer the appropriate treatment, which may or may not involve psychiatric referral [1].

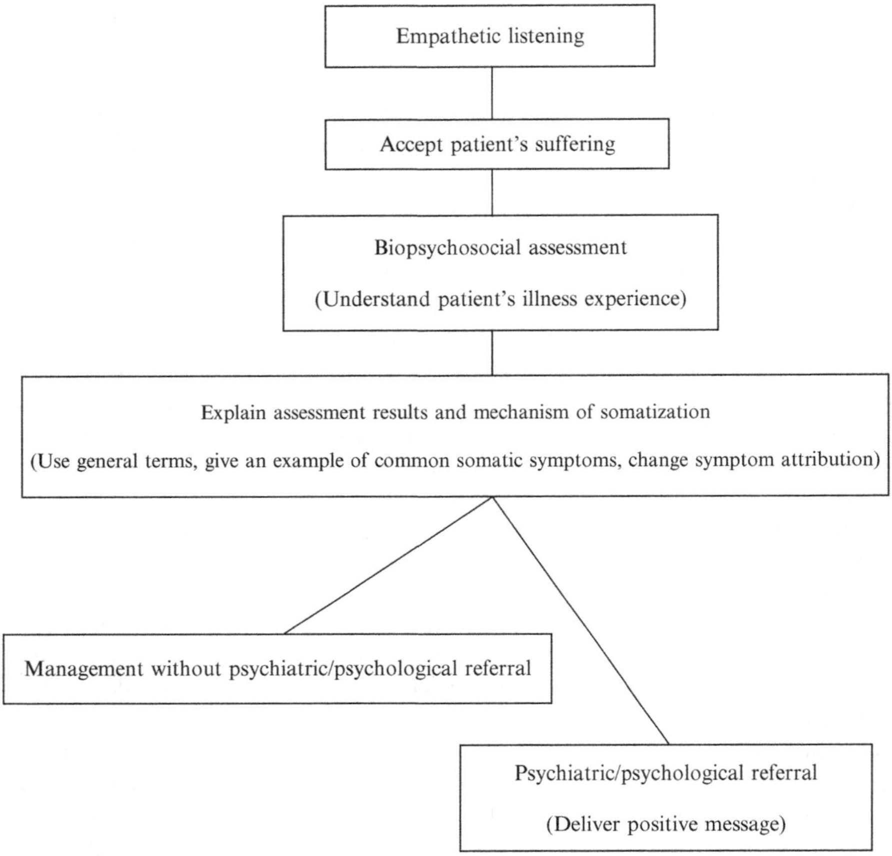

Fig. 9.2 An effective approach to somatization assessment and management for physicians

9.7.5 *How to Refer the Patient for Psychiatric or Psychological Assessment*

Physicians should learn how to refer somatizing patients for psychiatric or psychological assessment [1] because these patients show resistance to psychological explanations [9]. First, physicians should inform patients about their negative test results and provide explanations for the symptoms [1]. Second, medical students and physicians should be trained to give the patient positive messages based on positive experiences of the therapeutic process for somatizing patients during their clinical clerkship and based on practitioners' clinical experiences. For example, such statements may include "I've seen many patients get better after they were referred to specialists and received treatment." Finally, they should develop their skills for referral by practicing this experience or using role-playing.

The above-mentioned effective approach to somatizing patients for physicians is presented in the Fig. 9.2.

9.8 Clinical Outcomes of Training Primary Care Physicians

Some of the skills described in this chapter have been successfully taught to general practice trainees using videotaped learning packages [35]. Another education program including the reattribution model for primary care physicians has been tested in a 3-month, pre-post study and has reported positive effects on patients' physical functioning, psychiatric disorder symptoms [49], illness attributions, and satisfaction [50]. However, the training of primary care physicians was not found to have a significant effect on clinical outcomes and may not result in any significant improvement in patient satisfaction with care for those scoring high for somatization [51]. Further research is required to evaluate the effect of primary care interventions in somatizing patients in terms of the referral process, rather than clinical outcomes.

9.9 Evaluations of Management for Somatizing Patients

The treatment of somatizing patients has been evaluated in a number of studies, but few have focused on care administered by primary care physicians. A review of primary care interventions aimed at improving the treatment of mental disorders reported a positive effect on clinical outcomes in 8 of 16 studies, only 3 of which specifically targeted somatization [52]. Another review reported a consistent positive effect of CBT (71 % of 31 controlled trials) on physical health in somatizing patients. However, treatment was provided by mental health specialists in the reviewed studies [53].

Primary care treatment for somatization has taken two main directions. One approach is shared care, where mental health specialists offer patient assessment and treatment guidelines [54]. For example, a randomized controlled trial [55] of patients with medically unexplained physical symptoms showed that between 6 and 12 sessions of cognitive therapy resulted in significant improvement compared to medical care alone. Another approach is the education of primary care physicians to improve their management of somatization within their own setting by using the reattribution model [49, 50]. Clinical effects of such a program are mentioned in 9.8.

9.10 Education of Organizations

We need to educate organizations such as the Gastrointestinal and Heart Associations about the identification and successful management of irritable bowel syndrome and noncardiac chest pain. We also need to educate the lay organization about mind-body interactions. The results of current psychiatric research can influence its members, and this can in turn reduce both lay and medical prejudices about disorders with somatic symptoms [1]. There is a need for continuous development and evaluation of treatment strategies for patients with medically unexplained symptoms [51].

9.11 Conclusions

The importance of interviewing techniques has been stressed in the identification and management of somatizing patients. These patients require explanations and understanding from physicians beyond expectations for support, testing, and diagnosis. However, nonpsychiatric physicians should avoid mind-body dualism. Educational programs for physicians include review of diagnostic criteria for somatization; discussion of the role of stress, anger, and mood in somatization; skills training in biopsychosocial history taking; a general treatment model for somatization; and advice on the management of chronic cases. Teaching techniques, such as modeling, role-playing, and video feedback, are known to be effective in teaching psychological skills both to psychiatrists and general practitioners. From the beginning of assessment, equal attention should be devoted to each biopsychosocial factor that could affect somatizing patients. Additionally, nonpsychiatric physicians should learn to integrate aspects of cognitive therapy into medical care because such an approach to assessment, including diagnosis and explanation, is potentially a powerful form of treatment. Further, history taking, physical examinations, and testing can be used to confirm or refute patients' beliefs. Patient-centered care with its emphasis not just on the disease but also on the illness experience may be a good therapeutic framework for managing somatizing patients. Finally, medical students and primary physicians should learn how to refer such patient for psychiatric or psychological assessment. In particular, a positive explanation of possible causes, combined with an optimistic prognosis, may be effective in referral of medically unexplained patients.

References

1. Bass, C., & Benjamin, S. (1993). The management of chronic somatization. *British Journal of psychiatry, 162*, 472–480.
2. Toft, T., Fink, P., Oernboel, E., et al. (2005). Mental disorders in primary care: Prevalence and co-morbidity among disorders. Results from the functional illness in primary care (FIP) study. *Psychological Medicine, 35*, 1175–1184.
3. Fink, P., Sorensen, L., Engberg, M., et al. (1999). Somatization in primary care. Prevalence, health care utilization, and general practitioner recognition. *Psychosomatics, 40*, 330–338.
4. Arnold, I. A., de Waal, M. W., Eekhof, J. A., et al. (2006). Somatoform disorder in primary care: Course and the need for cognitive-behavioral treatment. *Psychosomatics, 47*, 498–503.
5. Kroenke, K., & Mangelsdorff, D. (1989). Common symptoms in ambulatory care: Incidence, evaluation, therapy and outcome. *The American Journal of Medicine, 86*, 262–266.
6. van Hemert, A. M., Hengeveld, M. W., Bolk, J. H., et al. (1993). Psychiatric disorders in relation to medical illness among patients of a general medical out-patient clinic. *Psychological Medicine, 23*, 167–173.

7. Goldberg, D., & Bridges, K. (1987). Screening for psychiatric illness in general practice: The general practitioner versus the screening questionnaire. *The Journal of the Royal College of General Practitioners, 37*, 15–18.
8. Aronowitz, R. A. (2001). When do symptoms become a disease? *Annals of Internal Medicine, 134*, 803–808.
9. Nettleton, S., Watt, I., O'Malley, L., et al. (2005). Understanding the narratives of people who live with medically unexplained illness. *Patient Education and Counseling, 56*, 205–210.
10. Price, J. R. (2000). Managing physical symptoms: The clinical assessment as treatment. *Journal of Psychosomatic Research, 48*, 1–10.
11. Koh, K. B. (2011). *Stress and psychosomatic medicine* (pp. 263–285). Seoul, Korea: Ilchokak.
12. Rhodes, L. A., McPhillips-Tangum, C. A., Markham, C., et al. (1999). The power of the visible: The meaning of diagnostic tests in chronic back pain. *Social Science & Medicine, 48*, 1189–1203.
13. Fink, P. (1992). Surgery and medical treatment in persistent somatizing patients. *Journal of Psychosomatic Research, 36*, 439–447.
14. Smith, G. R., Jr., Monson, R. A., & Ray, D. C. (1986). Patients with multiple unexplained symptoms. Their characteristics, functional health, and health care utilization. *Archives of Internal Medicine, 146*, 69–72.
15. Hahn, S. R., Thompson, K. S., Wills, T. A., et al. (1994). The difficult doctor-patient relationship: Somatization, personality and psychopathology. *Journal of Clinical Epidemiology, 47*, 647–657.
16. Sharpe, M., Mayou, R., Seagroatt, V., et al. (1994). Why do doctors find some patients difficult to help? *The Quarterly Journal of Medicine, 87*, 187–193.
17. Henningsen, P., Zipfel, S., & Herzog, W. (2007). Management of functional somatic syndromes. *Lancet, 369*, 946–955.
18. Aragones, E., Pinol, J. L., & Labad, A. (2007). Depression and physical comorbidity in primary care. *Journal of Psychosomatic Research, 63*, 107–111.
19. de Waal, M. W., Arnold, I. A., Eekhof, J. A., et al. (2008). Follow-up study on health care use of patients with somatoform, anxiety and depressive disorders in primary care. *BMC Family Practice, 9*, 5.
20. Gask, L., Sibbald, B., & Creed, F. (1997). Evaluating models of working at the interface between mental health services and primary care. *The British Journal of Psychiatry, 170*, 6–11.
21. Lieb, R., Meinlschmidt, G., & Araya, R. (2007). Epidemiology of the association between somatoform disorders and anxiety and depressive disorders: An update. *Psychosomatic Medicine, 69*, 860–863.
22. Hanel, G., Henningsen, P., Herzog, W., et al. (2009). Depression, anxiety, and somatoform disorders: Vague or distinct categories in primary care? Results from a large cross-sectional study. *Journal of Psychosomatic Research, 67*, 189–197.
23. Kessler, R. C. (2004). The epidemiology of dual diagnosis. *Biological Psychiatry, 56*, 730–737.
24. Faraone, A., Tsuang, M. T., & Tsuang, D. W. (1999). *Genetics of mental disorders. A guide for students, clinicians and researchers*. New York: Gilford Press.
25. Hotopf, M., Wadsworth, M., & Wessely, S. (2001). Is "somatisation" a defense against the acknowledgment of psychiatric disorder? *Journal of Psychosomatic Research, 50*, 119–124.
26. Williams, S., Weinman, J., Dale, J., et al. (1995). Patient expectations: What do primary care patients want from the GP and how far does meeting expectations affect patient satisfaction? *Family Practice, 12*, 193–201.
27. Matthews, D. A., Sledge, W. H., Lieberman, P. B., et al. (1987). Evaluation of intern performance by medical inpatients. *The American Journal of Medicine, 35*, 936–944.
28. Kerwick, S., Jones, R., Mann, A., et al. (1997). Mental health care training priorities in general practice. *The British Journal of General Practice, 47*, 225–227.
29. Reid, S., Whooley, D., Crayford, T., et al. (2001). Medically unexplained symptoms – GPs' attitudes towards their cause and management. *Family Practice, 18*, 519–523.
30. Fink, P., Rosendal, M., & Toft, T. (2002). Assessment and treatment of functional disorders in general practice: The extended reattribution and management model – an advanced educational program for nonpsychiatric doctors. *Psychosomatics, 43*, 93–131.

31. Koh, K. B., Kim, D. K., Kim, S. Y., et al. (2008). The relation between anger management style, mood, and somatic symptoms in anxiety disorders and somatoform disorders. *Psychiatry Research, 160*, 372–379.
32. Maguire, G. P., Goldberg, D. P., Hobson, R. F., et al. (1984). Evaluating the teaching of a method of psychotherapy. *The British Journal of Psychiatry, 144*, 575–580.
33. Goldberg, D. P., Smith, C., Steele, J. J., et al. (1980). Training family doctors to recognize psychiatric illness with increased accuracy. *Lancet, ii*, 521–523.
34. Gask, L., Goldberg, D. P., Lesser, A. L., et al. (1988). Improving the psychiatric skills of the general practice trainee: An evaluation of a group training course. *Medical Education, 22*, 132–138.
35. Gask, L., Goldberg, D., Porter, R., et al. (1989). The treatment of somatization: Evaluation of a teaching package with general practice trainees. *Journal of Psychosomatic Research, 33*, 697–703.
36. Craig, T. K. J., & Boardman, A. P. (1990). Somatization in primary care settings. In C. Bass (Ed.), *Somatization: Physical symptoms and psychological illness*. Oxford: Blackwell.
37. Grol, R. (1988). *To heal or to harm. The prevention of somatic fixation in general practice*. London: Royal College of General Practitioners.
38. Gorlin, R., & Zucker, H. D. (1983). Physician's reactions to patients: A key to teaching humanistic medicine. *The New England Journal of Medicine, 308*, 1059–1063.
39. Groves, J. E. (1978). Taking care of the hateful patient. *The New England Journal of Medicine, 298*, 883–887.
40. Mayou, R. A., Bass, C., & Sharpe, M. (1995). *Treatment of functional somatic symptoms*. Oxford: Oxford University Press.
41. Stewart, M., Brown, J., Weston, W., et al. (2003). *Patient-centered medicine transforming the clinical method*. Oxford: Radcliffe Medical Press.
42. Salmon, P. (2000). Patients who present with physical symptoms in the absence of physical pathology: A challenge to existing models of doctor-patient interaction. *Patient Education and Counseling, 39*, 105–113.
43. Salkovskis, P. M. (1989). Somatic problems. In K. Hawton, P. M. Salkovskis, J. Kirk, et al. (Eds.), *Cognitive behavior therapy for psychiatric problems. A practical guide*. Oxford: Oxford University Press.
44. Sharpe, M., Peveler, R., & Mayou, R. (1992). The psychological treatment of patients with functional somatic symptoms: A practical guide. *Journal of Psychosomatic Research, 36*, 515–529.
45. Thomas, K. B. (1987). General practice consultations: Is there any point in being positive? *BMJ, 294*, 1200–1202.
46. Fitzpatrick, R. M., & Hopkins, A. (1981). Referrals to neurologists for headaches not due to structural disease. *Journal of Neurology, Neurosurgery, and Psychiatry, 44*, 1061–1067.
47. van Dulmen, A., Fennis, J. F., Mokkink, H. G., et al. (1995). Doctor-dependent changes in complaint-related cognitions and anxiety during medical consultations in functional abdominal complaints. *Psychological Medicine, 25*, 1011–1018.
48. Sharpe, M., & Bass, C. (1992). Pathophysiological mechanisms in somatization. *International Review of Psychiatry, 4*, 81–97.
49. Morriss, R., Gask, L., Ronalds, C., et al. (1999). Clinical and patient satisfaction outcomes of a new treatment for somatized mental disorder taught to general practitioners. *The British Journal of General Practice, 49*, 262–267.
50. Morriss, R. K., & Gask, L. (2002). Treatment of patients with somatized mental disorder: Effects of reattribution training on outcomes under the direct control of the family doctor. *Psychosomatics, 43*, 394–399.
51. Rosendal, M., Olesen, F., Fink, P., et al. (2007). A randomized controlled trial of brief training in the assessment and treatment of somatization in primary care: Effects on patient outcome. *General Hospital Psychiatry, 29*, 364–373.
52. Kroenke, K., Taylor-Vaisey, A., Dietrich, A. J., et al. (2000). Interventions to improve provider diagnosis and treatment of mental disorders in primary care. A critical review of the literature. *Psychosomatics, 41*, 39–52.

53. Kroenke, K., & Swindle, R. (2000). Cognitive-behavioral therapy for somatization and somatic symptoms: A critical review of controlled clinical trials. *Psychotherapy and Psychosomatics, 69*, 205–215.
54. Smith, G. R., Jr., Rost, K., & Kashner, T. M. (1995). A trial of the effect of a standardized psychiatric consultation on health outcomes and costs in somatizing patients. *Archives of General Psychiatry, 52*, 238–243.
55. Speckens, A. E. M., van Hemert, A. M., Spinhoven, P., et al. (1995). Cognitive behavioral therapy for medically unexplained physical symptoms: A randomized controlled trial. *BMJ, 311*, 1328–1332.

Chapter 10
Role of Complementary and Alternative Medicine in Psychosomatic Medicine

Sae-il Chun

10.1 Introduction

"Medicine" itself is not exactly a science but rather an art – a healing art. Throughout history, humankind has used shamanism, witchcraft, religion, metaphysics, philosophy, science, and/or technology as tools in developing a better understanding of and further improving the healing arts [1, 2].

It can be said that Western culture has generally been more materially oriented, while Oriental culture has been more spiritually oriented. Western culture has made a greater contribution in the development of materialistic advancement because the West has received all the credit for achievements in science and technology, while Eastern culture has played a more important role in establishing spiritual advancement, because all of the world's major religions such as Judaism, Christianity, Islam, Hinduism, Buddhism, Confucianism, and Taoism were born in the Orient [2].

Our brain is characterized by lateralization with regard to the thinking processes. The left side of the brain (left hemisphere) tends to conduct more scientific, logic, mathematical, linear, and analytical ways of thinking, while the right side of the brain (right hemisphere) conducts intuitive, imaginative, comprehensive, metaphoric, and spiritual ways of thinking. In this line of thinking, Western culture seems to rely more on the left brain, and Oriental culture might rely more on right brain activity [1, 2].

Each nation or ethnic group in the world has their own unique background of culture, customs, tradition, philosophy, and sense of value. For example, Koreans maintain a unique way of perceiving life and death. In English "he passed away" has the same meaning as "he has died." This expression seems to indicate that "a life comes from one direction and goes away to the other direction," thus passing away. In Korea, the most polite way of saying "he has died" is to say as "he has gone

S.-i. Chun, M.D. (✉)
Department of Integrative Medicine, The Graduate School of Integrative Medicine, CHA University, 222 Yatapdong, Sungnam City 463-836, Kyeonggi Province, Korea
e-mail: chunscam@hanmail.net

K.B. Koh (ed.), *Somatization and Psychosomatic Symptoms*,
DOI 10.1007/978-1-4614-7119-6_10, © Springer Science+Business Media New York 2013

back." This expression implies that a life comes from somewhere and goes back to where it came from. Traditionally, Korean people believe that a home is a station of life to which a life arrives and from which a life leaves. In this view, a person should be born at home, and dying at one's own home has the same significance. To traditional Koreans, "being born" and "dying" in a place other than one's own home is considered to be a disgraceful thing. Because of this traditional belief, a dying patient in a hospital will go home to die instead of dying in the hospital [3].

Korea, as a nearly 4,400-year-old nation, like its neighboring countries, has had a long history of traditional medicine consisting of herbology, therapeutic exercise, and stimulation therapies. Stimulation therapies include Chim (acupuncture), Tdum (moxibustion), Jiahp (ischemic compression therapy, finger pressure therapy, shiatsu), and Buhang (negative pressure therapy, cupping, or tubing). The concept of "Qi or Chi (vital force)" is not merely popular in Korea but is also an essential part of daily living. The word "Qi" is used all the time in everyday conversation, and the practice of "Qi" is applied intentionally and subconsciously to the activities of daily living. For many Koreans, their reliance and dependence on traditional medicine is almost religious. The influence of traditional medicine on Korean society is very strong. Korea maintains a dual licensing system of medical doctors, including doctor of Western medicine (M.D.) and doctor of Oriental medicine (O.M.D.). There are 41 medical schools of Western medicine and 11 medical schools of Oriental medicine in Korea. The relatively large number of medical schools, medical students, and doctors in Oriental medicine per capita compared to Western medicine is greater than any other country in the world [4].

The recent trend of globalization has brought an information explosion and transcultural exchange of science, technology, arts, and medicine. There are many different kinds of traditional medicine, popular folk medicine, and various less recognized techniques and theories of healing arts. Some originate in Oriental culture, while others originate in Western culture. Experts in Western medicine claim that only evidence clarified or proven by objective and scientific methodology can be recognized as part of Western (orthodox or conventional) medicine. Excluding Western medicine, all other therapeutic modalities and theories of healing art within the framework of so-called traditional medicine and/or folk medicine are collectively labeled as "alternative medicine or complementary medicine."

In the United States and many other European countries, Oriental medicine is considered a part of alternative medicine, but in Korea, Oriental medicine is not included in alternative medicine. In Korea, anything other than orthodox conventional Western medicine and traditional Korean medicine is considered to be an alternative medicine [1, 2].

10.2 Complementary and Alternative Medicine

Complementary and alternative medicine is a relatively new terminology created in the 1970s to describe all forms of traditional and folk medicine other than Western medicine. Traditional medicine and folk medicine differ in that traditional medicine has its own unique system of knowledge, while folk medicine has no unique system of knowledge, but has simple and multiple therapeutic modalities. There are approximately 334 alternative medicine modalities known today, as listed in Table 10.1 [2, 5–16].

Table 10.1 Alternative medicine modalities

1.	Abdominal massage therapy
2.	Abhyanga
3.	Abjad
4.	Aboukra
5.	Absent healing
6.	ACCESS (access energy transformation)
7.	Acro-sage
8.	Active imagery
9.	Actualism bodywork
10.	Acuball pressure self-treatment
11.	Acu-diet
12.	Acumeridian energy transmission bodywork
13.	Acupoint bloodletting
14.	Acupoint therapy
15.	Acupowder treatment
16.	Acupressure
17.	Acupressure massage
18.	Acupuncture anesthesia
19.	Acupuncture cupping method
20.	Acupuncture imaging
21.	Acupuncture osteopathy
22.	Acupuncture therapy
23.	Acuscope therapy
24.	Acu-stop 2000
25.	Acu-Yoga
26.	Advanced dowsing
27.	Advanced energy healing
28.	Advanced Ingham method
29.	Advanced Kum Nye
30.	Advanced pranic healing
31.	Advanced Rolfing
32.	African holistic health
33.	Agape quest program
34.	Agartha program (Agartha personal life balancing program)
35.	Agni dhatu therapy
36.	Aikido
37.	AK/NOT program (Ferreri program)
38.	Alchemia heart breath
39.	Alchemical bodywork

(continued)

Table 10.1 (continued)

40.	Alchemical hypnotherapy
41.	Alchemical synergy
42.	Alchemical weight management
43.	Alexander technique
44.	Alliance method
45.	Alphabiotic alignment (unification process)
46.	Alpha calm therapy
47.	Alternative 12 steps
48.	Ama Deus
49.	American macrobiotics
50.	Advanced Ingham method
51.	Amplified energy therapy
52.	Angelic healing
53.	Anthroposophical medicine
54.	Apitherapy (bee sting therapy, bee venom therapy)
55.	Apple diet therapy
56.	Applied kinesiology
57.	Aqua acupuncture therapy
58.	Archetypal psychology
59.	Arhatic yoga system
60.	Arica movement
61.	Aroma behavior conditioning
62.	Aromatherapy (conventional aroma therapy)
63.	Art therapy
64.	Astanga yoga (Raja yoga)
65.	Aston-pattering technique
66.	Astromedicine (medical astrology)
67.	Attitudinal healing
68.	Aura analysis
69.	Auricular acupuncture
70.	Autogenic therapy
71.	Avatar therapy
72.	Ayurveda medicine
73.	Ayurvedic acupuncture
74.	Ayurvedic nutrition
75.	Bach flower therapy (flower essence therapy)
76.	Bamboo rod tapping
77.	Barbara Brennan health science
78.	Bates method
79.	BEST (Morter Bio Energetic Synchronization Technique)
80.	Bi-digital O-ring test
81.	Biodynamic psychology
82.	Bioelectronic diagnosis
83.	Bioenergetic healing
84.	Biofeedback therapy
85.	Biological dentistry
86.	Biomedical therapy

(continued)

Table 10.1 (continued)

87.	Biorhythm therapy
88.	Black Hat Tantric Buddhist Feng Shui
89.	Bleeding manipulation (bloodletting therapy)
90.	Blue water technique
91.	Body constitution herbology
92.	Body mapping technique
93.	Body-mind centering
94.	Body reflexology
95.	Bodywork therapy
96.	Bonnie Prudden myotherapy
97.	Bowen technique
98.	Breatharianism
99.	Breathwork
100.	Buddhist medicine
101.	Buddhist psychology
102.	Buhang therapy (air pumping cup method)
103.	Bush walk therapy
104.	Calligraphy therapy
105.	Cayce approach to health and healing
106.	Cayce diet
107.	Cayce-Reilly massage
108.	Cell salt therapy
109.	Cell therapy
110.	Chakra breathing
111.	Chakra yoga
112.	Chelation therapy
113.	Cherokee healing
114.	Chinese auricular therapy
115.	Chinese dietotherapy
116.	Chirognomy
117.	Chiropractics
118.	Chi therapy (Gestalt energy work)
119.	Clairvoyant diagnosis (psychic diagnosis)
120.	Colon therapy
121.	Color breathing
122.	Color therapy
123.	Core energetic therapy
124.	Coyote medicine (half-breed medicine)
125.	Craniosacral therapy
126.	Creative visualization
127.	Crude herb moxibustion
128.	Crystal therapy
129.	Curanderismo
130.	Dan breathing therapy (abdominal breathing technique)
131.	Dance therapy
132.	Detoxification therapy
133.	Diagnostic acupressure

(continued)

Table 10.1 (continued)

134.	Diamond approach
135.	Dietary therapy
136.	Digital ring therapy
137.	Distant pulse diagnosis
138.	Do in
139.	Dowsing
140.	Drama therapy
141.	Dream therapy
142.	Eagle medicine
143.	Eastern psychology
144.	Eight body constitution acupuncture
145.	Electric pulsating pill therapy
146.	Electroacupuncture according to Voll (EAV)
147.	Energetic bodywork
148.	Energy medicine
149.	Enneagram system
150.	Enzyme therapy
151.	Environmental therapy
152.	Ericksonian hypnosis
153.	Essene way of self-healing
154.	Eutonic therapy
155.	Facial diagnosis
156.	Faith healing (spiritual healing)
157.	Fasting therapy
158.	Feldenkrais method
159.	Feng Shui
160.	Five right lifestyle therapy
161.	Five rites of rejuvenation
162.	Five Tibetans
163.	Flower remedies
164.	Foot reflexology
165.	Functional craniospinal therapy (FCST)
166.	Functional integration
167.	Gerson diet therapy
168.	Gestalt therapy
169.	Glandular therapy
170.	Gnosis
171.	Guided imagery
172.	Hakomi method
173.	Hand acupuncture
174.	Hatha yoga
175.	Heller work
176.	Hemi-Sync
177.	HIFU therapy
178.	Hippocrates health program
179.	Holistic nursing
180.	Holotropic breathwork

(continued)

Table 10.1 (continued)

181.	Homeopathic medicine
182.	Horse riding therapy
183.	Horticulture therapy
184.	Hoshino therapy
185.	Human ecology program
186.	Hydrotherapy
187.	Hyperthermia therapy
188.	Hypnosis therapy
189.	Inner child therapy
190.	Integral counseling psychology
191.	Integrative therapy
192.	Integral yoga (Puma yoga)
193.	Intramuscular stimulation (IMS)
194.	Iridology
195.	Iroquois medical botany
196.	Iyengar yoga
197.	Jin Shin Do
198.	Juice therapy
199.	Kahuna healing
200.	Kinesio taping therapy
201.	Kneipp therapy
202.	Laughter therapy
203.	Lemonade diet
204.	Light therapy
205.	Living foods lifestyle (Hippocrates diet)
206.	Lymphasizing
207.	Macrobiotics
208.	Magic therapy
209.	Maggot therapy
210.	Magnetic field therapy (biomagnetic therapy)
211.	Maharishi Ayurveda
212.	Medical graphology
213.	Medical palmistry
214.	Mesotherapy
215.	Mind-body medicine
216.	Morter health system
217.	Moxibustion
218.	Mud therapy
219.	Muscle response testing (MRT)
220.	Music therapy
221.	Natural hygiene
222.	Natural salt therapy
223.	Naturopathic medicine
224.	Network spinal analysis
225.	Neural therapy
226.	Neurolinguistic programming therapy (NLP)
227.	Nichiren Buddhism

(continued)

Table 10.1 (continued)

228.	Nine Star Ki
229.	Nishi medicine
230.	Nutritional therapy
231.	Numerology therapy
232.	Nvwoti (Cherokee herbal medicine)
233.	Ogumhee therapy (animal motion therapy)
234.	Organismic psychotherapy
235.	Orgone therapy
236.	Oriental channel diagnosis
237.	Orthomolecular medicine
238.	Osteopathic medicine
239.	Oxygen therapy
240.	Panchakarma
241.	Phoenix rising yoga therapy
242.	Phytotherapy
243.	Planetary herbology
244.	Plant alchemy
245.	Pleiadian lightwork
246.	Podiatry
247.	Polarity therapy
248.	Postural and structural re-education therapy
249.	Pranic healing (bioplasmic healing, radiatory healing)
250.	Primal therapy (primal scream therapy)
251.	Psionic medicine
252.	Psychic surgery (etheric surgery)
253.	Psychogenetics
254.	Psychology of evil
255.	Psycho-neuro aligning (PNA)
256.	Psycho-neuro integration (PNI, psychic healing)
257.	Psychotherapeutic Reikism
258.	Pythagorean numerology
259.	Qigong
260.	Quantum healing
261.	Quan Yin method
262.	Qua Sha therapy
263.	Radiance breathwork
264.	Radionics (psionics)
265.	Rainbow diet
266.	Raktamoksa
267.	Raw juice therapy
268.	Ray method of healing
269.	Reading therapy
270.	Rebirthing (circular breathing, conscious breathing)
271.	Receptive imagery
272.	Reconstructive therapy
273.	Recreation therapy
274.	Reichian therapy (psychiatric orgone therapy)

(continued)

Table 10.1 (continued)

275.	Reiki therapy
276.	Remote diagnosis (distant diagnosis)
277.	Rife therapy
278.	Rolfing method
279.	Rosenfeld synergy method
280.	Rosen method (Rosen method psychospiritual bodywork)
281.	Rune casting
282.	Sacred psychology
283.	Scalp acupuncture therapy
284.	Schuessler biochemic system of medicine
285.	Sclerology (sclera diagnosis)
286.	Self-healing
287.	Shabda yoga
288.	Shadow sound therapy
289.	Shamatic counseling
290.	Shiatsu (acupressure)
291.	Shinkiko
292.	Shirodhara
293.	Siddha medicine
294.	Silva mind control
295.	Simonton method
296.	Sleep therapy
297.	Soaring Crane Qigong
298.	Somatic therapy
299.	Sotai therapy
300.	Soul-centered psychology
301.	Soul retrieval
302.	Sound therapy
303.	Spa therapy
304.	Spiritual healing
305.	Spiritual midwifery
306.	Spiritual psychology
307.	Sufi healing
308.	Tai Chi Chuan
309.	Tamang shamanism
310.	Tensegrity
311.	Thanato-spirituality
312.	Therapeutic touch
313.	Thought field therapy (TFT, Callahan technique)
314.	Tibetan herbal medicine
315.	Tibetan pulsing healing
316.	Tongue diagnosis
317.	Toning
318.	Torsion energy therapy
319.	Traditional acupuncture
320.	Traditional American Indian medicine
321.	Traditional herbal diagnosis

(continued)

Table 10.1 (continued)

322.	Transcendental meditation
323.	Transpersonal psychology
324.	Urine therapy
325.	Vedic astrology
326.	Vibrational medicine
327.	Wise woman healing
328.	Wu Ming Qigong
329.	Yagya
330.	Yantra yoga
331.	Zazen
332.	Zen dance therapy
333.	Zen macrobiotics
334.	Zone therapy (reflex zone therapy)

10.3 Differences Between Western Medicine and Oriental Medicine

There are no clear-cut delineations between the two medicines because in many areas they are similar and overlap. It cannot be said, however, that they are identical. Some of the most noticeable major differences between the two medicines are as follows [3, 4, 16–26]:

10.3.1 System of Knowledge

Western medicine is primarily based on science and technology, while Oriental medicine is based on philosophy and metaphysics. Oriental medicine strongly emphasizes the concepts of Qi (or Ch'i) which is a vital force or natural healing energy; Um-Yang (or Yin-Yang), which involves the relative establishment of balance and harmony; and the five elements of wood, fire, earth, metal, and water, which are the basic factors regulating the laws of change.

10.3.2 Perception

Western medicine emphasizes a logical and objective perception, whereas Oriental medicine emphasizes an intuitive and subjective perception. Western medicine emphasizes statistics which provide objective generalized information, but Oriental medicine emphasizes anecdotal reports which provide subjective and individualized information.

10.3.3 Understanding

In order to understand natural phenomena, Western medicine takes an eccentric (outgoing) and analytical approach. Western medicine emphasizes chopping things up into smaller pieces to investigate them so that specialization and subspecialization are the prevailing tendencies. This approach takes the view that the normal whole is the sum of normal pieces. On the other hand, Oriental medicine takes a concentric (incoming) and holistic approach. All phenomena are centered on oneness.

10.3.4 Observation

Western medicine observes and confirms phenomena by means of experiments, while Oriental medicine takes accumulated experience as a means of confirmation.

10.3.5 Treatment

Western medicine tends to emphasize an offensive therapeutic approach, while Oriental medicine focuses on a defensive therapeutic approach. An ancient teaching says "ordinary man tries to find the fault in others, while special man tries to find it in himself." This teaching applies to medical practice. Western medicine tries to identify the cause of disease from the outside, such as an infection caused by bacteria coming from the outside and requiring aggressive methods such as killing (antibiotics), cutting (surgery), or blocks. Oriental medicine tends to identify the problem from inside such as a lowered immune mechanism requiring defensive methods such as tonics (liver tonics, stomach tonics, etc.), dietary regimen, or self-trained exercises.

10.3.6 Measurement

Western medicine emphasizes accuracy, while Oriental medicine emphasizes adequacy. For example, 1 in. in Western culture is exactly the same length wherever it is applied. However, one body inch (tsun), as used in Oriental medicine, differs from one individual to the other. There are predetermined inch systems on body segments. For instance, the length between the elbow and the wrist is predefined as having 12 divisions (body inches) so that one body inch indicates 1 out of 12 divisions, and therefore one body inch in a tall adult is much longer than one body inch in a tiny child, and that one body inch falls on the same relative point regardless of the size of the individual. In other words, one is an “accurate inch,” and the other is an “adequate inch.”

10.3.7 Rapport Formation

The doctor-patient relationship is different between Western and Oriental medicine in that Western medicine takes a “technological” approach and Oriental medicine takes a “humanistic” approach. In Western medicine, the doctor is a “doer” and the patient is a “passive recipient,” while in Oriental medicine, the patient becomes a “doer” and the doctor plays a role as an “instructor.”

10.3.8 Study

Western medicine focuses on a study of “what,” and Oriental medicine focuses on a study of “why.” For example, Western medicine asks “What happens during sleep?” while Oriental medicine asks “Why do we have to sleep?”

10.3.9 Mechanism

Western medicine emphasizes “anatomy and physiology,” while Oriental medicine emphasizes “function and role.” The concepts of “meridian,” “acupuncture point,” “envelope of the heart,” and “triple burner” are nonexistent in Western medicine, although they are the most important functional units in Oriental medicine.

10.3.10 Orientation

Western medicine is “disease oriented,” while Oriental medicine is “health oriented.” In Western medicine, everything is centered around the disease with questions such as “where is the disease?” and “how do you eliminate the disease?” In contrast, in Oriental medicine, the main subjects are “how do you maintain health?” “how do you lose health?” or “how do you return to normal health?”

The human condition can be divided into three stages: a healthy stage, unhealthy stage, and diseased stage (Fig. 10.1). The first “healthy stage” is when the vital force (natural healing energy or Qi) is well balanced and harmonious. The second “unhealthy stage” is when the vital force has lost its balance and harmony, but there

Fig. 10.1 Health-related orientation in Oriental medicine and Western medicine

Health and Disease

I	II	III
Health	Unhealth (non-disease)	Disease

Oriental Medicine

Health	Unhealth

Western Medicine

Non-disease	Disease

is no mechanical damage yet. The third "diseased stage" is when there is actual mechanical damage to tissues (pathological changes).

To maintain health (Stage I): One may lose health by doing one of three things wrong. Doing the "don'ts," failing to do the "must," or doing things the "wrong way" can result in the loss of health. The five commandments to maintaining normal health are as follows: (1) eat right, (2) move right, (3) sleep right, (4) breathe right, and (5) mind right.

To reverse unhealth (Stage II) to health, the following methods are utilized: (1) natural substance therapy (herbal plant, animal, mineral), (2) practice therapy (Qi-Kong or Chi Kung exercises), and (3) stimulation therapy (heat, positive pressure, negative (suction) pressure, and needle).

To eliminate disease (Stage III), the following methods are utilized: (1) chemical treatment, (2) physical treatment, (3) psychological treatment, and (4) surgical treatment.

10.4 Complementary and Alternative Medicine as Applicable to Psychosomatic Medicine

Among more than 330 alternative medicine therapies known today, over 40 modalities are useful in research and can have a clinical application in the field of psychosomatic medicine, as listed below [1, 2, 5–12, 14–16]:

10.4.1 Alternative Medicine Similar to Western Medicine

1. Chelation therapy
2. Detoxification therapy
3. Hypnotherapy
4. Body-mind therapy
5. Energy medicine
6. Nutritional supplement
7. Orthomolecular medicine
8. Enzyme therapy
9. Environmental medicine
10. Oxygen therapy
11. Magnetic field therapy
12. Dream therapy
13. Recreation therapy
14. Magic therapy
15. Iridology
16. Autogenic therapy
17. Reichian therapy
18. Neurolinguistic programming
19. Guided imagery
20. Biofeedback therapy

10.4.2 Alternative Medicine Similar to Oriental Medicine

1. Acupuncture
2. Herbal medicine
3. Qigong therapy
4. Ayurvedic medicine
5. Naturopathic medicine
6. Transcendental meditation
7. Yoga
8. Flower therapies
9. Aromatherapy
10. Sound therapy
11. Horticulture therapy
12. Reflexology
13. Touching therapy
14. Psychic healing

10.4.3 Alternative Medicine with an Oriental-Western Mixture

1. Homeopathic medicine
2. Diet therapy
3. Fasting
4. Juice therapy
5. Colon therapy
6. Light therapy
7. Hydrotherapy
8. Quantum medicine
9. Art therapy
10. Dance therapy
11. Phytotherapy

10.5 Conclusions

Western culture has developed a "science and technology-oriented" Western medicine, while Oriental culture has developed "metaphysics and philosophy-oriented" Oriental medicine. There have been many unofficially recognized forms of traditional and folk medicine scattered all over the world in both Western and Oriental cultures. Recently, those medicines which do not belong to the orthodox conventional medicine have been labeled as "alternative medicine or complementary medicine." In the United States and European countries, alternative medicine includes Oriental medicine, but in the Far East region, particularly in Korea, Oriental medicine is not included in alternative medicine. In Korea, both Western and Oriental medicine are considered to be "conventional medicine." Accordingly, alternative medicine is "the medicine other than conventional medicine." There is clear evidence that Western medicine, Oriental medicine, and alternative medicine are all complementary to each other and that alternative medicine and psychosomatic medicine share much in common in terms of being "whole person oriented" and employing an "integrative approach." If and when all the complementary components existing in the various healing arts are integrated into one form of medicine, a new holistic medicine will be produced and will be useful in the field of psychosomatic medicine.

References

1. Chun, S. I. (2004). *Complementary alternative medicine*. Seoul, Korea: Kyechuk Munwhasa.
2. Chun, S. I. (2008). *Principle and practice of complementary alternative medicine*. Seoul, Korea: Gyechuck Munwhasa.

3. Chun, S. I. (1997). Similarities and dissimilarities between oriental medicine and western medicine. *Journal of the Korean Medical Association, 40*, 276–282.
4. Kim, J. Y., & Kim, W. J. (1994). *Comparative study of East–west medicine*. Seoul, Korea: Kyechuk Munwhas.
5. Goldberg, B. (1999). *Alternative medicine: The definitive guide*. Tiburon, CA: Future Medicine Publishing.
6. Bauman, E., Brint, A. I., Piper, L., et al. (1978). *The holistic health handbook: A tool for attaining wholeness of body, mind, and spirit*. Berkley, CA: AND/OR Press.
7. Bruce, D. F., & McIlwain, H. H. (1998). *Unofficial guide to alternative medicine*. New York: Simon & Schuster Macmillan.
8. Deepak, C. (1990). *Quantum healing: Exploring the frontiers of mind/body medicine*. London: Bantam Books.
9. Hastings, A. C., Fadiman, J., & Gordon, J. S. (1980). *Health for the whole person: The complete guide to holistic medicine*. Boulder, CO: Westview Press.
10. Kushi, M. (1987). *One peaceful world: Kushi's approach to creating a healthy and harmonious mind. Home and world community*. New York: St. Martins Press.
11. Pelletier, K. R. (1977). *Mind as healer, mind as slayer: A holistic approach to preventing stress disorders*. New York: Delacorte & Delta.
12. Sierpina, V. S. (2001). *Integrative health care*. Philadelphia, PA: FA Davis.
13. Sharma, C. H. (1976). *A manual of homeopathy and natural medicine*. New York: Dutton.
14. Stalker, D., & Glymour, C. (1985). *Examining holistic medicine* (pp. 107–125). Buffalo, NY: Prometheus Books.
15. Williams, R. J. (1973). *Nutrition against disease*. New York: Bantam.
16. Kaptchuk, T. J. (1983). *The web that has no weaver*. New York: Congdon & Weed.
17. Chun, S. I. (2005). *Acupuncture medicine*. Seoul, Korea: Gyechuck Munwhasa.
18. Chu, L. S. W., Yeh, S. D. J., & Wood, D. D. (1979). *Acupuncture manual: A western approach*. New York: Marcel Dekker.
19. Aristide, H., & Dong, P. (1990). *Chi Kung: The ancient Chinese way to health*. New York: Paragon House.
20. Chung, T. H. (1997). Educational perspectives in coordinating East–west medicine. *Journal of the Korean Medical Association, 40*, 291–297.
21. Choi, Y. K. (1997). Problems of clinical practices in coordinating East–west medicine. *Journal of the Korean Medical Association, 40*, 298–303.
22. Chang, S. T. (1986). *Complete system of self-healing: Internal exercises*. San Francisco: Tao Publishing.
23. Diamond, J. (1985). *Life energy*. New York: Dodd, Mead and Co.
24. MoJahnke, R. (1990). *Profound medicine*. Santa Barbara, CA: Health Action Books.
25. Lee, J. C. (1997). Meeting point of concepts of diseases in eastern and western medicine. *Journal of the Korean Medical Association, 40*, 283–287.
26. Lim, J. K. (1995). *Clinical coordination in East–west medicine*. Seoul: Hansungsa.

Chapter 11
Family Assessment and Intervention for Physicians

Gabor I. Keitner

11.1 Introduction

Most symptoms or illnesses evolve in a social context: understanding the social context of the presenting problem is critical to biopsychosocial formulation and treatment planning. Families (including nonrelative significant others) can help in identifying history, precipitants, and potential future obstacles to the management of presenting problems and thereby significantly impact ongoing treatment. How a patient with an illness interacts with his or her significant others and how they in turn interact with the patient has a significant impact on the duration of the presenting problems, their likelihood of resolving and recurring over time.

There are many reasons why physicians do not assess or treat families. Meeting with families is often not cost effective given current reimbursements. Equally important is a lack of sufficient training for physicians in meeting with families, not only to gather information but also to help them to learn how to deal with each other and their loved one's illness.

Family interventions can be implemented successfully at all phases of illness: to prevent disease, to reduce chronicity, and to improve functioning in the chronic phase. Families can be involved in the assessment and treatment of the patient at all stages of care and to varying degrees, ranging from participating in psychoeducational programs to intensive family treatment that aims to change relational functioning.

G.I. Keitner, M.D. (✉)
Department of Psychiatry, Rhode Island and Miriam Hospitals,
Brown University, Providence, RI, USA
e-mail: gkeitner@lifespan.org

K.B. Koh (ed.), *Somatization and Psychosomatic Symptoms*,
DOI 10.1007/978-1-4614-7119-6_11,

11.2 The Significance of the Family in Illness

Families have a powerful influence on health equal to traditional medical risk factors [1]. Improved healthcare has led to prolonged periods of living with disease. Longer periods of illness increases strain on patients and their significant others leading to caregiver burden which in turn impacts on the ability of caregivers to provide support for ill family members [2]. Emotional support [being listened to, cared for, and empathized with] is the most important and influential type of support provided by families. Negative, critical, or hostile family relationships, in turn, have a stronger, detrimental, influence on health than positive or supportive relationships [1].

Families can influence health by direct biological pathways, health behavior pathways, and psychophysiological pathways. Examples of direct biological pathways include spreading of infectious agents, sharing similar toxic environments and genetic vulnerabilities. Health behavior pathways include lifestyle behaviors such as smoking, exercise, diet, and substance abuse. Healthcare behaviors include adherence to treatment as well as family caregiving. Pathophysiological pathways refer to the effects of family environment on neuroendocrine and psychoimmunological pathways [1].

There are a large number of family-based risk factors that adversely influence the onset and course of illness. These include poor conflict resolution, low relationship satisfaction, high interpersonal conflict, criticism and blame, intrafamilial hostility, lack of congruence in disease beliefs and expectations, poor problem-solving, extra-familial stress, lack of extra-familial support systems, poor organization, inconsistent family structure, family perfectionism and rigidity, low cohesion and closeness, and presence of psychopathology in family members [3]. Conversely, there are many protective relational factors. These include good communications, good problem-solving skills, adaptability, clear roles, achievement of family developmental tasks, mutual support, open expression of appreciation, commitment to the family, extra-familial social connections, spending time together, and religious and spiritual orientation [4].

Not all families of patients are dysfunctional. In fact, many families deal very effectively with recurring, chronic, and severe illnesses. Even well-functioning families, however, can benefit from information about the illness, validation of effective ways of coping, and reinforcement of resilience in the face of major stressors. Being clear about what constitutes functional or dysfunctional families and about normal versus pathological ways of dealing with difficult situations is an important base from which to be able to evaluate the functionality of any family.

11.3 Family Assessment

The essential task in meeting with family members for the first time in family assessment is to assess their functioning in the context of understanding their presenting problems. Family assessment is the first step in determining both the need for further interventions and the specific areas of family life that might need to be addressed. Family assessment should focus on adjustments related to the diagnosis of medical illness, clarification of treatment options, and collaboration in carrying out the treatment plan. A proper assessment should also identify family strengths [5].

An indispensable first step in meeting with the family is to establish connection with them. The family needs to feel understood, respected, and validated. They do not want to be blamed for their loved one's problems or judged for their perceived deficiencies. It is the job of the clinician to put families at ease and to make them feel comfortable enough to participate openly in the assessment process. The assessment is used to gain a better understanding of how everybody sees the problem(s) at hand, to gather information to allow for a more comprehensive formulation, and to provide an opportunity for all members involved in trying to cope with the illness to ask questions and to solicit the help of all involved in setting up a meaningful treatment plan.

There are many different ways to assess a family and many different kinds of information that can be gathered. Some clinicians begin with a long history of the family's life, connections, and evolution as a unit. They gather information on families of origin and may develop a genogram. Other clinicians are more interested in a here-and-now view of how the family functions and the current problems they are dealing with. Still other clinicians focus primarily on process issues in the family session. They address what they observe as the current family interactional pattern and assume that this is representative of the way in which the family deals with issues outside of the assessment session. All three approaches have merit and they are not mutually exclusive. The challenge for the clinician is to integrate these three approaches in such a way as to meet the goals of the evaluation without getting unduly sidetracked by peripheral issues or taking so long to complete the evaluation that the family loses interest.

The assessment process consists of four identifiable components: orientation, data gathering, problem description, and problem clarification.

11.3.1 Orientation

The orientation explains the purpose of the evaluation and establishes goals for the assessment process. It is often helpful to start off the meeting with introductions of the participants. The meeting is normalized with an explanation that family meetings are a regular part of the assessment and treatment of most patients. The family can be further oriented by clarifying why they came for help, what they expected would happen, and what they would like to get out of the meeting.

The clinician explains that the goal of the meeting is to provide an opportunity for all family members to identify what they see as problems and to bring up any areas of concern. The family's cooperation in the assessment process is enhanced by letting them know that they will also have an opportunity to ask questions of the therapist and to have input into the development of a treatment plan.

The clinician should obtain information about family members' names, ages, relationships within the family, and living arrangements. It is also helpful to ascertain the correct phase of the family life cycle to anticipate the kinds of problems and issues that the family may be struggling with in addition to the presenting problems.

11.3.2 Data Gathering

The clinician begins by asking family members what they think are the problems in the family. Each family member is given the opportunity to express his or her concerns without being interrupted by others. The challenge for the clinician at this stage is to not get sidetracked by beginning to deal with problems before everybody has had an opportunity to present their perspectives. The clinician also has to make sure that the problems are not described in such great detail as to leave no time for the exploration of other problems and the concerns of other family members. Once the presenting problems are clearly delineated by the various family members and once the clinician has summarized his or her understanding of these problems with consensus of all participants that the problems are understood and agreed upon, the therapist moves on to assess broader dimensions of family functioning [6].

11.3.3 Overall Family Functioning

The clinician orients the family to this new stage of the assessment process by letting them know that he or she will be asking a series of questions about different aspects of their family's life. These include problem-solving, communication, affective involvement, affective responsiveness, roles, and behavior control [6].

11.3.3.1 Problem-Solving

Problem-solving refers to a family's ability to resolve problems to a level that maintains effective family functioning. A family problem is one that threatens the integrity and functional capacity of the family and the family has difficulty solving.

The following questions may be helpful in exploring the family's effectiveness in managing problems: Who first notices problems? What was done after the problem was noticed? Did you discuss it with anybody? What did you decide to do about the problem? Did you think of any alternatives? Did you review how you dealt with the problem once you had taken care of it? How do you handle practical problems? How do you handle problems that involve emotions?

11.3.3.2 Communication

Communication refers to the verbal exchange of information within the family. Nonverbal communication is very important as well, but it is more difficult to quantify and monitor.

The following are questions that can be used to assess communication in a family: Do you talk with one another? Can you talk about practical things with each other? Can you talk about emotional issues with each other? Do you feel that you can say what you want or do you have to be guarded about what you say? Can you tell things to each other directly or do you have to use someone else to let others know how you feel and think?

11.3.3.3 Affective Involvement

Affective involvement refers to the extent to which the family shows interest in and values the activities of individual family members.

The following questions can help explore aspects of affective involvement: Who cares about what is important to you? Do you think that other family members are interested in you? Do they ever show too much interest? Do you think that others are truly interested in you because it is important to you or only because they think that they should be? Do you feel that other members of the family go their own way and do not care or notice what happens to you?

11.3.3.4 Affective Responsiveness

Affective responsiveness refers to whether family members are able to respond to the full spectrum of feelings experienced in emotional life and whether the emotion experienced is consistent or appropriate with the stimulus, situation, or context. It refers to the person's capacity to experience particular kinds of emotions.

The following questions can elicit information regarding emotional responsiveness: Are you a family that responds to situations with a lot of feeling? Do you feel that you are a family that does not respond with enough emotions? Which kinds of emotions do you think that you overrespond or underrespond to? Do others sense that you do not experience feelings that you should feel? Are there any feelings that you experience more intensely than you think is reasonable given the situation?

11.3.3.5 Roles

Roles are the repetitive patterns of behavior by which family members fulfill family functions. Family functions include the provision of resources, nurturance and support, sexual gratification, personal development, and maintenance and management of the family system. These include decision making, boundaries and membership functions, as well as household finances and management.

Questions to explore roles in the family include the following: How do you divide responsibilities? Who works and for how many hours? Who handles the money? Who buys the groceries and prepares the meals? Who does the housework? Who looks after the home and cars? Who oversees what happens with the children's education? Who gets involved with the schools? Who is involved in major decisions? Who has the final say? How do you decide who does what job? Do you feel that some people have too many jobs? Do any of you feel overburdened by your jobs? Are the responsibilities fairly shared between family members? If not, how would you like to see it done differently?

11.3.3.6 Behavior Control

The behavior control dimension evaluates the ways in which a family establishes rules about acceptable behavior related to physically dangerous situations, situations involving meeting and expressing psychological needs and drives, and situations involving socializing behavior between family members and people outside the family. It concerns parental discipline toward children as well as standards and expectations of behavior that adults set for each other.

The following questions can be used to explore the behavior control dimension of family functioning: Do you have rules in your family about how to handle different situations? How do you handle dangerous situations? Do you have rules for table manners and for bedtime? Do you allow hitting or yelling at each other? Do you know what is expected of you in terms of behavior with people outside the family? Do you have rules about drinking? Driving too fast? Letting people know where you are when away from home? Are the rules clear? Are the rules the same for everybody? Can you discuss the rules to change them? Do you always know what the family expects? Do you know what to expect if the rules are broken?

It is important not to get side tracked by a particular problem before understanding the whole system. Often, further exploration of the family system allows the identification of dysfunctional patterns in which a similar problem surfaces in other areas of family functioning.

11.4 Problem Description

After the thorough assessment described above, family problems are likely to be clear to the clinician and to the family. It is helpful to group a variety of different problems into related clusters in order to focus the family and to avoid the risk of getting bogged down in excessive detail. What may seem to be many different problems often emanate from a few core problems.

11.5 Problem Clarification

The final step in the assessment process is to obtain agreement between the clinician and family members on the problems identified. If the clinician has been careful to listen to each family member and has checked out his or her understanding of the problems with the family, there should be good agreement on the final problem list. If there are disagreements about the problem list between the clinician and various family members, these should be resolved before proceeding to any recommendations for treatment.

11.6 Tools for Family Assessment

A variety of instruments are available to evaluate families systematically. Family assessment instruments allow for numerical quantification of family functioning, so as to track change over time, make comparisons with other families, and carry out quantitative research. There are subjective and objective family assessment tools.

11.6.1 Subjective Family Rating Scales

These scales are self-report paper and pencil or computer touch screen instruments filled out by individual family members. They elicit individual family members' views of their own family's functioning. Self-report instruments are cost effective as family members can fill them out at their leisure and the assessment does not require trained interviewer time. Most questionnaires can be filled out in less than 30 min.

There are a number of useful self-report measures of marital adjustment/satisfaction and family functioning. Family members can fill these out in the waiting room or at home, before the first session or during a course of treatment as a way of monitoring progress. The following are examples of commonly used instruments.

11.6.1.1 Dyadic Adjustment Scale

Measures satisfaction, cohesion, consensus, and affectional expression in couples [7].

11.6.1.2 Family Environment Scale

Assesses relationship [cohesion, expressiveness, conflict], personal growth [independence, achievement, mortality/religion], and system maintenance (organization, control) [8].

11.6.1.3 Family Assessment Device

Assesses the dimensions of the McMaster Model of Family Functioning—problem-solving, communication, role allocation, affective responsiveness, affective involvement, behavior control, and general functioning [9]. Available in more than 25 different languages.

11.6.2 Externally Rated Instruments of Family Functioning

These instruments are administered by trained interviewers and provide a more objective view of the family's functioning. These structured or semi-structured interview instruments are independent of the family's tendency to want to see themselves in a particular way. They provide more reliable assessments for comparisons between different families and comparisons with established population norms. A disadvantage of externally rated family assessment instruments is their relative expense. Interviewers have to be trained to rate families reliably, and these instruments take a longer time to administer. The following are some of the commonly used instruments.

11.6.2.1 Global Assessment of Relational Functioning

The Global Assessment of Relational Functioning (GARF) scale is similar to the individual-focused Global Assessment of Functioning (GAF) but focuses instead on relational adjustment and also on the quality of the family environment [10]. The GARF measures relational functioning on a scale of 1 to 99. Three areas are assessed: interactional problem-solving, organization, and emotional climate.

11.6.2.2 Beaver's Interactional Styles Scale

The Beaver's Interactional Styles Scale [11] evaluates a family's competence and style. It also assesses power, parental coalitions, clarity of expression, conflict, negotiation, responsibility, and empathy.

11.6.2.3 McMaster Clinical Rating Scale

The McMaster Clinical Rating Scale [12] is an interviewer assessment (with the aid of the McMaster Structured Interview of Family Functioning, if desired) of a family's communications, problem-solving, affective involvement, affective responsiveness, roles, behavior control, and general functioning.

11.7 General Assessment Issues

In case of a crisis [suicidality, homicidality, spousal abuse, acute substance abuse], a comprehensive assessment may need to be suspended until the acute crisis has been contained and managed.

Some family members may be overly talkative and controlling. It is important for the clinician not to become engaged in a power struggle with family members about the direction of the assessment. The clinician needs to respectfully focus the assessment to ensure that all family members have an opportunity to express their own perspectives.

Some families, in contrast, are very quiet and reluctant to participate in a family discussion. The clinician has to be careful in this situation to not fill in the vacuum by taking on too much responsibility for defining the family's problems. The clinician should identify that one of the problems in the family is a lack of ability or willingness to contribute to the understanding and exploration of their problems. If the family is still unwilling to participate, the clinician has to outline the reality that without their participation and help, it will not be possible to arrive at a clear understanding of the issues at hand and a family assessment cannot continue. The clinician may have to be more directive if the family members are unable to engage more fully in the assessment process because of limitations in social competence and/or intellectual capacity.

The challenge for the clinician is to maintain control of the family meeting without being authoritarian or inhibiting a family's willingness to express their concerns. The family usually responds well if the clinician stays focused and provides a structure for the assessment.

11.8 Family Intervention

A wide variety of family interventions have been developed and tested for many medical illnesses including dementia, cardiovascular diseases, cancer, diabetes, arthritis, stroke, chronic pain, traumatic brain injury, systemic lupus erythematosis, and AIDS [13]. In spite of the differences, most family approaches can be divided into two broad categories, psychoeducational and relationship focused. The goals of psychoeducational interventions are to increase knowledge about the illness and to teach patients and family members more effective ways of managing it. Skills training include lifestyle modifications relating to diet and exercise, learning skills to monitor the illness such as blood pressure monitoring, and supporting compliance with medical treatment [14]. Relationship-focused interventions attempt to directly improve family functioning by helping families to communicate more effectively, solve problems, resolve conflicts, and develop a greater sense of cohesiveness. These interventions also include some degree of education about the illness and discussion of more effective coping skills.

Two meta-analyses of family/psychosocial interventions for adult patients with chronic illnesses have been published [15, 16]. Martire et al. [15] concluded that family interventions led to family members feeling less depressed and less burdened. Family interventions also enhanced patients' survival particularly for patients with cardiovascular disease. There was no evidence that the family interventions reduced anxiety or disability in patients or that they increased their relationship satisfaction.

Hartmann et al. [16] concluded that family interventions led to significantly better physical health of patients compared to standard treatment. Both psychoeducational- and relationship-focused interventions showed a significant positive effect. Family interventions also lead to improved mental health of the patient compared to standard treatment. Family member's health issues such as caregiver burden, depression, anxiety, quality of life, and self-efficacy were all improved by family interventions.

These reviews show that many different types of family interventions are effective in helping to deal with a wide range of medical illnesses. They do not provide information on what specific interventions may be the most helpful for a given illness at a particular point in time nor what the mechanisms that lead to change are.

11.9 Family Therapy

There are many different schools of family therapy. These include strategic family therapy, structural family therapy, experiential family therapy, narrative therapy, cognitive behavioral family therapy, solution-focused therapy, emotionally focused family therapy, integrative family therapy, and problem-centered family therapy [17–19].

Clinicians would be advised to learn a family treatment model that addresses a wide range of family problems: it should not be rigid, encourage a broad assessment of the family's needs, and enlist the open collaboration of the family in working toward mutually agreed-upon goals in treatment. The Problem-Centered Systems Therapy of the Family (PCSTF) [6] is one such model of family treatment. The PCSTF was developed to help families clearly identify their needs and concerns, to assess obstacles in the way to addressing their concerns, and to work with them to develop more effective ways of functioning as a family.

11.9.1 Problem-Centered Systems Therapy of the Family (PCSTF)

The PCSTF is a problem-focused, behaviorally directed family therapy model that empowers families to work effectively on resolving their distressing situation [20]. The PCSTF has been empirically validated as a useful adjunct in the treatment of patients with mood disorders [21–23]. The PCSTF emphasized the need for a comprehensive understanding of the family system, including its problems and strengths, as fully as possible. In addition to the presenting problems, the assessment includes understanding the structure, organization, and transactional patterns within the family. The assessment process includes reviewing multiple dimensions of family life as described earlier in this chapter.

The emphasis is on stages of treatment. These stages are assessment, contracting, treatment, and closure. The PCSTF focuses on these stages and steps in therapy and depends less on the particular personality of the therapist. It accommodates therapists with a variety of clinical styles.

The therapist models open and direct communication with the family by explaining his or her formulations and actions with the family along each step of the therapy process and makes sure that family members clearly understand and agree. The PCSTF assumes that family members understand their problems and are interested in changing them and that they have the capacity to do so with support and guidance. Family members are directly involved in identifying, clarifying, and resolving their difficulties. The role of the therapist is that of a catalyst, clarifier, and facilitator. The therapist provides a safe environment in which family members can be more open with each other, communicate more clearly with each other, and be more active in their problem-solving. The goal is to help families develop effective problem-solving methods that can be generalized to resolve future difficulties.

The PCSTF focuses mostly on the current problems. When appropriate, it may be necessary to review past issues to obtain a full understanding of how the current problems came about, what it means to the individual family members, and what attempts have been made at resolution, but once the meaning of the problem is understood, the focus is on what the family wants to do about it now.

Treatment is generally time limited, taking six or eight sessions spaced over a period of weeks or months. The length of each individual session or the time between them will vary depending on the issues involved, the stage of treatment, and the urgency of the situation. The assessment session[s] may take longer [up to an hour or an hour and a half], while later task setting treatment sessions may range from 15 min to 45 min.

11.9.1.1 Stages of Treatment

The stages of treatment are assessment, contracting, treatment, and closure.

Assessment

The assessment stage is made up of orientation, data gathering, problem description, and problem clarification. The assessment stage is the most important of the macro stages. It is the stage during which information and observations are gathered so as to be able to develop a comprehensive and meaningful biopsychosocial formulation which is the roadmap for effective treatment. This process has been described earlier in this chapter.

Contracting

The goal of this stage is to prepare a contract that delineates the expectations, goals, and commitments regarding therapy between family members and the therapist. The steps in this stage include orientation, outlining options, negotiating expectations, and drawing up a contract. The therapist orients the family to the stage of deciding what they want to do about the problems and solicit their agreement to move forward.

Although there are many options for how to deal with a variety of different problems, in fact there are generally four broad options which family members can choose in dealing with problems: the family can continue to function as before without attempting to bring about any change; the family can attempt to work out their problems on their own without the help of the therapist; the family can choose another type of treatment; the family can agree to engage with the therapist in the current treatment format.

The therapist should not try to persuade or entice the family into treatment. The only exception to this general rule is when a dangerous situation exists such as physical abuse, suicidality, or a behavior pattern which can significantly worsen illness in a family member.

The goal of the contracting stage is to formulate a set of expectations that each family member wants to see occur in order for the problems to be resolved successfully. The expectations should be stated in concrete, behavioral terms to allow for clearly identifying and assessing change. The main technique for establishing treatment goals is that family members negotiate what they would like from each other and how they want each other to change. The therapist may also need to raise additional problems that are not addressed by the family during the negotiating process particularly if the therapist feels those problems may be central to the ongoing difficulties the family is experiencing. It is useful to limit to two or three at a time the number of changes that any family member expects from others. It is helpful to write down the list of expectations from each family member in order to decrease the likelihood of misunderstandings in subsequent meetings.

Treatment

The goals of the treatment stage are to develop and employ problem-solving strategies to change the identified problems. Evaluation of the success or failure of the family in accomplishing tasks becomes the main focus of the work in subsequent family sessions. The treatment stage consists of orientation, clarifying priorities, setting tasks, and task evaluation.

The first step, as usual, is to orient the family to this new stage and to obtain their permission and collaboration to proceed. Clarifying priorities involves listing problems in order of importance. In general, priorities should be given to problems that involve communications and behavioral control, because problems in these areas can lead to difficulties in solving other problems. If family members are unable to come up with reasonable tasks and expectations from each other, the therapist may have to make some suggestions, checking with the family to ensure that these are agreeable to everyone.

Task evaluation is a critical process. This is the crux of the therapeutic work. It is in the review of the family's success or failure in carrying out the tasks that the real issues in the family become manifest. The tasks, apart from their intrinsic value, are a stimulus for core family issues to emerge and become more evident, not only to the therapist but also to the family members through the eyes of the therapist. Obstacles in carrying out agreed-upon tasks become stimuli and catalyst for bringing about subsequent changes. Failure to accomplish tasks should not be seen by the therapist or the family as an obstacle to change but as an opportunity to gain a much clearer insight into the problems of the family in a more immediate, nonintellectual, and affective manner.

If the agreed-upon tasks are accomplished, the therapist provides positive reinforcement, reviewing and highlighting the positive aspects of the family's performance to ensure that the family members understand what worked so they can continue to resolve problems in the future. If the tasks are not accomplished or only partially accomplished, the therapist needs to go through the particular steps in some detail to find out what went wrong.

A failed task may also mean that the family is not interested in working to bring about change. If noncompliance is a key reason for the failure of tasks, this needs to be addressed with the family directly to determine if they are invested enough in the treatment process to make treatment succeed. In general, unless there is a dangerous situation involved, it should be more important for the family to obtain good results in therapy than it should be for the therapist. If they are not ready to commit to the treatment process, they should be offered the opportunity to return to the therapist at some future date if and when they decide they are ready for the effort they will need to put into the treatment.

During the treatment stage, the major part of each session is devoted to reviewing previously assigned tasks and developing and negotiating new tasks. There are, however, other specific intervention tools that can help the therapist and family negotiate their way to bring about meaningful change. The therapist can be helpful in clarifying problems. The therapist can provide feedback on his or her perception of the family's functioning. The therapist can also label and interpret transactional processes and unacknowledged affect. Labeling and interpreting the process is based on observable behaviors that occur during the therapy sessions, therefore making them more immediate and real. The therapist can also provide education to modify incorrect assumptions, expectations and information about their illness, its consequences, and treatment options.

Closure

The final macro stage of closure consists of orientation, summary of treatment, long-term goals, and follow-up. During the orientation step, the therapist points out to the family that the goals of treatment have been met. If the family wants to continue with further therapy, this needs to be renegotiated. It is expected that families should be able to resolve new issues that come up using their newly learned coping skills. They should return for treatment only if they run into significant problems that they could not resolve on their own. It is important not to make professional patients out of families by keeping them too dependent on the therapist. Family members should be asked to summarize what they have learned during treatment. The therapist confirms or elaborates on their perceptions and adds any insights that may have been overlooked. The family is encouraged to discuss and set long-term goals. They should identify issues they anticipate might come up or prove problematic in the future. The therapy ends at this point, although for some families, an intermittent follow-up scheduled may be appropriate. This could be at 3, 6, or 9 months. If needed, the follow-up session should support and monitor progress rather than rehash issues that have already been dealt with.

11.10 Conclusions

A systematic assessment of the family is central to understanding the pertinent issues in the family and its potential role in shaping a patient's presenting problem. This understanding contributes to a comprehensive biopsychosocial formulation leading to a treatment plan that is likely to address most of the variables that may need and could benefit from clinical interventions. The clinician needs a consistent, broadly based, and structured assessment template to be able to perform a systematic family assessment. Such a template ensures that a wide range of family dimensions are assessed and helps the clinician stay on track. There are also subjective and objective assessment instruments, in addition to the standard clinical interview, to help in the evaluation process. These instruments complement the clinical evaluation. A good family assessment can be therapeutic in and of itself even if the decision is made that no further family intervention is indicated.

References

1. Campbell, T. (2003). The effectiveness of family interventions for physical disorders. *Journal of Marital and Family Therapy, 29*, 263–281.
2. Molloy, G. J., Johnston, D. W., Johnston, M., et al. (2005). Extending the demand-control model to informal caregiving. *Journal of Psychosomatic Research, 58*, 243–251.
3. Fisher, I. (2006). Research on the family and chronic disease among adults: Major trends and directions. *Families, Systems & Health, 24*(4), 373–380.
4. Fisher, L., & Weihs, K. (2000). Can addressing family relationships improve outcomes in chronic disease? Report of the national working group on family-based interventions in chronic disease. *The Journal of Family Practice, 49*, 561–566.

5. Keitner, G. I., Ryan, C. E., & Epstein, N. B. (2006). Family assessment. In D. Goldbloom (Ed.), *Psychiatric clinical skills* (pp. 327–338). Maryland Heights, MO: Mosby Elsevier.
6. Ryan, C. E., Epstein, N., Keitner, G. I., et al. (2005). *Evaluating and treating families: The Mcmaster approach*. New York: Routledge Taylor & Francis Group.
7. Spanier, G. B. (1976). Measuring dyadic adjustment: New scales for assessing the quality of marriage and similar dyads. *Journal of Marriage and the Family, 38*, 15–28.
8. Moos, R., & Moos, B. (1981). *Family environment scale manual*. Palo Alto, CA: Consulting Psychologists Press.
9. Epstein, N. B., Baldwin, L. M., & Bishop, D. S. (1983). The mcmaster family assessment device. *Journal of Marital and Family Therapy, 9*, 171–180.
10. Rosen, K. H., Mccollum, E. E., Middletown, K., et al. (1997). Interrater reliability and validity of the global assessment of relational functioning (GARF) scale in a clinical setting: A preliminary study. *American Journal of Family Therapy, 4*, 357–360.
11. Beavers, R., & Hampson, R. B. (1990). *Successful families: Assessment and intervention*. New York: Norton.
12. Miller, I. W., Kabacoff, R. I., & Keitner, G. I. (1994). The development of clinical rating scale for the McMaster model of family functioning. *Family Process, 33*, 53–69.
13. Chesla, C., Fisher, L., Mullan, J., et al. (2004). Family and disease management in African-American patients with type 2 diabetes. *Diabetes Care, 27*, 2850–2855.
14. DiMatteo, M. (2004). Variations in patients' adherence to medical recommendations: A quantitative review of 50 years of research. *Medical Care, 42*, 200–209.
15. Martire, L., Lustig, A., Schultz, R., et al. (2004). It is beneficial to involve a family member? A meta-analysis of psychosocial interventions for chronic illness. *Health Psychology, 23*, 599–611.
16. Hartmann, M., Bazner, E., Wild, B., et al. (2010). Effects of interventions involving the family in the treatment of adult patients with chronic physical diseases: A meta-analysis. *Psychotherapy and Psychosomatics, 79*, 136–148.
17. Nichols, M. (2010). *Family therapy concepts and methods* (9th ed.). Boston: Allyn & Bacon.
18. Gurman, A. S., & Jacobson, N. S. (2002). *Clinical handbook of couple therapy* (3rd ed.). New York: The Guilford Press.
19. Pisani, A., & McDaniel, S. (2005). An integrative approach to health and illness in family therapy. In J. L. Lebow (Ed.), *Handbook of clinical family therapy* (pp. 569–590). Hoboken, NJ: Wiley.
20. Keitner, G. I., Heru, A. M., & Glick, I. D. (2010). Family assessment. In *Clinical manual of couples and family therapy* (pp. 63–92). Washington, DC: American Psychiatric Publishing.
21. Miller, I. W., Keitner, G. I., Ryan, C. E., et al. (2005). Treatment matching in the post hospital care of depressed patients. *The American Journal of Psychiatry, 162*, 2131–2138.
22. Miller, I. W., Keitner, G. I., Ryan, C. E., et al. (2008). Family treatment for bipolar disorder: Family impairment by treatment interactions. *The Journal of Clinical Psychiatry, 69*, 732–740.
23. Solomon, D. A., Keitner, G. I., Ryan, C. E., et al. (2008). Preventing recurrence of bipolar 1 mood episodes and hospitalizations: Family psychotherapy plus pharmacotherapy versus pharmacotherapy alone. *Bipolar Disorders, 10*, 798–805.

Part V
Specific Psychosomatic Symptoms

Chapter 12
Pain, Depression, and Anxiety: A Common Language of Human Suffering

Tatjana Sivik and Matteo Bruscoli

Nietzsche: "Did you ever say yes to a pleasure?
Oh my friends, then you also said yes to all pain.
All things are linked, entwined, in love with one another."

12.1 Introduction

The framework of this chapter is psychosomatological. This represents an attempt to integrate different theoretical approaches, including psychodynamic theories of human development, complex systems theory, psycho-neuro-endocrino-immunology (PNEI), and biosemiotics, in studying the pain-depression-anxiety complex [1].

According to such a paradigm, the human being is an entity that simultaneously and constantly is feeling, thinking, and behaving in both physical and psychological-existential sense.

12.2 Complex System Theory and PNEI

According to complex system theory, human organism itself can be viewed as a suprasystem, consisting of interrelated subsystems in constant interaction within the environment. This complex web of interactions (*connectivity*) is in action, using

T. Sivik, M.D., Ph.D. (✉)
Department of General Medicine, Institute of Psychosomatic Medicine, University of Göteborg, Fridkullagatan 14, 41262 Göteborg, Sweden
e-mail: t.sivik@ipsoma.se

M. Bruscoli, M.D.
Societa Italina Medicina Psichosomatica, Italy, Affiliated to Institute of Psychosomatic Medicine, Sweden, Borgo Ognissanti, 38, Florence 50123, Italy
e-mail: m.bruscoli@evolutivamente.com

K.B. Koh (ed.), *Somatization and Psychosomatic Symptoms*,
DOI 10.1007/978-1-4614-7119-6_12, © Springer Science+Business Media New York 2013

cross-subsystem information and feedback loops for self-regulation (*plasticity*), and reacting when perturbed by any kind of injury (*irritability*) – physical as well as psychological.

Major interrelated subsystems are the nervous/mental, the immunological, and the endocrinological ones, and together these constitute the PNEI system. There is a constantly ongoing reciprocal communication (unconscious, preconscious, and conscious), and this takes place on all levels: molecular, cellular, and psychophysiological/functional. This is actually a prerequisite for all actions and responses of a living (human) organism. In direct connection with the PNEI system, however, are all the other subsystems of a living body, such as the cardiovascular, dermatological, muscular, visceral, and connective tissue. All these subsystems relate to and communicate within and between each other and the environment, following all the intricate psychophysiological "*memories,*" interactions, and activation pathways available. Memory in this context is to be seen as the process of storing all the experiences, both psychosocial and biological that a living creature has encountered both phylogenetically and ontogenetically as well as during the individual life span. In that sense, the DNA molecule as well as all its expressions (i.e., through immune cells, endocrine peptides, neural signal substances) stores and carries the information necessary for the maintenance of life.

A balanced and meaningful interaction between the different *memory and communication subsystems* of the organism is in fact necessary for survival, as well as for the preservation of health. A continuously ongoing exchange of information within and between each of these subsystems is, as pointed out, always activated at all times. In other words, we could say that "the body is a swarm…" [2].

12.3 Health, Growth, Memories, and Communication

In concordance with the definition above, health is the result of optimal energy consumption and interdependent interaction between human organism and the environment. Disease, on the other hand, is a result of an acute injury/hurt or prolonged allostatic load, leading to dysregulation of the communication and the psychophysiological memory processes, as well as exuberant energy usage. Therefore, health and disease are determined by the integration of and interaction between genetic vulnerability, epigenetic feedback loops, previous life stress experiences, and coping strategies and personality styles of the individual. The "pure" biochemistry behind any condition or occurrence is meaningless if not perceived and interpreted in a meaningful way by the individual (organism) within which it occurs.

At the moment of birth, the infant carries biological predispositions (both inherited and acquired "memories") from previous generations. These predispositions underlie the reaction patterns of the organism. Throughout life, those predispositions interact with each other and with external stimuli, evolving into reaction patterns specific to the individual. These are then carried on to the next generation, together with everything that came before.

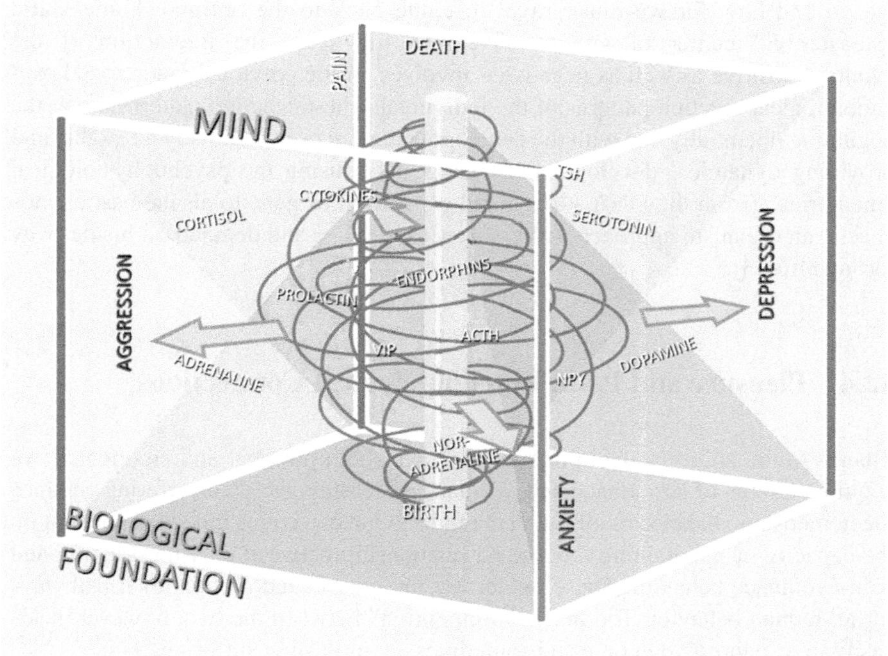

Fig. 12.1 The cube of life: a schematic presentation of a theoretical concept of psychosomatology. From the very moment of conception, all inherited biopsychological "memories" interact with all the acquired experiences and "memories" through constant ongoing interdependent processes. The "ideal" growth, presented as a *yellow* column in the *middle* of the figure, represents a homeostatic state, an experience-free process (i.e., even a slightest experience/demand on the system results in an allostatic load. In other words, there is no "ideal" growth since that would be a life without experiences, that is an "un-born life"!) and an ultimate pleasure. Life itself, through environmental demands, hurts and causes injuries, brings along developmental changes, making different gene expressions possible. Over the life span, the interaction between the events – positive as well as negative – involves all the previously acquired psychobiological reaction patterns of the individual. With the development, these reaction patterns – from being a potential – become more or less actively adaptable and provide dynamical developmental changes. By using the psychophysiological "memories" (from the DNA storage and expression of genes to all the past experiences), an organism approaches every new experience and demand in his/her specific way. A variety of expressions of life (pleasure as well as pain, depression, anxiety, and aggression) are present on all the levels – cells, tissues, and organs – through the biological, nonverbal language. The "translation" from this bodily language to our mental apparatus is going on constantly, even though we hardly understand anything of it and mostly never listen to it. If the "translation" proceeds smoothly, the contact between our living and our perceiving body is mainly positive, without creating too much allostatic load, and we remain "healthy." If, on the other hand, the demands put upon us from the environment are overwhelming our (individual) resources, we become ill or develop a disease that eventually may end in a (premature) death. The "ideal" life would, on the other hand, last as long as our genetic predispositions would make it possible

We start experiencing life events early and that pushes us toward the corners of life, where fear, anxiety, aggression, pain and depression abide – as well as pleasure. The perception and interpretation of life events, including insults (physical as well as emotional), determines how far out in the corners of the "life cube" (Fig. 12.1) we go and how far we must travel to come back to the optimal, homeostatic (pleasurable) center of growth. Over the life span, the interaction of the events – positive as well as negative – involves all the previously mentioned psychobiological reaction patterns of the individual. These reaction patterns are at the beginning potentially and with the development more or less actively adaptable and providing dynamical developmental changes. By using the psychophysiological "memories" (from the DNA storage and expression of gene to all the past experiences), an organism approaches every new experience and demand on his/her way through life [3].

12.4 Pleasure and Pain: Psychobiological Connections

Thanks to the ability to feel pleasure and pain (both physical and emotional), we acquire patterns of acceptance and avoidance. Pleasure and pain/suffering enhance the homeostatic balance of all living creatures. Our survival is indeed dependent on the capacity of maintaining a balanced relationship between pleasure-seeking and pain-avoidance behavior. These two create the interrelated motivational pathways for all human behavior. Too much "competition" between the two, however, leads easily to a "painful" outcome and sometimes a long-lasting suffering.

The notion of the interwoven connection between pain and pleasure has been obvious to the mankind since we became conscious of our selves. In psychobiological research, it has only been recognized recently that the connection of the two indeed is very strong. The biological "language" of neural circuitry and biochemistry of pain and pleasure are more or less the same and/or overlapping. Well-designed controlled studies have, for instance, demonstrated the interrelated role played by dopamine and opioids in both pain and pleasure. Opioids are necessary for hedonic experience, "liking", and dopamine motivates for the "wanting" [4, 5]. Both pain and pleasure elicit opioid release in several brain areas, such as orbitofrontal cortex, nucleus accumbens, ventral pallidum, and amygdala [6]. In particular, amygdala registers and "reads" both positive and negative value of reward and punishment signals. All the regions mentioned release endogenous opioids during painful stimulation in an effort to maintain the homeostasis of the pain-pleasure reward system. Feedback-dependent regulatory processes and stress responses cross the nervous, endocrine, and immune system boundaries and thereby contribute to overall system regulation.

12.5 Pain and PNEI

Allostatic load engages the activities in all the subsystems of the PNEI suprasystem by interdependently *detecting* the threat and *anticipating* the danger (cognition, appraisal) in the external environment and *organizing* fight, flight, or freezing. Through a common chemical language comprising neurotransmitters, peptides, endocannabinoids, cytokines, and hormones, an ensemble of interdependent nervous, endocrine, and immune processes operates in concerto to cope with any kind of injury or/and distress. Since nervous, endocrine, and immune systems are interdependently connected in constant reciprocal communication, they react to any stressor in a highly orchestrated manner where – in a metaphoric sense – the performing "musicians" simultaneously are the "conductors."

Endocrino-immune reciprocal interactions involve hypothalamus, pituitary gland, adrenal cortex, and adrenal medulla as well as multiple immune cells, which have adrenoceptors and receptors for various peptides. Neural structures initiate hormonal responses and provide the mechanisms of feedback-controlled regulation of corticotropin-releasing hormone, epinephrine, norepinephrine, endorphin, etc., which take the role of neurotransmitter in the nervous system and the role of hormone in the endocrine system [7]. All the "words" of the PNEI language are pleiotropic substances. The PNEI suprasystem is "thinking and behaving"; it *evaluates* and *differentiates* (i.e., self vs. nonself); it *makes decisions* (i.e., cell trafficking) and *takes action* (i.e., inflammatory response, cell trafficking, endocrino-immune reactivity), that is, it "*behaves.*" More so, it *learns* from the past experience (adaptive immunity and conditioning), and it "*remembers*."

12.6 Living and Perceiving Body Concept

As stated above, PNEI, besides being a suprasystem itself, is also a system within a higher suprasystem structure of the human organism within the environment. One of the most prominent and (probably) exclusively human characteristics is the capacity of simultaneously being an object (a *living* body) and an observing/reflecting subject (a *perceiving* body). That capacity implies some specific mental processes where emotion, cognition, and behavior are constantly interwoven and interdependent and give us the bless and the curse of remembering the past, observing the present, and anticipating the future [8].

12.7 Perception and Processing

Recent neuroscientific research demonstrates that affects constitute the base of our consciousness. Affects involve all the levels of the human brain – from brainstem, over limbic, to neocortical level [9, 10]. Affects first emerge on a subcortical level, i.e., brainstem and midbrain periaqueductal and not – as assumed in cognitive scientific approach – on a neocortical level [11]. The "drive" for the development of the perceptual and higher self-reflecting consciousness emerges from the lower, subcortical brain areas common to all the mammals. Consequently, the (affective) perceptual experiences initiated at the brainstem, called *primary processes*, create the ground for the limbic, *secondary processes*, of learning, and together they constitute the bases of all higher, neocortical, *tertiary processes*, of cognitions and emotions [12].

The capacity to think, feel, and behave while observing and reflecting over one's thoughts, feelings, and actions is the representation of the neocortical tertiary processes (supposedly) reserved for humans. Still, all the three processes are all the time (onto-, phylo-, and epigenetically as well as during the lifespan) interrelated and interwoven and should not and cannot be considered as separate entities. So, the process of cognition starts prior to the neocortical consciousness (recognition) thus making us – in the same way as with other mammals – "conscious" of both negative and positive experiences before we become conscious of our consciousness. Our living body "knows" before the perceiving body realizes the knowledge [8, 12].

12.8 Acute Versus Chronic Pain Process

Acute pain is "now" and as such shared by humans and other mammals as well as the rest of animal world. It involves basal ganglions (preconscious processes) and limbic brain areas (conditional learning conscious processes). Acute pain elicits fear and action: flight, fight, or freezing reactions. Chronic pain is "then," it includes neocortical, reflective consciousness and as such evokes anxiety and depression [11, 13].

12.9 Prediction and Expectation of Life and Pain

Parallel to the development of language, our capacity to grasp the concept of time evolves. With that, the capacity of reflective consciousness (neocortical process) and the painful insight of mortality emerge (both in an explicit and implicit sense). Regardless of our *belief* system, we do not *know* what, if anything, is "waiting" for us. Knowing and believing are actually two different aspects of reality. Our knowledge about the objective reality is primarily circumscribed by the limitations of our senses. Just because of this (painful) insight, we sometimes are willing to do almost anything to deny it and lure ourselves into believing that we can anticipate what is coming. Consequently we "create" our future, both in "real" and in "spiritual" life. Certain amount of this "creative" attitude toward the uncertainties of life is necessary for a balanced life. Mostly, we are creating the future on our (perception of) past experiences, as well as on our appraisal of the narratives of experiences of the others. Possibly, the greatest differences between people's behaviors and their feelings are based on the differences in their appraisal of the past and how one projects it onto the future [14].

12.9.1 The Loop of Pain Prediction: Certainty Versus Uncertainty

To predict pain or other unpleasant events by learning from prior experiences is an important adaptive behavior for all living healthy organisms [14]. At the same time, predictability can elicit and reinforce disabling fear, anxiety, depression, and avoidance in patients with chronic pain [15]. A very common reason for the transmission from acute pain to chronic state of pain and distress is the belief that the pain will never end. Thus, future not only becomes unbearably insecure it also becomes infinitely painful, and the remaining period of one's life is seen as an unending suffering.

12.9.2 Pain Prediction: Fear Versus Anxiety Responses

It is important, however, to distinguish between the experienced (subjective) certainty and uncertainty. Being *certain* that a specific negative event is impending ("certain" expectation) is associated with the emotional state of fear. Particularly, in acute phases after an injury, fear mobilizes the organism to take action (fight or flight) or, if these options are not available, to minimize the impact of the aversive event (e.g., by cognitive distraction) [16, 17]. In addition, fear has an impact on pain perception itself; numerous experimental studies with animals (and some with humans) have shown that fear leads to decreased pain sensitivity or hypoalgesia [18–21]. In contrast, *uncertainty* about the nature of the impending event ("uncertain" expectation) has very different consequences. It is associated with the emotional state of anxiety (rather than fear) which is characterized by risk assessment behavior or behavioral inhibition and by increased attention to the body and environment (rather than by distraction as in the case of fear) with elevated muscular tension and inhibited breathing [22]. Compared with fear, anxiety has the opposite effect on pain perception; it leads to increased pain sensitivity or hyperalgesia [20, 21]. Uncertain expectation and anxiety indeed increase pain sensitivity [22, 23].

12.10 Link Between Chronic Pain, Anxiety, and Depression

In a situation of acute threat – that might lead to pain – fear is an adequate response, leading to flight or fight response. In chronic pain, no "logical" response is possible, so anxiety (i.e., response to an unknown enemy when there is no known defense strategy available) becomes a "natural" response. A vicious circuit is established, with pain and anxiety reinforcing one another leading to less and less diversity of both emotion and motion. Depression, as a psychobiological "capitulation" becomes a more and more stable state of the mind-body complex. The longer the pain continues, it usually leads to more uncertainty and suffering. One of the predominant characteristics of patients suffering from long-term pain is the specific *pain-prone behavior pattern* and the development of a stable pain-related "sense of self." Patients with long-term pain often describe themselves as *governed by the pain*, so eventually we are not dealing with "the patient who has the pain," but rather with "the pain that has the patient" [20].

12.10.1 Chronic Pain, Anxiety, and Depression in Medical Settings

Consequently, comorbidity between chronic pain, anxiety, and depression is often observed in most medical settings [24]. Particularly, the relationship between low back pain and emotional instability has been reported in several studies [25–32].

Patients suffering from a triad of pain-anxiety-depression are difficult to handle and are usually labeled as "somatizers" (about 30 % of primary care patients) [33]. When a patient is very difficult to deal with and the symptoms are abundant, concepts of somatoform and even multisomatoform disorders are used in an attempt to describe the complexity of the problem [33–35]. A great number of papers on the comorbidity between pain, depression, and anxiety demonstrate that the problem is indeed huge and that it causes troubles in medical settings, particularly so in primary health-care settings [32, 36–45]. This triad involves a reduction in the ability of chronic pain sufferers to enjoy everyday pleasures (anhedonia). This reduction in pleasure leads to further reinforcement of the vicious circuit where both negative mood and lack of pleasure result in exacerbated pain, leading to more negative mood and more severe anhedonia [23]. Measuring biological correlates of this state reveals that the normal interaction between the dopamine system and pain gets disrupted in patients suffering from chronic pain. Patients suffering from chronic pain – for various reasons (related to past experiences and epigenetic predisposition) – often are lacking conscious, meaningful contact with the original experience, so the symptom becomes "meaningless" [46–48].

Often the medical society, sometimes even including psychosomatically oriented doctors and therapists, gets involved in more or less fruitful attempts to "take the symptom away," instead of seeing it as a sign (in biosemiotic terms) of something beyond the symptom and as an attempt to communicate a disrupted discourse [47].

In the "somatizer" the capacity to feel pain, sadness/loss, and fear is distorted into undesirable symptoms of anxiety, depression, and chronic pain [48–50]. With growing uncertainty of a distorted (unconscious or misunderstood) psychophysiological message, the symptom grows, and the sense of control and understanding of one's own life shrinks. Adaptive behavior gets more and more stereotypic, focus of attention narrows, and perception gets more and more distorted. Distortion itself is experienced on all levels of the psychophysiological functioning of the organism: emotional, behavioral, cognitive, musculoskeletal, circular, and neuronal (as exhibited in the altered neural pathways) [48].

12.11 Somatization and Patient-Doctor Relationship

The label "somatization," however, should be used with caution. It is easily misinterpreted for a more or less conscious process of transformation of a psychic symptom into a somatic complaint. This may sometimes, but very seldom indeed, be the case. Any symptom has both psychic and somatic representation. We perceive a discomfort in our bodies, but how we interpret and communicate them to our social environment (including the doctor) is an entirely different matter [47, 50]. Since pain, as any other symptom, is a carrier of a sign which is representing something other than itself and is forming a link between the injury (psychological and/or physical) and a system of interpretation (i.e., a patient and the doctor), the doctor cannot be excluded from the effects of the interactions [51–54]. Behind any sign (i.e., pain), there is a (often hidden) potentiality and an internal experience (Peirce's "firstness"), thereby placing the creation of a sign into the position of "secondness," a materialization of the "firstness." So the symptom presentation itself, as an actuality presented by the patient, is a result of an interaction within the interpretation system (the patient and doctor complex). Such an interaction influences (changes) both patient's and doctors' perceptions and emotions. Finally, the process of normalization, generalization, and habit formation (i.e., verbal communication, examinations, assessment, treatment plans), the "thirdness" emerges. Therefore, the process of "thirdness" includes the presentation and possibilities of the future and predictability. All the three levels – just as the three levels of brain activities (brainstem, limbic, and cortical levels), as unconscious, preconscious, and conscious processes – coexist and are always present at the same time and space and mutually interdependent [52, 55, 56].

12.12 Pain from the Perspective of Chaos and Complex Adaptive System

The interactions of sensory, autonomic, endocrine, and immune responses to tissue injury as well as to psychosocial insult are both complex and adaptive. Complex systems perspective can facilitate understanding and answering difficult questions, such as how pain becomes chronic and how different expressions of pain and suffering (physical as well as emotional) are mutually interdependent.

Traumatic life events can permanently alter the set point of an individual's feedback-dependent hypothalamic-pituitary-adrenal and sympathetic-adrenomedullary axis and lead to difficulties in coping with future life experiences. Particularly, during the acute phase after an insult or injury, the human organism moves toward chaos which increases the energy usage and entropy. Over time, however, the organism starts moving toward the best possible reorganization and will emerge into a new adaptation, sometimes resulting in chronic pain. When encountering a patient, it is of utmost importance to realize that he/she always expresses the best possible self-organization of the system in the actual (memory) context, i.e., time, space, environment, and history [57].

12.13 Multimodal and Integrative Treatment Approach

The question of which organ or function level is most involved is dependent on a whole array of (biopsychosocial) factors. The most obvious factor should *never* a priori be considered as the only or even the most important – component.

This implies that the treatment *may* be symptom-oriented, but *should not* necessarily be so [8].

Health is not a "non-painful" state; it is the result of a non-linear complex dynamic and adaptive state where interdependent and dynamic relationships generate various kinds of behavior patterns which are often simple but never *completely* predictable. Therefore, the outcome can vary considerably from time to time, even though the different incoming parts are seemingly the same. The web of non-linear interactions determine that even minimal changes in initial input can exit in extremely different outcome because every change results in a feedback or feed-forward loop leading to new conditions creating a new adaptive complexity. Chaotic systems, opposite to the complex ones, have not yet reached organized patterns of behavior. They have potentially all the possible outcomes in themselves, but we could say that they "deny" their history, having difficulties in adapting to new (more complex) demands and in developing complex organized response. Therefore, entering into a pattern of stereotypic responses such as pain, anxiety, and depression until new input will lead to a new chaotic but potentially evolving state toward a better adaptation. The organism, in this case, will develop toward the edge of chaos, a new complex order. So a healthy organism "balances" at the edge of chaos. Such an organism, the person, is (reflectively) conscious of the irreversibility of the past and the unpredictability of the future.

An ill system fixated in a stereotypic communication through pain, depression, and anxiety is characterized by a rigid and more predictable pattern of response, mainly disconnected from its earlier experiences and unable to use the complex variability and adaptability of a healthy non-linear system. Such system makes these individuals vulnerable to demands from the environment, since without the living, flexible (biopsychological) capacity of adaptability, and learning, it is difficult to cope with the uncertain, unpredictable future [57, 58].

A complex system is robust and as such possessing the potential for radical and qualitative change, while retaining systemic integrity. To adapt, to change, and to lose (anything and/or anybody) without losing oneself is the core characteristic of a (robust) complex system. A person characterized in such a way experiences pain, sadness, loss, and fear. He/she can have pain but pain can never have him/her. Consequently, the subjective (emotional) judgment and appraisal of all life events (on unconscious, subconscious, and conscious level simultaneously) is interdependently related, in a web of self-sustaining and coherent connections, to the "objective" reality of the events themselves that create and give sense to all human experience, including pain. [52, 59].

12.14 Reductionism Versus Holism in Research and Treatment

In Western medical research as well as in education and medical practice, it is the biological paradigm that has dominated in the tradition of empiricism, monism, realism, materialism, and positivism. The search for a universal truth and general laws (in our case, the truth about the nature of diseases) has been believed to be the most fruitful. In many instances, this approach is indeed helpful. But, unfortunately, because of the successes achieved, we still often continue to look for the lost key under the biomedical "lamp" even when such approach not only cannot help us finding what we look for, but it may even hinder us from daring to go into the darkness where we perhaps might be able to find not only the key itself but also develop a 'lamp' with substantially better light [46].

The objectivist's postulates presuppose many things. First, it is supposed that there is only *one (*objective*) reality* independent of consciousness, and by dividing and studying its parts, the whole can be understood (*reductionism*). Secondly, it is presumed that "the knower" can stand outside what is to be known and not influence what is observed (*positivism*). Thirdly, it is assumed that the knower's own values and opinions can be suspended (*objectivism*). Fourthly, it is concluded that an event that comes before another event can be said to cause the first event (*determinism*). And, lastly, it is considered evident that explanations from one time and place can be generalized to other times and places (*inference*).

These postulates, though astonishingly still often taken for granted, are actually hardly applicable in any science at all. At least one of them, namely, the fantasy that an observer is never influenced by his/her own belief system, prejudices, and feelings, is in fact nothing more than just a fantasy. This belief of being totally objective, however, has advantages in many biomedical fields. But, as soon as human emotions are involved, as in dealing with pain, depression, and anxiety, and any other psychological symptom, such an approach is not only unfruitful but even harmful. Pain does indeed follow C-fiber activation, but pain *is* not C-fiber activation. Pain is subjective and has a strongly individual meaning for the patient. Loneliness and vulnerability connect physical pain with psychic pain such as anxiety, depression, and mourning. However, physical pain is an overpowering body experience that might lead us to the point of "losing the mind." Psychic pain, on the other hand, may imprison us in our minds and make us "loose" the body.

Working with patients suffering from pain-depression-anxiety triad forces us to deal with multiple and subjective "realities" that form the "whole" complex; therefore the observer (doctor) and the observed (patient) are interdependent (as in quantum theory), values influence and create what is perceived and understood, and events relate with each other by multidirectional relationships across time and space (chaos theory and emergence) [6, 8, 48, 55–60].

When a narrow biomedical paradigm is applied to persons with pain, depression, and anxiety, with its expectation that patients will follow deterministic paths and that pain in one patient will normatively predict pain in another, it does very seldom match the clinical reality. Pain cannot be separated from the person experiencing it, and the human experience cannot be omitted from a scientific explanation of how the mind works [56, 59]. The same is basically also valid for all the symptoms, including anxiety and depression, since the experiences a person has are always subjective. Considering that the vast majority of symptoms presented to the medical society by patients are pain, depression, and anxiety, this biomedical strategy appears extremely fruitless. Still it prevails mostly because the alternative requires that the doctors become interdependently involved co-actors. *However, it is indeed important that we teach young students that a doctor cannot be an objective, detached non-involved observer since he/she is a part of the integrated complex system.*

12.15 The Misconception of Assessing Objective Pain

It takes lots of energy to continue preserving the misconception or "lie" (a common subconscious belief) of pain being objectively observable and measurable. Every "lie" is consuming energy, and when this "lie" on the part of the doctor gets interwoven with the "lie" of the patient (that the symptom is something that has nothing to do with himself/herself but just "happened"), the result is commonly disastrous. Assessing pain – as well as depression and anxiety – is causing lots of problems because it is actually – in spite of lots of efforts – still mostly relying on self-assessing psychometric instruments such as visual analog scales [61–63]. Even when an attempt is made to get access to preconscious or even unconscious levels of the (emotional) experience, as performed by means of projective test, we are still assessing patients' subjective experience [64–68]. Indeed, as described several thousand years ago by Tao te Ching: "Pain is felt by all but it cannot be touched. It cannot be seen or directly measured, but its patterns can be recognized. Elusive and ill defined yet it has substance and specific characteristics" [58].

12.16 Psychosomatology and Psychosomatic Medicine Perspective

Psychosomatic medicine has developed in counterreaction to the traditional biomedicine. The psychophysiology of emotion is one cornerstone of psychosomatic medicine. The American Psychosomatic Society was launched by the publication of *Emotions and Bodily Changes* by H. Flanders Dunbar [69]. The journal *Psychosomatic Medicine* was to be "devoted not to the isolated problems of the diseased mind or the diseased body, but to the interrelationships between emotional life and bodily processes" [70]. Psychosomatology is an integrative research approach that studies the *simultaneous* interaction between all the internal (genetic, neuroendocrine, immunological, etc.) and external memory and communication systems (societal, cultural, psychosocial, ecological, etc.) of the human organism [1].

To this day, a majority of papers in various psychosomatic journals involve emotion and emotional regulation. Unfortunately, in spite of abundant excellent research results, most of the findings are only marginally being applied to medical settings. Majority of the health-care institutions still dwell in the reductionistic cause-effect approach and blindly search for the key under the strictly biomedical and narrowly illuminating lamp.

The development of psychosomatic medicine has itself been influenced by all the different scientific paradigms that have emerged since its history, initially from psychoanalysis, over phenomenological, psychosocial, existential, behavioral points of view, all the way to the neurochemical coloring of today [71].

The discussions concerning the meaning of a symptom (i.e., pain) have been changing with the shifts in paradigms and perspectives. The emphasis has been fluctuating from the concept of conversion (a symptom representing a hidden emotion that has to be disclosed and interpreted), over social causation of the (reactive, psychosomatic) symptom, behavioral reinforcement of a (random?) physical reaction, to neuroendocrionological overexcitation due to allostatic imbalance.

The conflict on whether a symptom should be considered as conscious or unconscious has consumed lots of energy among the researchers. Most of us do persist in exploring "interrelationships between emotional life and bodily processes." However, in our endeavor to get access to the scientific society (which still is mainly reductionistic), an ambivalent attitude sometimes emerges. Even though it is broadly acknowledged that reality is complex and that an integrative, psychosomatic approach, and inclusive scientific paradigm is to be applied to both research and clinical settings, reductionistic research methods still often prevail. This has, unfortunately, been noticeable even in pain research [1, 72].

Understanding pain in relation to human suffering demands a multilevel scientific approach. The level of the investigators' understanding for the patient suffering from chronic pain depends very much on his/her capacity to recognize that he/she is an interacting part of the doctor-patient complex. His/her intersubjectivity and life experiences are interwoven with that of a patient, in concordance with the basic concepts of biosemiotics [51–56].

The need for understanding all the levels of the psychobiological (PNEI) organization of pain is adding still more to the complexity of the problem. Particularly, so when we are forced to realize that our knowledge of these processes – just as the above mentioned intersubjectivity – is still in its cradle.

Multidisciplinary research, to incorporate knowledge from many different scientific areas needs to be included in biopsychosocial framework. Fantastic research opportunities to connect different branches of science have emerged through new techniques mainly used in neuroscience. In 2012, at the 101st Annual Meeting of the American Psychoanalytic Association, a revolutionary, empirical, and experimental research demonstrated a neurophysiological link between unconscious conflicts and conscious anxiety disorder symptoms. These findings and the interdisciplinary methods used – which draw on psychoanalysis, cognitive psychology, and neuroscience – demonstrate that it is possible, or even mandatory, to develop an interdisciplinary science drawing on psychoanalytic theory [73].

Philosophy (primarily studies of consciousness and mentality), physics (particularly quantum mechanics), and ecological phenomenology should be included in research on human emotions and its bodily representations. Last but far from least, expressive arts (literature, music, theater, and painting) would broaden our perspective still more.

In addition, the treatment programs are requested to have a multimodal approach, with teams consisting of several professionals that possess knowledge and techniques based on both western and eastern frame of knowledge as well as on expressive arts. Such teams have been slowly emerging over the last years in several countries, for example, in Sweden where a political decision concerning multimodal treatment teams has been made and also implemented by governmental financing.

12.17 Conclusions

Pain, anxiety, and depression represent the three major, interrelated "languages" of human distress. Any symptom has both psychic and somatic representation. Understanding pain-anxiety-depression complex demands a psychosomatological and multilevel scientific approach, including psychodynamic theories of human development, complex systems theory, psycho-neuro-endocrino-immunology, and biosemiotics.

To predict pain/suffering by learning from prior experiences is an important adaptive behavior. Still, predictability can elicit and reinforce disabling fear, anxiety, depression, and avoidance in patients with chronic pain. A very common reason for the transmission from acute pain to chronic state of pain and distress is the belief that the pain will never end.

In order to better help patients suffering from pain-anxiety-depression complex, a variety of professionals need to collaborate over the borders of different disciplines and create multimodal treatment programs, using techniques based on both western and eastern frame of knowledge as well as on expressive arts.

References

1. Sivik, T., & Schoenfeld, R. (2006). Psychosomatology as a theoretical paradigm of modern psychosomatic medicine. *International Congress Series, 1287*, 23–28. Elsevier.
2. Hoffmeyer, J. (1996). *Signs of meaning in the universe*. Bloomington, IN: Indiana University Press.
3. Sivik, T. (2000). Den lyckliga kroppen (the happy body). *Forskning och Framsteg, 35*, 9–24.
4. Berridge, K. C. (2003). Pleasures of the brain. *Brain and Cognition, 52*, 106–128.
5. Barbano, M., & Cador, M. (2007). Opioids for hedonic experience and dopamine to get ready for it. *Psychopharmacology, 191*, 497–506.
6. Leknes, A., & Tracey, I. (2008). A common neurobiology for pain and pleasure. *Neuroscience, 316*, 314–318.
7. Goldstein, D. S., & McEwen, B. (2002). Allostasis, homeostats, and the nature of stress. *The International Journal on the Biology of Stress, 5*, 55–58.
8. Chapman, C. R., Tuckett, R. P., & Song, C. W. (2008). Pain and stress in a systems perspective: Reciprocal neural, endocrine, and immune interactions. *The Journal of Pain, 92*, 122–145.
9. Panksepp, J., & Solms, M. (2012). The "Id" knows more than the "Ego" admits: Neuropsychoanalytic and primal consciousness perspectives on the inference between affective and cognitive neuroscience. *Brain Sciences, 2*, 147–175.

10. Panksepp, J. (1992). A critical role for "affective neuroscience" in resolving what is basic about basic emotions. *Psychological Review, 99*, 554–560.
11. Panksepp, J. (1998). *Affective neuroscience: The foundations of human and animal emotions*. New York: Oxford University Press.
12. Damasio, A. R. (1999). *The feeling of what happens: body and emotion in the making of consciousness*. New York: Harcourt.
13. Van den Stock, J., Tamietto, M., Sorger, B., et al. (2011). Cortico-subcortical visual, somatosensory, and motor activations for perceiving dynamic whole-body emotional expressions with and without striate cortex. *Proceedings of the National Academy of Sciences of the United States of America*. Washington, DC: PNAS.
14. Ploghaus, A., Becerra, L., Borras, C., et al. (2003). Neural circuitry underlying pain modulation: Expectation, hypnosis, placebo. *Trends in Cognitive Sciences, 7*, 197–200.
15. Crombez, G., Vlaeyen, J. W., Heuts, P. H., et al. (1999). Pain-related fear is more disabling than pain itself: Evidence on the role of pain-related fear in chronic pain disability. *Pain, 80*, 329–339.
16. Barlow, D. H., Chorpita, B. F., & Turovski, J. (1996). Fear, panic, anxiety and disorders of emotion. In D. A. Hope, et al. (Eds.), *Nebrasca Symposium on Motivation* (pp. 251–328). Lincoln: University of Nebrasca Press.
17. Blanchard, R. J., Yudko, E. B., Rodgers, R. J., et al. (1993). Defense system psychopharmacology: An ethological approach to the pharmacology of fear and anxiety. *Behavioural Brain Research, 58*, 155–165.
18. Rhudy, J. L., & Meagher, M. W. (2000). Fear and anxiety: Divergent effects on human pain thresholds. *Pain, 84*, 65–75.
19. Ploghaus, A., Narain, C., Beckmann, C. F., et al. (2001). Exacerbation of pain by anxiety is associated with activity in a hippocampal network. *Journal of Neuroscience, 21*, 9896–9903.
20. Ploghaus, A., Tracey, I., Gati, S., et al. (1999). Dissociating pain from its anticipation in the human brain. *Science, 284*, 1979–1981.
21. Chua, P., Krams, M., Toni, I., et al. (1999). A functional anatomy of anticipatory anxiety. *NeuroImage, 9*, 563–571.
22. Miller, S. M. (1981). Predictability and human stress: Toward a clarification of evidence and theory. In L. Berkowitz (Ed.), *Advances in experimental social psychology* (pp. 203–256). Amsterdam: Academic Press Elsevier.
23. Simpson, J. R., Jr., Drevets, W. C., Snyder, A. Z., et al. (2001). Emotion-induced changes in human medial prefrontal cortex: II. During anticipatory anxiety. *Proceedings of the National Academy of Sciences of the United States of America, 98*, 688–693.
24. Maier, W., & Falkai, P. (1999). The epidemiology of co-morbidity between depression, anxiety and somatic diseases. *International Clinical Psychopharmacology, 14*(suppl. 2), 51–56.
25. Sivik, T (1992). *Diagnoses and treatment of patients with idiopathic back pain*. Doctoral Thesis (pp. 34–37). Department of Primary Health Care, University of Göteborg.
26. Sivik, T., Röjwall, S., Gustafsson, E., et al. (1992). Relationship between back pain and personality. Psychological vulnerability as risk factors for development of chronic back pain. *Nordic Journal of Psychiatry, 46*, 188–193.
27. Sivik, T., & Delimar, D. (1994). Characteristics of patients who attribute chronic pain to minor injury. *Scandinavian Journal of Rehabilitation Medicine, 26*, 27–31.
28. Lansinger, B., Nordholm, L., & Sivik, T. (1994). Characteristics of low back pain patients who do not complete physiotherapeutic treatment. *Scandinavian Journal of Caring Sciences, 8*, 163–167.
29. Hellzén-Ingemarsson, A., Nordholm, L., & Sivik, T. (1997). Risk for long-term disability among patients with back pain. *Scandinavian Journal of Rehabilitation Medicine, 4*, 205–212.
30. Sivik, T. (1991). Personality traits in patients with acute low-back pain. A comparison with chronic low-back pain patients. *Psychotherapy and Psychosomatics, 56*, 135–140.
31. Pincus, T., Santos, R., Breen, A., et al. (2002). A systematic review of psychological factors as predictors of chronicity/disability in prospective cohorts of LBP. *Spine, 27*, 109–120.
32. Bair, M. J., Robinson, R. L., Katon, W., et al. (2003). Depression and pain comorbidity: A literature review. *Archives of Internal Medicine, 163*, 2433–2445.

33. Fink, P., Jensen, J., & Sorensen, L. (1999). Somatization in primary care: Prevalence, health care utilization and general practitioner recognition. *Psychosomatics, 40*, 330–338.
34. Guggenheim, F. G. (2000). Somatoform disorder. In B. J. Sadock & V. A. Sadock (Eds.), *Comprehensive textbook of psychiatry* (7th ed., pp. 1504–1532). Baltimore, MD: Lippincott Williams & Wilkins.
35. De Waal, M. W., Arnold, I. A., Eekhof, J. A., et al. (2004). Somatoform disorders in general practice: Prevalence, functional impairment and comorbidity with anxiety and depressive disorders. *The British Journal of Psychiatry, 184*, 470–476.
36. McWilliams, L. A., Goodwin, R. D., Cox, B. J., et al. (2004). Depression and anxiety associated with three pain conditions: Results from a nationally representative sample. *Pain, 111*, 77–83.
37. Jitender, S., Cox, B. J., Clara, I., et al. (2005). The relationship between anxiety disorder and physical disorders in the U.S. national comorbidity survey. *Depression and Anxiety, 21*, 193–202.
38. Bair, M. J., Wu, J., Damush, T. M., et al. (2008). Association of depression and anxiety alone and in combination with chronic musculoskeletal pain in primary care patients. *Psychosomatic Medicine, 70*, 890–897.
39. Kato, K., Sullivan, P. F., Evengård, B., et al. (2006). Chronic widespread pain and its comorbidities. A population-based study. *Archives of Internal Medicine, 166*, 1649–1654.
40. Gatchel, R. J. (2004). Comorbidity of chronic pain and mental health disorders: The biopsychosocial perspective. *American Psychologist, 59*, 795–805.
41. Tsang, A., von Korff, M., Lee, S., et al. (2008). Common chronic pain conditions in developed and developing countries: Gender and age differences and comorbidity with depression-anxiety disorders. *The Journal of Pain, 9*, 883–891.
42. Nicolson, S. E., Caplan, J. P., Williams, D. E., et al. (2009). Comorbid pain, depression and anxiety: Multifactorial pathology allows for multifaceted treatment. *Harvard Review of Psychiatry, 17*, 407–420.
43. Gerrits, M. M., Vogelzangs, N., van Oppen, P., et al. (2012). Impact of pain on the course of depressive and anxiety disorders. *Pain, 153*, 429–436.
44. Mostoufi, S. M., Ahumada, S. M., Reis, V., et al. (2012). Health and distress predictors of hearth rate variability in fibromyalgia and other forms of chronic pain. *Journal of Psychosomatic Research, 72*, 39–44.
45. Gore, M., Brandenburg, N. A., Dukes, E., et al. (2005). Pain severity in diabetic peripheral neuropathy is associated with patient functioning, symptom levels of anxiety and depression, and sleep. *Journal of Pain and Symptom Management, 30*, 374–385.
46. Sivik, T. (1999). Psychosomatic research in relation to theory of science. *Journal of Advances in Body and Mind Medicine, 15*, 148–153.
47. Sivik, T. (1998). Since we have both body and mind we are all psychosomatic. *Journal of Advances in Body and Mind Medicine., 14*, 223–233.
48. Ploghaus, A., Becerra, L., Borras, C., et al. (2003). Neural circuitry underlying pain modulation: Expectation, hypnosis, placebo. *Trends in Cognitive Science, 7*, 197–200.
49. Sivik, T. (1998). More on somatization. *Advances in Mind-Body Medicine, 14*, 223–230.
50. Sivik, T. (1992). Tendency to somatize, personality traits and low back pain – Psychological vulnerability as risk factor for the development of chronic back pain. In E. Ernst, M. Jayson, & M. Pope, et al. (Eds.), *Proceedings of advances in idiopathic low back pain* (pp. 191–195). Vienna: Blackwell-MZV.
51. von Uexkull, J. (1982). The theory of meaning. *Semiotica, 42*, 25–82.
52. Peirce, C. S. (1977). Semiotic elements and classes of signs. In C. H. Hardwick (Ed.), *Semiotics and significs*. Bloomington, IN: Indiana University Press.
53. Collier, J. D. (1998). Information increase in biological systems: How does adaptation fit? In G. van de Vijver et al. (Eds.), *Evolutionary systems: Biologocal and epistemological perspectives on selection and self-organization*. Dodrecht, The Netherlands: Kluwer.
54. Salthe, S. N. (2007). Semiotics in biology: Inside neodarwinism. In M. Barbieri (Ed.), *Biosemiotic research trends* (pp. 255–268). Hauppauge, NY: Nova.

55. Hoffmeyer, J. (2008). *Biosemiotics. An examination into signs of life and the life of signs*. Scranton, PA: University of Scranton Press.
56. Long, T. L. (2011). *Pain as sign and symptom*. New York: Biomedical Research.
57. Cilliers, P. (1998). *Complexity and postmodernism: Understanding complex systems*. London: Routledge.
58. Notcutt, W. (1998). The Tao of pain. *Pain reviews, 5*, 203–215.
59. Cahana, A. (2007). Pain and philosophy of mind. *Pain, Clinical Updates, 25*, 1–4.
60. Sivik, T. (2000). The difference between taking an anamnesis and listening to a (life) story. *Advances in Mind-Body Medicine, 16*, 182–184.
61. Turk, D. C., & Melcack, R. (2011). *Handbook of pain assessment*. New York: Guilford Publications.
62. Sivik, T., Gustavsson, E., & Klingberg-Olsson, K. (1992). Differential diagnosis of low-back pain patients; a simple quantification of the pain drawing. *Nordic Journal of Psychiatry, 46*, 55–62.
63. Sivik, T., & Hösterey, U. (1992). The thematic apperception test as an aid in understanding the psychodynamics of development of chronic idiopathic pain syndrome. *Psychotherapy and Psychosomatics, 57*, 57–60.
64. Sivik, T., Delimar, N., & Schoenfeld, R. (2007). Sivik psychosomaticism test and test of operational style – construct validity: Relationship with Toronto Alexithymia Scale (TAS-R). *Psychological Topics, 1*, 251–258.
65. Sivik, T., Delimar, N., & Schoenfeld, R. (1999). Construct validity of the sivik psychosomaticism test and test of operational style: Correlations with four Minnesota Multiphasic Personality Inventory (MMPI) subscales. *Integrative Physiological and Behavioural Science, 34*, 79–84.
66. Sivik, T., Delimar, N., & Schoenfeld, R. (1999). Construct validity of the sivik psychosomaticism test and test of operational style: Correlations with karolinska scheme of personality. *Integrative Physiological and Behavioural Science, 34*, 71–78.
67. Sivik, T., Delimar, N., & Schoenfeld, R. (1999). Sivik psychosomaticism test and test of operational style: Relationship with state-trait anxiety inventory and Beck's depression inventory. *Revista Portugisa de Psicossomatica, 2*, 71–81.
68. Sivik, T., Delimar, N., & Schoenfeld, R. (2002). Sivik psychosomaticism test and test of operational style: Relationship with a Swedish Mood Adjective Check List -MACL. *Revista Portugisa de Psicossomatica, 4*, 31–38.
69. Dunbar, H. F. (1935). *Emotions and bodily changes: A survey of literature on psychosomatic relationships* (pp. 1910–1933). New York: Columbia University Press.
70. Lane, R. (2008). Neural substrates of implicit and explicit emotional processes: A unifying framework for psychosomatic medicine. *Psychosomatic Medicine, 70*, 213–230.
71. Sivik, T. (2000). Psychosomatic medicine: Why fix it if it ain't broken? *Psychotherapy and Psychosomatics, 69*, 178–180.
72. Sivik, T. (1999). Integrative medicine, loving openness, and the need for wisdom. *Advances in Mind-Body Medicine, 15*, 29–32.
73. Shevrin, H. (2012, June). *Freud's theory of unconscious conflict linked to anxiety symptoms ScienceDaily*. Presented at 101st Annual Meeting of the American Psychoanalytic Association, Chicago.

Chapter 13
Psychosomatic Aspects of Fibromyalgia

Masato Murakami and Woesook Kim

13.1 Introduction

In the field of psychosomatic medicine, there are many patients who report muscle and joint pain. In some patients who report chronic general pain and autonomic dysfunction, the underlying pathological condition is difficult to understand. Fibromyalgia is a chronic pain disorder characterized by long-lasting generalized pain of the fibromuscular system and has historically been studied as a model of chronic pain.

Although the etiology of fibromyalgia is unidentified, various factors including viral infection, endocrine abnormality, immune dysfunction, or psychogenesis have been suggested. Fibromyalgia patients often report psychogenic and neurogenic symptoms such as anxiety, strain and depression, and various symptoms of autonomic nerve dysfunction. Fibromyalgia is considered one of psychosomatic disorders because this disorder is affected by psychosocial stressors [1, 2].

Fibromyalgia has primarily been studied in Europe and the United States. However, as objective and disease-specific findings have been difficult to obtain, no consensus has been reached on a disease concept of fibromyalgia or its diagnosis and treatment. The Japanese College of fibromyalgia Investigation was established in 2009, and practice guidelines for fibromyalgia in Japan were published for the first time in 2011 [3] and revised in 2013 [4]. In this chapter, we are going to focus on the psychosomatic aspects of fibromyalgia and the clinical issues relevant to diagnosis and treatment of fibromyalgia.

M. Murakami, M.D., Ph.D. (✉)
Department of Psychosomatic Internal Medicine, Nihon University Hospital,
Oyaguchi-kamicho, Itabashi-ku, 173-8610 Tokyo, Japan
e-mail: mmasato@med.nihon-u.ac.jp

W. Kim, Ph.D.
Clinical Psychology, College of Nursing Art and Science, University of Hyogo,
13-71 Kitaoji-cho, Akashi, 673-8588 Hyogo, Japan
e-mail: woesook_kim@cnas.u-hyogo-ac.jp

K.B. Koh (ed.), *Somatization and Psychosomatic Symptoms*,
DOI 10.1007/978-1-4614-7119-6_13, © Springer Science+Business Media New York 2013

13.2 Definition and Prevalence of Fibromyalgia

Fibromyalgia is a syndrome characterized by pain (algia) of muscles (my) and connective tissue (fibro) such as ligaments and tendons. The pathological condition of fibromyalgia is well recognized in Europe and America, where it has historically been described as a non-articular rheumatism, soft tissue rheumatism, muscular rheumatism, fibrositis, and primary fibromyalgia syndrome. It is a syndrome with various symptoms including diffuse pain and stiffness of the connective tissue of the whole body, including the periarticular tissue, muscles, tendons, and ligaments. The presence of clear tender points is an objective symptom of fibromyalgia.

It is important to note that fibromyalgia is neither an acute pain nor an organic disease but is characterized by chronic pain and functional impairment. Approximately 85–90 % of fibromyalgia patients are women. Fibromyalgia is diagnosed in women of all ages, but often develops between the age of 40 and 50, the middle of the climacteric period in Japan [3]. Approximately 15 % of the outpatients at a rheumatic clinic are considered to have fibromyalgia [5, 6], and the number of fibromyalgia patients in the United States is estimated to be three to five million. The Ministry of Health, Labor and Welfare of Japan reported that there were approximately two million latent fibromyalgia patients in Japan in 2004 [7]. However, only 7–8 % of these individuals are supposed to visit a medical institution [7].

13.3 Diagnosis of Fibromyalgia

Diagnosis of fibromyalgia is usually based on a precise history and physical examination. There are no specific abnormalities in the laboratory studies of fibromyalgia patients. In particular, it is important to differentiate fibromyalgia from other diseases. In 1990, the American College of Rheumatology (ACR) proposed criteria for fibromyalgia that require widespread pain that has been present for more than 3 months and identified 18 bilateral tender points in muscles of bilateral trapezius, sternocleidomastoid, major pectoralis, the gluteal region, the trochanteric region, and inside the knee, among others [5]. If tenderness is detected at more than 11 points, fibromyalgia can be diagnosed with more than 90 % sensitivity and specificity. However, these criteria were revised in 2010 [8]. In the new criteria, a widespread pain index (WPI) is quantified by assessing the levels of pain at 19 sites over the body, and a symptom severity (SS) index is quantified according to the severity of malaise, sleep, cognitive dysfunction and general physical symptoms. These symptoms must persist for more than 3 months.

In primary fibromyalgia, there are no changes in inflammatory markers, including erythrocyte sedimentation rate and C-reactive protein (CRP), and no abnormal rise in antinuclear antibodies, rheumatoid factors, or specific autoantibodies of individual collagen diseases. X-ray, magnetic resonance, and ultrasonic images do not show any joint inflammation or destruction. The etiology of fibromyalgia is considered to be unidentified because of the lack of abnormal findings in muscle and articular biopsies [9].

To diagnose fibromyalgia it is necessary to differentiate many rheumatic diseases including rheumatoid arthritis, systemic lupus erythematous, polymyositis rheumatica, Sjögren's syndrome, and sacroiliitis. In addition, many orthopedic diseases, including osteoarthritis, axial skeleton disease, spinal column stenosis, lumbago, and herniated disk should be differentiated. In the case of primary fibromyalgia, laboratory findings and imaging examinations, sometime tissue biopsy, are useful for differentiating it from other diseases. In secondary fibromyalgia, however, close medical observation is needed to differentiate it from the underlying diseases [9].

13.4 Clinical Manifestations of Fibromyalgia

Descriptions of the pain experienced by fibromyalgia patients are various: "the pain is sometimes intense like burning or fulgurant," "the pain persists even after termination of noxious stimulus," and "the pain is accompanied by an unpleasant sense (dysesthesia)." These patients report that pain is caused by light contact (allodynia), another pain, and repeated noxious stimulus. Accompanying symptoms include malaise, headache, dizziness, tinnitus, temporomandibular joint arthralgia, chest pain, a functional dyspepsia-like symptom, irritable gastrointestinal symptoms, peroneal muscle convulsions (leg cramps), and dysmenorrhea. Due to the comorbidity with these symptoms, fibromyalgia is regarded as a functional somatic syndrome [10].

Sometimes, fibromyalgia patients report anxiety, tension, insomnia, and depressive mood, and some patients have psychiatric disorders such as major depressive and anxiety disorders. Among our cases (48 cases), we have found a tendency of dysautonomia in 87.5 %; irritable gastrointestinal symptoms in 36 %; typical irritable bowel syndrome in 48 %; sleep disorders in 84 %; and headache, primarily tension headache, in 62 %. Ninety percent of fibromyalgia patients are women, and 80 % of the female patients with fibromyalgia reported difficultly with menstruation, menstrual irregularity, or amenorrhea [11]. In addition to extreme generalized pain, chronic fatigue, slight fever, and pharyngitis symptoms are regarded as primary symptoms of fibromyalgia. Of 16 cases with fibromyalgia, 32 % met the diagnostic criteria for chronic fatigue syndrome [11].

13.5 Pathophysiology of Fibromyalgia

13.5.1 Factors Underlying Onset of Fibromyalgia

Various factors including viral infection, endocrine, or immunological abnormalities have been proposed to underlie the onset of fibromyalgia. Prior to the onset of fibromyalgia, there is often an episode of physical overload induced by diseases, surgery, trauma, delivery, and sports. Among our cases, 30 % reported physical overwork or injury at the time of onset of fibromyalgia [11]. It has been suggested that anaerobic metabolism caused by laborious work or exercise may be an etiological factor of

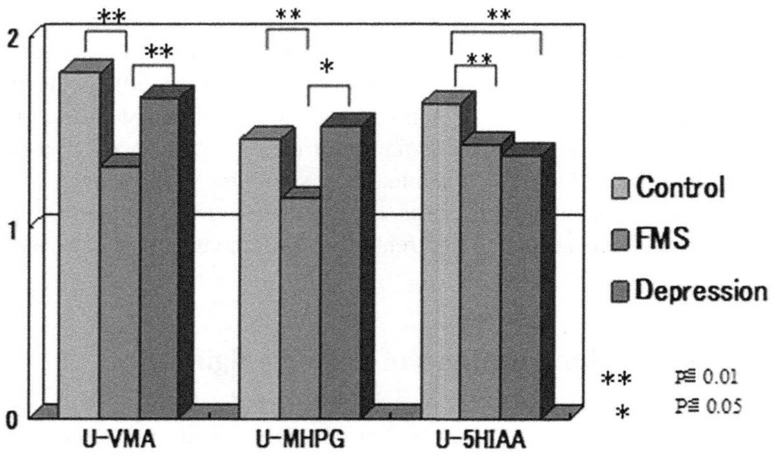

Fig. 13.1 Monoamine change in patients with fibromyalgia ($n = 12$) and depression ($n = 9$) compared with healthy controls ($n = 10$). *FMS* fibromyalgia syndrome (From Murakami et al. [11], reprinted by permission of Japanese Society of Psychosomatic Medicine)

fibromyalgia. Arousal of sympathetic nervous system may cause anaerobic metabolism through the intramuscular vascular constriction and disturb the peripheral microcirculation and internal endocrine environment [12–14].

The reasons why fibromyalgia persists for many years are unknown, but central sensitivity and chronic stressors are thought to create a vicious circle of pain.

13.5.2 Physiological Changes Associated with Fibromyalgia

The concentration of substance P in the cerebrospinal fluid is significantly higher, and the concentration of 3-methoxy-4-hydroxyphenylglycol (MHPG) and 5-hydroxyindoleacetic acid (5HIAA) is significantly lower in fibromyalgia patients than in rheumatoid arthritis patients [15]. It is known that 60 % of MHPG is of central nervous system origin and that MHPG concentration indicates the activity of the central sympathetic nervous system. 5HIAA is a metabolite of serotonin and is associated with depression, anxiety, chronic pain, and various autonomic nerve symptoms. Our study [11] found that MHPG and 5HIAA concentration in the 12 h urine of fibromyalgia patients was lower than that in healthy individuals, and similar findings were obtained in patients with depression (Fig. 13.1).

Acylcarnitine, involved in the glycolysis of the mitochondrial system, is engaged in energy production of skeletal muscle and plays an important role in the neuronal activity of the brain. A decrease in serum acylcarnitine levels is associated with lassitude, fatigability, forgetfulness, and poor concentration in patients with chronic fatigue syndrome (CFS) [16]. Our study found that patients with fibromyalgia, CFS, and depressive disorders had lower levels of serum

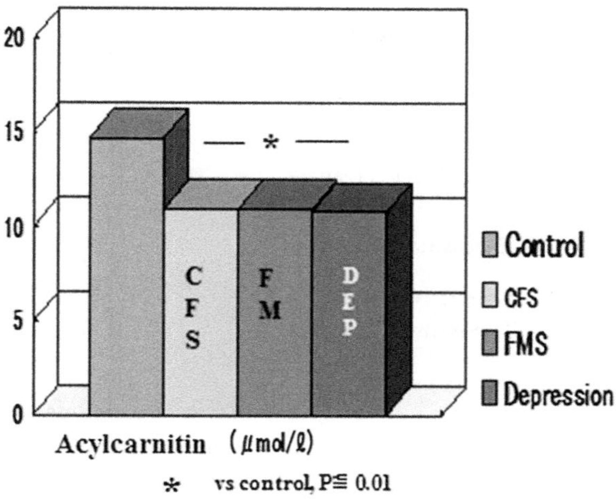

Fig. 13.2 Serum acylcarnitine concentration in patients with fibromyalgia ($n=12$), chronic fatigue syndrome ($n=10$) and depression ($n=9$) compared with healthy controls ($n=10$) (From Murakami et al. [11], reprinted by permission of Japanese Society of Psychosomatic Medicine)

acylcarnitine concentration compared to healthy individuals, which suggests that there is a commonality between pain, fatigue, and depression (Fig. 13.2) [11].

13.6 Psychosomatic Aspects of Fibromyalgia

13.6.1 Comorbidity with Mental Disorders

Diagnosis and management of comorbid psychiatric disorders is important because most patients with fibromyalgia have various psychosocial stressors and mental symptoms [17–21]. Hudson et al. [21] reported that 71 % of fibromyalgia patients have history of depression, compared to only 13 % of patients with rheumatoid arthritis, and 64 % experienced depression more than 1 year prior to onset. Our study found that 92 % of fibromyalgia patients showed psychosocial episodes of physical strain and mental stress [18]. In addition, patients with fibromyalgia were sometimes observed during the clinical course of mental disorders.

Because of the pain, all patients felt troubles and inconvenience in their daily lives and visited multiple medical facilities for consultations. Various symptoms of fibromyalgia are susceptible to environmental changes such as weather, temperature, atmospheric pressure, humidity, physical conditions such as labor, and psychological variables such as sleep state and emotional trouble. Therefore, psychogenic rheumatism has been alternatively used for fibromyalgia. In Japan, many nonpsychiatric physicians have negative ideas about such concept of fibromyalgia. Especially psychiatrists assume that fibromyalgia can be classified as a mental disorder such as persistent somatoform disorder (ICD-10) [22], pain disorder, somatization disorder (DSM-IV) [23], conversion disorder, or depressive disorders, but not classified as a physical disease. The disease concept of fibromyalgia remains controversial between psychiatrists and nonpsychiatric physicians.

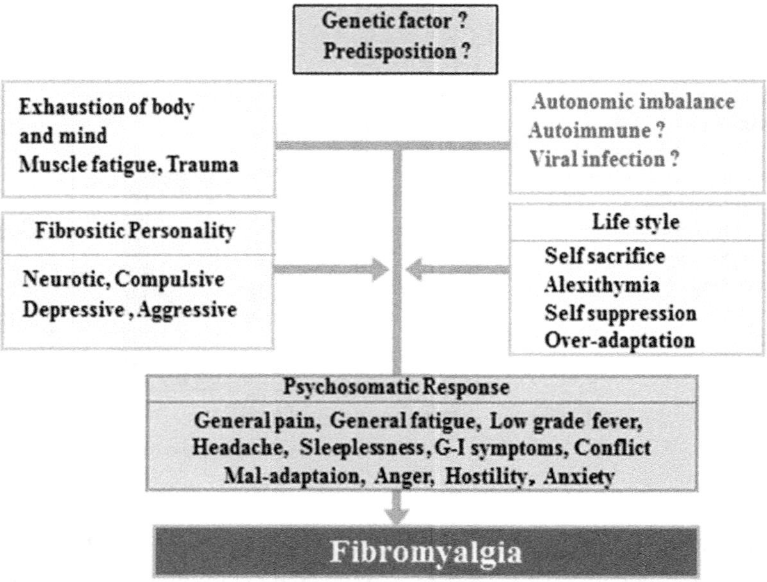

Fig. 13.3 Multiple pathological factors in patients with fibromyalgia (From Murakami et al. [11], reprinted by permission of Japanese Society of Psychosomatic Medicine)

13.6.2 Fibromyalgia as a Psychosomatic Disorder

A variety of factors are involved in the pathogenesis of fibromyalgia, including genetics and physical health, mental and physical exhaustion and stress, viral infections or injuries, personality, and lifestyle [18]. These factors may cause dysfunction of neurological, endocrine, and immunological systems and result in fibromyalgia. Fibromyalgia can be regarded as a psychosomatic disease of the musculoskeletal system. Therefore, a combination of biological factors and psychosocial factors are likely to be involved in the pathogenesis of fibromyalgia, as presented in the schema (Fig. 13.3).

13.7 Treatment of Fibromyalgia

Many methods of treatment for fibromyalgia have been suggested, because the pathogenesis is complicated and multifactorial. However, the evidence for treatment is insufficient, so large-scale randomized controlled trials are required. In 2011, study groups from the Ministry of Health, Labor and Welfare and the members of the Japanese College of Fibromyalgia Investigation collaborated to publish the practical guidelines for the diagnosis and treatment of fibromyalgia [3].

13.7.1 Pharmacological Treatment

Before selecting the drugs, therapists should check the clinical characteristics of fibromyalgia such as chronic pain, peripheral neuropathic pain, muscle cramps, autonomic seizure, arousal of sympathetic nervous system, and depression. Analgesics such as nonsteroidal anti-inflammatory drugs or corticosteroids are effective for early or mild stage of fibromyalgia, but the efficacy declines in the moderate or chronic stages of fibromyalgia [24, 25]. It is necessary to select the appropriate therapeutic drugs according to the patients' current clinical condition.

Tricyclic antidepressants such as amitriptyline have been conventionally used as a therapeutic drug for chronic pain [26]. In recent years, selective serotonin reuptake inhibitors (SSRI), serotonin noradrenaline reuptake inhibitors (SNRI), and noradrenergic and specific serotonergic antidepressants (NaSSA) were introduced to clinical fields [27, 28]. It is assumed that these drugs show analgesic effects by affecting the descending pain inhibitory system independently of their antidepressant effects, and such an effect can be expected even at a small doses compared to those used in depression.

Clonazepam or gabapentin are anticonvulsants conventionally used to treat fibromyalgia. Pregabalin has been used recently to inhibit neural transmission of pain and exerts an analgesic effect by binding to $\alpha_2\delta$ subunits of the voltage-dependent Ca^{2+} channel [29, 30]. Anticonvulsants improve peripheral muscle tone and blood circulation in patients with fibromyalgia. Because these drugs also inhibit the fear circuit of anxiety, they are effective for panic disorder or other anxiety disorders.

Tramadol shows strong analgesic effect. Tramadol has effects on both opioid system and monoamine system in a μ receptor and works by stimulating the descending pain inhibitory systems. Recently, a combination of tramadol and acetaminophen has been used for the treatment of fibromyalgia in Japan [31].

Neurotrophin (trade name) is an inflammation-derived agent extracted from rabbit skin inoculated with vaccinia virus and is a unique drug that has been developed in Japan. It is administered by mouth, intravenous infusion, or local injection on a trigger point. The efficacy of neurotrophin in the treatment of fibromyalgia has not yet been established, but it is assumed to activate the descending pain inhibitory system [32].

Benzodiazepine anxiolytics improve tension, irritation, and excitability. However, the evidence for pain relief of the anxiolytics is insufficient. Because of the increased risk of falls in elderly people and of dependency with chronic administration, these drugs should only be used as an adjunctive drug.

Chinese herbal medicine (Kampo medicine) is another option we should consider in the treatment of fibromyalgia [33]. Keishi-bukuryo-gan, Kami-shoyo-san, Unkei-to, and Shakuyaku-kanzo-to may be effective for the treatment of fibromyalgia symptoms that fluctuate with the menstrual cycle. Sokei-kakketsu-to, Gosha-jinki-gan, Keishi-ka-jitsubu-to, or processed aconite root are effective in relieving muscle ache, myotonia, and blood circulation, and Yokukan-san or Kamikihi-to are often used to treat anxiety or excitement. In Japan, a combination of Kampo medicines with antidepressants or antispasmodic agents is used to treat fibromyalgia patients.

13.7.2 Nonpharmacological Therapy

Guidance for living, exercise therapy, relaxation, or psychotherapy can be used to treat fibromyalgia. Patient education is important to enable the patients to understand that fibromyalgia is a functional disease that does not involve physical impairment. Patients with catastrophic thoughts should be taught that pain of fibromyalgia is not at all a hopeless symptom. Patients should also be educated that continuing physical activity or physical exercise is essential to avoid secondary muscle atrophy or joint contracture.

Moderate aerobic exercise at 65–70 % of maximal heart rate, such as aqua-exercise or Tai chi chuan, has a high therapeutic efficacy for fibromyalgia, equivalent to pharmacotherapy [34, 35]. Physical therapy, including thermotherapy, traction, and massage, is also reported to be effective for fibromyalgia, but the evidence is insufficient because the quality of studies is poor. Cognitive-behavioral therapy is also effective for fibromyalgia, because fibromyalgia patients often have obsession, compulsion, or aggressiveness [36, 37]. Patients with fibromyalgia are apt to fall into exhaustion from physical or psychological excessive load. In such patients, it is important to correct their thoughts and egomania and alter the behavioral pattern of over-adaptation. Therefore, collaboration between psychiatrists, nonpsychiatric physicians, and clinical psychologists is essential for effective management of patients with fibromyalgia.

13.8 Conclusions

Although the concept of fibromyalgia remains controversial between psychiatrists and nonpsychiatric physicians, the term “fibromyalgia” is still used broadly. This disorder is characterized by long-lasting generalized pain of the fibromuscular system. The onset and clinical course of fibromyalgia are affected by psychosocial stressors, and it is important to check the psychosomatic background of fibromyalgia patients before treatment. Patients with fibromyalgia experience physical strains such as surgery, accident, trauma, delivery, physical overload, and excessive exercise prior to the onset of fibromyalgia. Personality traits such as anxiety, fear, anger, obsession, depression, and sorrow are observed in many patients with fibromyalgia. Physiological characteristics in fibromyalgia patients are similar to those in patients with depression. Dysfunction of the serotonin- and noradrenalin-mediated descending pain control system, and the contraction of muscular and vascular systems following circulatory disorders, may be involved in fibromyalgia. Analgesics are not effective in treating fibromyalgia, but antidepressants and anticonvulsants often show remarkable effect. Therefore, biopsychosocial care including counseling and psychotherapy may be more effective for fibromyalgia than treatments based on the medical model. Comorbidity with psychiatric disorders such as depressive disorders or somatoform disorders should be always considered for diagnosis and treatment of fibromyalgia. Multidisciplinary collaboration between psychiatrists, nonpsychiatric physicians, and clinical psychologists is essential for effective treatment of fibromyalgia.

Acknowledgment Our research was supported in part by the grants from Japanese Ministry of Health, Labor and Welfare for Health Science Research. Authors would like to thank Toshio Matsuno, Ayako Aoki, Mitsuko Isii, Shuichiro Maruoka, and Katsuhiro Miura for technical assistance.

References

1. Murakami, M., Takei, M., Matsukawa, Y., et al. (2004). Psychosomatic approach for fibromyalgia. *Clinical Rheumatology and Related Research, 16*, 362–367.
2. Murakami, M., Matsuno, T., & Koike, K. (2005). *Research on the establishment of disease concept of fibromyalgia syndrome* (pp. 162–164). Annual Report on Assigned Research for Health Science Research Grants from the Ministry of Health, Tokyo: Labour and Welfare.
3. Japan College of Fibromyalgia investigation. (2011). *Practice Guidelines for Fibromyalgia 2011*. Tokyo: Nihon Iji Shimpo.
4. Japan College of Fibromyalgia investigation. (2013). *Practice Guidelines for Fibromyalgia 2013*. Tokyo: Nihon Iji Shimpo.
5. Wolfe, F., Smythe, H. A., Yunus, M. B., et al. (1990). The american college of rheumatology 1990, criteria for the classification of fibromyalgia. *Arthritis and Rheumatism, 33*, 160–172.
6. Yunus, M. B., Masi, A. T., Aldag, J. C., et al. (1989). Preliminary criteria for primary fibromyalgia syndrome (PFS): Multivariate analysis of a consecutive series of PFS, other patients and normal subjects. *Clinical and Experimental Rheumatology, 7*, 63–69.
7. Matsumoto, Y., Maeda, S., Tamakoshi, A., et al. (2005). *Study on elucidation of the clinical epidemiology of fibromyalgia in Japan* (pp. 156–158). Annual Report on Assigned Research for Health Science Research Grants from the Ministry of Health, Tokyo: Labor and Welfare.
8. Wolfe, F., Clauw, D. J., Fitzcharles, M. A., et al. (2010). The American College of Rheumatology preliminary diagnostic criteria for fibromyalgia and measurement of symptom severity. *Arthritis Care & Research, 62*, 600–610.
9. Wolfe, F., & Cathy, M. A. (1983). Prevalence of primary and secondary fibrositis. *Journal of Rheumatology, 10*, 965–968.
10. Wessely, S., Nimnuan, C., & Sharp, M. (1999). Functional somatic syndrome: One or many ? *Lancet, 354*, 936–939.
11. Murakami, M., Matsuno, T., & Kim, W. (2009). How to evaluate the pain of fibromyalgia syndrome: FMS as a typical model of chronic pain. *Japanese Journal of Psychosomatic Medicine, 49*, 893–902.
12. Elert, J. E., Rantapää, S. B., Henriksson-larsén, K., et al. (1992). Muscle performance, electromyography and fibre type composition in fibromyalgia and work-related myalgia. *Scandinavian Journal of Rheumatology, 21*, 28–34.
13. Morf, S., Amann-Vesti, B., Forster, A., et al. (2005). Microcirculation abnormalities in patients with fibromyalgia measured by capillary microscopy and laser flowmetry. *Arthritis Research & Therapy, 7*, R209–R216.
14. Elvin, A., Siösteen, A. K., Nilsson, A., et al. (2006). Decreased muscle blood flow in fibromyalgia patients during standardized muscle exercise: A contrast media enhanced color doppler study. *European Journal of Pain, 10*, 137–144.
15. Russell, I. J., & Larson, A. A. (2009). Neurophysiopathogenesis of fibromyalgia syndrome: A unified hypothesis. *Rheumatic Diseases Clinics of North America, 35*, 421–435.
16. Reuter, S. E., & Evans, A. M. (2011). Long-chain acylcarnitine deficiency in patients with chronic fatigue syndrome. Potential involvement of altered carnitine palmitoyl transferase-I activity. *Journal of Internal Medicine, 270*, 76–84.
17. Lesley, M., & Arnold, M. D. (2008). Management of fibromyalgia and comorbid psychiatric disorders. *The Journal of Clinical Psychiatry, 69*(Suppl. 2), 14–19.
18. Murakami, M., Matsno, T., Kim, W., et al. (2010). Fibromyalgia and negative emotion. *Japanese Journal of Psychosomatic Medicine, 50*, 1157–1163.

19. Wassem, R., McDonald, M., Racine, J., et al. (2002). Fibromyalgia patient perspectives on symptoms, symptoms management, and provider utilization. *Clinical Nurse Specialist, 16*, 24–28.
20. Fietta, P., Fietta, P., & Manganelli, P. (2007). Fibromyalgia and psychiatric disorders. *Acta Bio-Medica, 78*, 88–95.
21. Hudson, J. I., Hudson, M. S., Pliner, L. F., et al. (1985). Fibromyalgia and major affective disorder: A controlled phenomenology and family history study. *The American Journal of Psychiatry, 142*, 441–446.
22. Toru, M., Nakane, Y., & Komiyama, M. (1994). *The ICD-10 classification of mental and behavioral disorders* (p. 170). Tokyo: Igaku Shoin.
23. Takahashi, S., Ono, Y., & Someya, T. (1995). *Quick reference to the diagnostic criteria from DSM-IV*. Tokyo: Igaku Shoin.
24. Reilly, P. A., & Littlejohn, G. O. (1990). Current thinking on fibromyalgia syndrome. *Australian Family Physician, 19*, 1505–1516.
25. Häuser, W., Thieme, K., & Turk, D. C. (2010). Guidelines on the management of fibromyalgia syndrome – a systematic review. *European Journal of Pain, 14*, 5–10.
26. Carette, S., McCain, G. A., Bell, D. A., et al. (1986). Evaluation of amitriptyline in primary fibrositis. *Arthritis and Rheumatism, 29*, 655–659.
27. O'Malley, P. G., Balden, E., Tomkins, G., et al. (2000). Treatment of fibromyalgia with antidepressants: A meta-analysis. *Journal of General Internal Medicine, 15*, 659–661.
28. Arnold, L. M., Keck, P. E., Jr., Welge, J. A., et al. (2000). Antidepressant treatment of fibromyalgia. A meta-analysis and review. *Psychosomatics, 41*, 104–113.
29. Dooley, D. J., Taylor, C. P., Donevan, S., et al. (2007). Ca^{2+} channel alpha 2 delta ligands: Novel modulators of neurotransmission. *Trends in Pharmacological Sciences, 28*, 75–82.
30. Crofford, L. J., Rowbotham, M. C., Mease, P. J., et al. (2005). Pregabalin for the treatment of fibromyalgia syndrome: Results of a randomized, double blind, placebo-controlled trial. *Arthritis and Rheumatism, 52*, 1264–1273.
31. Bennett, R. M., Kamin, M., Karim, R., et al. (2003). Tramadol and acetoaminophen combination tablets in the treatment of fibromyalgia pain: A double-blind, randomized placebo-controlled study. *American Journal of Medicine, 114*, 537–545.
32. Nakamura, H., Hoshi, K., Kato, T., et al. (2003). Clinical feature of fibromyalgia syndrome in Japan and novel strategy in the treatment by bioproduct (Neurotropin). *Arthritis Research & Therapy, 5*(Suppl. 3), 170.
33. Murakami, M. (2008). Therapeutic evidence of Kampo treatment for psychosomatic diseases and stress related diseases. *Journal of Japanese Association of Oriental Psychosomatic Medicine, 23*, 100–102.
34. Goldenberg, D. L., Burckhardt, C., Crofford, L., et al. (2004). Management of fibromyalgia syndrome. *Journal of the American Medical Association, 292*, 2388–2395.
35. Wang, C., Schmid, C. H., & Rones, R. (2011). A randomized trial of tai chi for fibromyalgia. *The New England Journal of Medicine, 363*, 743–754.
36. Rossy, L. A., Buckelew, S. P., Dorr, N., et al. (1999). A meta-analysis of fibromyalgia treatment intervention. *Annals of Behavioral Medicine, 21*, 180–191.
37. Goldenberg, D. L., Burckhard, C., Crofford, L., et al. (2004). Management of fibromyalgia syndrome. *Journal of the American Medical Association, 292*, 2388–2395.

Chapter 14
A Psychosomatic Approach to the Treatment of the Difficult Chronic Pain Patient

Jon Streltzer

14.1 Introduction

Chronic pain is an enigmatic condition that defies understanding by a traditional biomedical model [1, 2]. In chronic pain conditions, the particular type of anatomical pathology present does not tend to predict the level of pain reported nor the extent of associated suffering or disability [3–5]. Rather, chronic pain is a medical condition that perfectly exemplifies the biopsychosocial model. Biologically, a great deal is understood about mechanisms of nociception. Psychologically, pain perception can vary immensely, depending on the meaning of the painful stimulus, including the potential for secondary gain. The patient's cognitive style and tendency toward catastrophizing and underlying emotions, particularly fear, anxiety, and depression, all critically influence the perception of pain. Socioculturally, the communication of a painful state will vary according to the context. Pain may be minimized by soldiers in battle, athletes during a crucial contest, and during childbirth in some cultures. It naturally follows, then, that treatment of chronic pain should take into account its biopsychosocial nature.

This chapter will focus on a biopsychosocial approach to the difficult chronic pain patient who is opioid dependent. Such patients have become common in some countries (e.g., the United States and Canada) and could potentially become common in other countries if emphasis on pain management increases.

J. Streltzer, M.D. (✉)
Department of Psychiatry, University of Hawaii at Manoa, John A. Burns School of Medicine, 1356 Lusitana Street, 4th Floor, Honolulu, Hawaii 96813, USA
e-mail: streltzerj@dop.hawaii.edu

K.B. Koh (ed.), *Somatization and Psychosomatic Symptoms*,
DOI 10.1007/978-1-4614-7119-6_14, © Springer Science+Business Media New York 2013

14.2 Historical Background

In the United States, pain has been recognized as a symptom with implications for mental health for more than 50 years. In a classic paper, George Engel described "the pain prone patient" [6]. Psychological factors and personality traits were recognized as contributing to the symptomatic expression of pain in some patients. Current research confirms that psychological factors are prominent in many chronic pain syndromes. Recent emphasis has been on cognitive constructs, including catastrophizing, and fear of reinjury. The most complex and controversial issue in chronic pain management, however, has much to do with the role of opioid analgesics in treatment.

Historically, medical appreciation for the benefits of opioids has been tempered by the dangers that become obvious with chronic use. In the United States, the problem became widely recognized as a result of the American Civil War of 1861–1865, when pain from battle injuries was treated with injections of morphine, utilizing the newly available hypodermic syringe. The treatment of painful injuries leads to such frequent dependence that morphine addiction became known as "the soldier's illness" [7].

In the latter part of the nineteenth century, narcotic preparations were available without prescription, primarily for women's ailments. Many middle and upper class women became addicted, and the percentage of narcotic dependent individuals was estimated to have been much higher than it is today. Subsequent to legislation taxing narcotics in 1914, however, narcotic use became associated with prescriptions from physicians or else with the illicit drug trade [8]. Complications from dependence on prescription pain medications were well described [9], although probably widely tolerated.

In the 1960s and 1970s, drug abuse became a rapidly increasing phenomenon in the United States, subject to immense societal concern. Medical culture reflected attitudes prevalent in the society at that time with regard to fears of addiction. Opioid narcotics were prescribed in lower doses, and they were given much less frequently, even for severe pain [10, 11]. Consultation-liaison psychiatrists came to recognize undertreatment of acute pain as a cause of mental distress in hospitalized patients. In recent years, however, it has become widely accepted to vigorously treat acute pain and cancer pain. In these situations, when opioid treatment is time limited, it is thought that addiction is rarely a problem complicating opioid use; however, recent evidence suggests that it is not so rare [12]. Simultaneously, there has been an increasingly popular, but controversial, movement to apply similar principles to the long-term treatment of chronic nonmalignant pain [13].

In the 1980s and 1990s, much attention was given to the medication management of chronic pain. In particular, opioids, which had previously not been thought to be appropriate for chronic use, came into vogue. Opinion started to accumulate that opioid pain medication would remain effective in producing analgesia even with long-term use, and the major problem to worry about was addiction [14]. Since chronic pain patients receiving prescribed opioids did not behave the same as street drug abusers using illicit opioids, the incidence of addiction in chronic pain patients was thought to be extremely low.

In the 1990s and into the twenty-first century, the percent of chronic pain patients treated with daily opioids grew rapidly. New, higher dose formulations of opioids were developed and vigorously marketed by pharmaceutical companies, and doses were escalated to levels far beyond what had previously been considered acceptable. Complications from these therapies grew rapidly. Hospital emergency room visits related to prescribed opioids grew exponentially, and, alarmingly, unintentional deaths from prescribed opioids are also growing exponentially [15–17].

In recent years, improvements in the treatment of acute pain and terminal cancer pain have been substantial, but the treatment of chronic nonmalignant pain remains difficult both diagnostically and in terms of therapeutic options. Management of the chronic pain patient dependent on prescription opioids is the most difficult and controversial area of pain management, because of conflicting interpretations of the literature and because of the need to set limits, a process in which physicians often have little training [18].

14.3 Efficacy Versus Addiction: The Controversy

The literature provides anecdotes and research studies that conflict and fail to clarify the proper use of opioids in chronic pain. Studies have substantial limitations, due to small sample sizes, short follow-up periods, or questionable selection, intervention, and evaluation procedures [19]. Thus, substantial controversy exists regarding the treatment of the chronic pain patient [20].

One school of thought distinguishes "dependence" from "addiction," suggesting that only the latter needs to contraindicate chronic opioid treatment because of behavior problems. However, even addictive behaviors such as uncontrolled dose escalation, claims to have lost prescriptions, and obtaining opioids from more than one physician have been considered "pseudoaddiction" [13, 21] due to undertreatment of pain (with opioids). Opioids are believed to be efficacious for persistent, severe pain just as they are for acute pain. This leads to a willingness to treat with high doses in response to complaints of pain, such as 15–20 tablets per day or several 100 mg of methadone per day. Often this occurs without clear objective medical findings to substantiate a painful condition. Perhaps, this is because there is no direct relation between objective medical findings and the degree of subjective pain [4, 22–24].

A contrary school of thought believes patients will have less pain and disability with non-opioid pain management [25]. The psychology of opioid dependence is powerful in that each dose is associated with less pain temporarily but with failure to improve, and possibly more pain, in the long run. Because patients commonly deny the deterioration caused by opioids (a denial sometimes shared by the prescribing physician) [26], strict limits must be set to counteract opioid-dependent behaviors while simultaneously providing psychological support.

A middle ground suggests that only a minority of chronic pain patients with severe, persistent pain from an objective medical condition and no history of substance abuse may be appropriate for and responsive to chronic opioid therapy [14, 27]. Such patients must be managed with strict limits so that failure to improve or failure to comply would end the opioid treatment.

14.4 Animal Studies

Recent research calls into question the assumptions that chronic opioids are effective for chronic pain. Animal studies, utilizing standardized models of pain, show that not only does chronic morphine administration result in tolerance to its analgesic effects but also heightened pain sensitivity, compared to placebo, actually develops [28, 29]. If rats are given morphine by continuous infusion for a week and then they are subjected to a painful stimulus, a large bolus of morphine will protect them less from the pain than will rats which have been pretreated with saline. Furthermore, the rats pretreated with morphine actually become more pain sensitive. Mechanisms responsible for this are being elucidated [30, 31], including the release of newly discovered peptides, termed "anti-opioids" [32]. If these peptides are isolated and then administered to an opioid-naive animal, enhanced pain sensitivity occurs. For example, chronic morphine administration increases the levels of dynorphin, a kappa agonist, in the dorsal horn of the spinal cord [33]. Dynorphin is associated with increased pain [34]. These studies demonstrate that enhanced pain sensitivity is a response to chronic morphine, and not just due to brief withdrawal effects when blood levels fall.

Viewed from another perspective, nerve injury can produce changes in the nervous system leading to hyperalgesia. Chronic morphine administration produces the same changes [35]! In sum, the evidence that chronic opioid administration causes changes leading to hyperalgesia in animals is now consistent and convincing at the molecular, cellular, physiological and behavioral levels. Presumably, similar mechanisms occur in humans, with individual variation.

14.5 Basic Science

Basic science studies are increasingly providing the explanations for this phenomenon. Chronic stimulation of the mu receptor by exogenous opioids suppresses cyclic AMP. The cell responds to this ongoing suppression by upregulating the systems that lead to the synthesis of cyclic AMP. This leads to an upregulation of cyclic AMP response element binding protein, which causes RNA to produce more dynorphin in the cells that are capable of doing so [36]. These include cells in the dorsal horn of the spinal cord that are involved in pain transmission. This increase in a dynorphin is associated with increased pain. Chronic morphine also activates mechanisms that occur through the NK1 receptor, which is stimulated by substance P, and this also enhances the transmission of pain [37]. In fact, biochemical and physiological mechanisms are multiple and overlapping in response to the reception of chronic opioids.

14.6 Methadone Patients

In the United States, patients who become addicted to heroin often are treated in methadone maintenance programs. By giving them daily methadone in high doses, they become so tolerant to opioids that an injection of street heroin will have little to no effect. The methadone patient also does not experience opioid withdrawal symptoms. Methadone treatment is helpful because these patients are more likely to stop using illicit drugs and to reenter normal society. Many of these patients take daily doses of methadone that would be lethal to an opioid-naive individual.

Does this high daily dose of a powerful analgesic protect them from pain? No! If they have a painful injury or are recovering from surgery, their pain is more difficult to treat and requires higher than normal doses over and above their daily methadone. When pain is administered experimentally, methadone patients demonstrate enhanced pain sensitivity [38] compared to normal controls. Furthermore, methadone patients report a high degree of chronic and severe pain; the more so, the longer they have been taking methadone [39].

Methadone, in contrast to other opioids, blocks *N*-methyl-D-aspartate (NMDA) receptors [40], which may explain why it seems to remain efficacious for pain longer than other opioids. Nevertheless, tolerance does develop, and methadone maintenance patients have demonstrated enhanced pain sensitivity perhaps because of the multiple, overlapping, counteradaptive mechanisms that seem to be involved. The use of NMDA antagonists to potentiate opioid analgesia has also proven disappointing in pain patients [41].

Thus, chronic opioids are not analgesic, but actually hyperalgesic. They enhance pain sensitivity. Despite this, it is very difficult for chronic pain patients to stop taking opioids. If they are stopped suddenly, the withdrawal effects on the body are stressful, and a mental craving for them is induced. Thus, the subjective response is that despite ongoing and increasing pain, and often disability, the patient thinks that he or she would be worse off without the opioids. The patient will appreciate the doctor that prescribes the opioids and may be unhappy with the doctor that tries to stop them. Thus, despite the increasing evidence that chronic opioids in high doses are not effective or safe for chronic pain [42], many physicians believe that this is an effective treatment.

14.7 Prescription Drug Abuse

The street addicts may or may not present with legitimate pain. Addicts commonly seek prescription narcotics from physicians to satisfy their habit, and some learn to fabricate or exaggerate pain to this end. Certain physicians tend to collect these patients.

Case Example 1

A family practitioner frequently prescribed high-dose preparations of extended release oxycodone for pain. He accepted complaints of chronic pain at face value, and he was influenced by literature promoting chronic opioid treatment. His patients seemed pleased, and his practice grew. Soon his name became known in the drug-abusing community. Drug abusers would seek him out to obtain prescriptions of narcotics. Several of his patients were admitted to the hospital in a short period of time having taken accidental overdoses. In the hospital, it became clear that these patients greatly exaggerated any pain problem and had a history of illicit drug abuse as well as prescription drug abuse. Feedback to the physician resulted in his changing the way he managed chronic pain.

Case Example 2

A 44-year-old man had a history of being in a motor vehicle accident when he was 30 years old. He sustained multiple injuries requiring several surgical procedures. After 2 years of recovery and rehabilitation, he had no disability other than chronic pain. He was treated with opioid analgesics from the beginning. Over the years, his opioid use increased, ultimately reaching the highest doses that any of his physicians had ever seen. He would take 140 mg of methadone at a time, as frequently as every hour, averaging more than 1,400 mg per day. When he was 30, he was married and owned a home. Over the years, he lost his family, lost his house, and then became homeless.

He was admitted to the hospital after passing out in a shopping mall after visiting his physician that day and receiving his prescription for methadone. In the hospital, he at first insisted that he required this medication to function normally. He was confronted, however, with the fact that his life had steadily deteriorated, and now he focused only on obtaining his pain medications. He acknowledged that he was stuck on his medications but was unwilling to stay in the hospital to do anything about it. His physician was contacted. He said that he had been trying to lower the medication dose for this patient but had been unsuccessful. He would appreciate any help the patient could be given in the hospital. He continued to prescribe methadone as desired by the patient, however, until he was investigated leading to the loss of his medical license.

Assessment of these patients is difficult and should be on the basis of objective medical findings. If one accepts that opioids are not magic bullets for pain and tolerance and hyperalgesia result from chronic opioid intake, then the patient can be told that opioids are not a good way to treat chronic pain. The legitimate pain patient is likely to be interested in other types of treatment, while the addict will focus entirely on the goal of obtaining opioids.

14.8 Hyperalgesia

Hyperalgesia has been acknowledged when opioid doses are very large or when doses are reduced. It has been suggested that opioid rotation can reverse this problem, at least temporarily, and the use of either long-acting or controlled-release opioids prevents it. Frequently, patients whose doses are increased or who are switched to long-acting preparations report substantial short-term improvement [43]. Clinically, however, such patients may gradually add in more "breakthrough" doses, and eventually their condition becomes similar to what it had been, but they are at greater risk for adverse reactions because they are now maintained at a higher dosage. Thus, these strategies may help in the short run but are likely harmful in the long term.

Hyperalgesia may explain the pain behavior of many opioid-dependent patients. The patient tends to experience pain all the time, feels some relief when blood levels go up, and learns to fear decreasing blood levels. Typically, these patients describe opioid medications as "taking the edge off" and "I have to take something."

Case Example 1

A 39-year-old man suffered from chronic back pain for many years. The patient was a well-to-do sales professional and active in the community. The back pain had gradually increased despite surgery 4 years previously. A physician friend, who would often supply him with oxycodone or codeine preparations for his pain, suggested he might be developing an addiction and referred him for a psychiatric pain evaluation. He had recently been treated by a pain specialist and given tramadol. When he supplemented this with opioids prescribed by his physician friend, the pain specialist refused to see him any further.

The patient had a past history of alcoholism but had been sober since his back surgery. He went to Alcoholic Anonymous regularly and often led the meetings. He acknowledged, however, that he felt some guilt about his use of opioid pain medicine which, at times, he may have used more than necessary for his back pain. He was taking an average of 10–12 narcotic tablets per day plus 10–20 mg of diazepam. He had resisted periodic temptations to increase his doses for over 3 years. He acknowledged that he had several physician and dentist friends who were supplying him with these medications without the knowledge of the others.

He was treated by giving him low-dose methadone for his back pain and told to take no other opioid medications. The dose was tapered off over 3 weeks, and non-opioid analgesics and 10 mg of imipramine were prescribed as needed for back pain. Diazepam was also slowly tapered off. Despite some initial anxieties requiring frequent visits and phone calls, he soon became opioid-free. He agreed to tell his physician sources not to supply him anymore.

After 1 year, he still had back pain, but it was much improved and manageable with the occasional non-opioid analgesic. He was exercising regularly. His relationship with his wife had improved since his moods were more stable, no longer influenced by varying doses of opioids. He was extremely grateful for the treatment. After 3 years, he had continued to do well.

14.9 Somatoform Pain Disorder

Patients who develop multiple sites of pain or spread of pain following minor injury are likely to have psychological factors providing the major influence on their pain. These patients may have a much higher propensity to become dependent on opioids and benzodiazepines than those with more serious injury [22]. In the author's experience, a DSM-IV defined somatoform pain disorder is typically present in the opioid-dependent chronic pain patient. Rarely do objective findings fully explain the pain.

14.10 Treatment

We have had success in treating such patients [44–46] utilizing a biopsychosocial approach. We start by explaining the rationale behind why chronic opioids actually contribute to pain. The patient is then detoxified from opioids, and the pain is treated with non-opioid analgesics. Crucial in this treatment is psychological support through this process. It is commonplace to find that chronic pain patients improve in function, and often in subjective sense of pain, when weaned off opioids. This can be more difficult than it sounds due to patient resistance. The following guidelines are recommended in treating the opiate-dependent chronic pain patient.

14.10.1 Use a Pain-Oriented History to Assess the Extent of Dependence

The patient may report the history evasively if he senses the physician is seeking to find drug dependence [47]. If asked how many pain pills are taken daily, the patient may minimize the amount, knowing he or she is taking more than he or she should. If asked how many pills it takes to relieve the pain and how long do they last, the patient is likely to give more accurate answers.

14.10.2 Explain the Role of Opioids in Maintaining Pain and Enhancing Pain Sensitivity

> You are not at fault for seeking to relieve your pain. You have been unsuccessful, however, despite vigorous use of opioids. In fact, this has contributed to your chronic painful condition. Your body needs to recover from the changes induced by chronic opioids, and it is likely that you will become stronger and feel better as a result.

This approach, when given confidently, inspires hope. For many patients, this makes sense and relieves them because they have suspected that the medication is a problem and they have become dependent upon it.

Other patients are convinced that they need opioids and cannot live without them. This is similar to the cigarette smoker, who believes this is something that cannot be stopped, despite all the warnings about the health consequences. These patients may argue that opioids are not the problem but the solution. Such a patient will resist change but may do well if the physician is supportive but strict in eliminating opioids. The physician does best by not focusing on addiction but rather the most efficacious long-term solution for the pain.

14.10.3 Detoxify While Providing Psychological Support

Once the level of opioid dependence is estimated, the dose can be fixed and steadily reduced. Buprenorphine works particularly well if the opioid-dependence level is not too high. Opioid substitution with methadone works well if the dependency is at a high level. Methadone metabolism changes with use, and duration of action lengthens each day [48, 49]. A technique that works well for inpatients recovering from acute pain on top of a chronic opioid dependence (other than methadone) is to give methadone every 4 h for three doses, then every 6 h for three doses, then every 8 h, which allows the patient to sleep through the night. For outpatients, three times daily dosing is satisfactory. This may be done when treating pain, but if the patient only needs detoxification for a substance abuse problem, it must be done at a specially licensed clinic. Methadone is surprisingly potent in a patient naive to this drug, perhaps because of its NMDA blocking effect [40], so care must be taken not to start with too high a dose. Mild constriction of the pupils [50] indicates an appropriate methadone effect.

Compared to methadone, short-acting opioids are less comfortable for the patient during detoxification because of fluctuating blood levels, and they do not allow a comfortable sleep through the night. Extended-release morphine does not have a buildup effect and may be immediately given every 12 h, but it is much less reliably absorbed, and dosing is more difficult to predict [48]. Extended-release oxycodone has less flexibility in dosing schedules, and if the patient uses up the prescription too rapidly, withdrawal symptoms are intense, stimulating substantial pain behaviors.

During detoxification, time must be spent with the patient, and this may involve supportive psychotherapy [46], including attention to concurrent issues. The patient must be supported through that critical stage where long-established drug-taking habits are changing [45]. This change in habits is usually associated with anxiety, even in highly motivated patients. Frequent visits and reassurances can go a long way toward relieving this anxiety.

14.10.4 Treat the Pain Independently of Detoxification with Nonnarcotic Analgesics (Such as Acetaminophen and Ibuprofen)

Supplemental medications, such as tricyclics, antihistamines, or neuroleptics, may also be given as needed, in doses small enough to minimize adverse effects. Many patients become very anxious if they do not have "as needed" medications for backup.

These medications will help somewhat with somatic pain [51, 52], although this will rarely be noticed by the patient dependent on higher dose opioids. When the opioid dose reaches low levels, these medications often are recognized as helpful by the patient.

14.10.5 Coordinate Care with Other Providers and with Key Family Members

The physician(s) who had been prescribing high-dose opioids to the patient need to be contacted to enlist support for this treatment plan and to make sure they do not inadvertently sabotage it by prescribing as usual.

Spouses or other family members frequently recognize opioid-related problems when the patient does not. They can help the patient comply with his alternative medications, and they can encourage increased functionality. The encouragement and appreciation of family members can help solidify and sustain the patient's improvement.

14.10.6 Promote Healthy Behaviors in General (Diet, Exercise, Smoking, Attitude)

This demonstrates the physician's concern for the well-being of the patient, not just a moral judgment about addiction, as the patient may fear. This tends to increase the likelihood that the patient will develop trust in the physician.

14.11 Conclusions

For the opioid-dependent chronic pain patient, opioids are typically ineffective with chronic opioid intake actually *enhancing* pain sensitivity. Opioid treatment is very seductive, however, in that each dose helps momentarily, even when the long-term course involves deterioration. For the patient, it is difficult to resist the immediate relative increase in comfort. For the doctor, providing opioids seems to offer a fast, simple solution to what may be a very complex problem. In the long-term, however, chronic opioid treatment of pain is associated with substantial risks, including accident proneness, unnecessary invasive procedures and tests, adverse health consequences, impaired judgment and cognitive function, decline in occupational and social functioning, and strained family relationships. If the opioid-dependent patient does not seek outside sources of opioids, a biopsychosocial approach that eliminates the opioids can result in gratifying improvements in pain and function.

References

1. Spiro, H. (1995). The problems of pain. *Social Science & Medicine, 5*, 6–7.
2. Shorter, E. (1997). Somatization and chronic pain in historic perspective. *Clinical Orthopedics and Related Research, 336*, 52–60.
3. Deyo, R. A., & Weinstein, J. N. (2001). Low back pain. *The New England Journal of Medicine, 344*, 363–370.
4. Turk, D. C., & Rudy, T. E. (1991). Persistent pain and the injured worker: Integrating biomedical, psychosocial, and behavioral factors in assessment. *Journal of Occupational Rehabilitation, 1*, 159–177.
5. Awerbuch, M. S. (1992). Whiplash in Australia: Illness or injury? *The Medical Journal of Australia, 157*, 193–196.
6. Engel, G. L. (1959). 'Psychogenic pain' and the pain-prone patient. *American Journal of Medicine, 26*, 899–918.
7. Quinones, M. A. (1975). Drug abuse during the civil war (1861–1865). *International Journal of the Addictions, 10*, 1007–1020.
8. Musto, D. F. (1992). Historical perspectives on alcohol and drug abuse. In J. H. Lowinson, P. Ruiz, R. B. Millman, et al. (Eds.), *Substance abuse a comprehensive textbook* (2nd ed.). Baltimore, MD: Williams & Wilkins.
9. Hawkins, J. A. (1937). *Opium addicts and addictions*. Danville, V. A. & Townes, J. T. (Reprint ed. 1981). New York: Arno Press).
10. Marks, R. M., & Sachar, E. J. (1973). Undertreatment of medical inpatients with narcotic analgesics. *Annals of Internal Medicine, 78*, 173–181.
11. Streltzer, J., & Wade, T. C. (1981). Cultural factors in the undertreatment of postoperative pain. *Psychosomatic Medicine, 43*, 397–403.
12. Alam, A., Gomes, T., Zheng, H., et al. (2012). Long-term analgesic use after low-risk surgery: A retrospective cohort study. *Archives of Internal Medicine, 172*, 425–430.
13. Collett, B. J. (1998). Opioid tolerance: The clinical perspective. *British Journal of Anaesthesia, 81*, 58–68.
14. Portenoy, R. K., & Payne, R. (1992). Acute and chronic pain. In J. H. Lowinson, P. Ruiz, R. B. Millman, et al. (Eds.), *Substance abuse a comprehensive textbook* (2nd ed.). Baltimore, MD: Williams & Wilkins.

15. Drug abuse related ED visits involving narcotic analgesics. *The Dawn Report*, Office of Applied Studies, SAMHSA, September 2004
16. Increase in poisoning deaths caused by non-illicit drugs – Utah, 1991–2003. Centers for Disease Control, (2005, January 21). *MMWR*.
17. Von Korff, M., Kolodny, A., Deyo, R. A., et al. (2011). Long-term opioid therapy reconsidered. *Annals of Internal Medicine, 155*, 325–328.
18. Longo, L. P., Parran, T., Jr., Johnson, B., et al. (2000). Addiction: Part II. Identification and management of the drug-seeking patient. *American Family Physician, 61*, 2401–2408.
19. McQuay, H. J. (1997). How should we measure the outcome? In E. Kalso, H. J. McQuay, & Z. Wiesenfeld-Hallin (Eds.), *Opioid sensitivity of chronic noncancer pain*. Seattle, WA: IASP Press.
20. Stein, C. (1997). Opioid treatment of chronic nonmalignant pain. *Anesthesia & Analgesia, 84*, 912–914.
21. Eriator, I. (1998). Narcotic analgesics for chronic pain management. *Current Review of Pain, 2*, 193–200.
22. Streltzer, J., Eliashof, B. A., Kline, A. E., et al. (2000). Chronic pain disorder following physical injury. *Psychosomatics, 41*, 227–234.
23. Hadler, N. M. (1997). Workers with disabling back pain. *The New England Journal of Medicine, 337*, 341–343.
24. Jensen, M. C., Brandt-Zawadzki, M. N., Obuchowsi, N., et al. (1994). Magnetic resonance imaging of the lumbar spine in people without back pain. *The New England Journal of Medicine, 331*, 69–73.
25. Schofferman, J. (1993). Long term use of opioid analgesics for the treatment of chronic pain of nonmalignant origin. *Journal of Pain and Symptom Management, 8*, 279–288.
26. Johnson, B. (1999). Three perspectives on addiction. *Journal of the American Psychoanalytic Association, 47*, 791–815.
27. Portenoy, R. K. (1996). Opioid therapy for chronic nonmalignant pain: A review of the critical issues. *Journal of Pain and Symptom Management, 11*, 203–217.
28. Ibuki, T., Dunbar, S. A., & Yaksh, T. L. (1997). Effect of transient naloxone antagonism on tolerance development in rats receiving continuous spinal morphine infusion. *Pain, 70*, 125–132.
29. Celerier, E., Laulin, J. P., Corcuff, J. B., et al. (2001). Progressive enhancement of delayed hyperalgesia induced by repeated heroin administration: A sensitization process. *Journal of Neuroscience, 21*, 4074–4080.
30. Vanderah, T. W., Suenaga, N. M., Ossipov, M. H., et al. (2001). Tonic descending facilitation from the rostral ventromedial medulla mediates opioid-induced abnormal pain and antinociceptive tolerance. *Journal of Neuroscience, 21*, 279–286.
31. Li, X., Angst, M. S., & Clark, J. D. (2001). A murine model of opioid-induced hyperalgesia. *Brain Research. Molecular Brain Research, 86*, 56–62.
32. Stinus, L., Allard, M., Gold, L., & Simmonet, G. (1995). Changes in CNS neuropeptide FF-like material, pain sensitivity, and opiate dependence following chronic morphine treatment. *Peptides, 16*, 1235–1241.
33. Vanderah, T. W., Gardell, L. R., Burgess, S. E., et al. (2000). Dynorphin promotes abnormal pain and spinal opioid antinociceptive tolerance. *Journal of Neuroscience, 20*, 7074–7079.
34. Ossipov, M. H., Lai, J., Malan, T. P., Jr., et al. (1999). In E. Kalso, H. J. McQuay, & Z. Wiesenfeld-Hallin (Eds.), *Opioid sensitivity of chronic noncancer pain*. Seattle, WA: IASP Press.
35. Mayer, D. J., Mao, J., Holt, J., et al. (1999). Cellular mechanisms of neuropathic pain, morphine tolerance, and their interactions. *Proceedings of the National Academy of Sciences of the United Stated of America, 96*, 7731–7736.
36. Nestler, E. (2004). *Neuropharmacology, 47*(Supp. 1), 24–32.
37. King, T., Gardell, L. R., Wang, R., et al. (2005). Role of NK-1 transmission in opioid-induced hyperalgesia. *Pain, 116*, 276–288.

38. Doverty, M., White, J. M., Somogyi, A. A., et al. (2001). Hyperalgesic responses in methadone maintenance patients. *Pain, 90*, 91–96.
39. Rosenblum, A., Joseph, H., Fong, C., et al. (2003). Prevalence and characteristics of chronic pain among chemically dependent patients in methadone maintenance and residential treatment facilities. *Journal of the American Medical Association, 289*, 2370–2378.
40. Gorman, A. L., Elliott, K. J., & Inturrisi, C. E. (1997). The *d*- and *l*- isomers of methadone bind to the non-competitive site on the *N*-methyl-D-aspartate (NMDA) receptor in rat forebrain and spinal cord. *Neuroscience Letters, 223*, 5–8.
41. Wadhwa, A., Clarke, D., Goodchild, C. S., et al. (2001). Large-dose oral dextromethorphan as an adjunct to patient-controlled analgesia with morphine after knee surgery. *Anesthesia and Analgesia, 92*, 448–454.
42. Ballantyne, J. C., & Mao, J. (2003). Opioid therapy for chronic pain. *The New England Journal of Medicine, 349*, 1943–1953.
43. Roth, S. H., Fleischmann, R. M., Burch, F. X., et al. (2000). Around-the-clock, controlled-release oxycodone therapy for osteoarthritis-related pain. *Archives of Internal Medicine, 160*, 853–860.
44. Streltzer, J. (1994). Chronic pain and addiction. In H. Leigh (Ed.), *Consultation-liaison psychiatry: 1990 and beyond*. New York: Plenum Press.
45. Streltzer, J. (1980). Treatment of iatrogenic drug dependence in the general hospital. *General Hospital Psychiatry, 2*, 262–266.
46. Anooshian, J., Streltzer, J., & Goebert, D. (1999). Effectiveness of a psychiatric pain clinic. *Psychosomatics, 40*, 226–232.
47. Buckley, F. P., Sizemore, W. A., & Charlton, J. E. (1986). Medication management in patients with chronic non-malignant pain. A review of the use of a drug withdrawal protocol. *Pain, 26*, 153–165.
48. Gourlay, G. K., Cherry, D. A., & Cousins, M. J. (1986). A comparative study of the efficacy and pharmacokinetics of oral methadone and morphine in the treatment of severe pain in patients with cancer. *Pain, 25*, 297–312.
49. Mercadante, S., Sapio, M., Serretta, R., et al. (1996). Patient-controlled analgesia with oral methadone in cancer pain: Preliminary report. *Annals of Oncology, 7*, 613–617.
50. Verebely, K., Volavka, J., Mule, S., et al. (1975). Methadone in man: Pharmacokinetic and excretion studies in acute and chronic treatment. *Clinical Pharmacology & Therapeutics, 18*, 180–190.
51. Breivik, H., & Rennemo, F. (1982). Clinical evaluation of combined treatment with methadone and psychotropic drugs in cancer patients. *Acta Anaesthesiologica Scandinavica, Supp. 74*, 135–140.
52. Schreiber, S., Backer, M. M., Weizman, R., et al. (1997). Augmentation of opioid induced antinociception by the atypical antipsychotic drug risperidone in mice. *Neuroscience Letters, 228*, 25–28.

Part VI
Specific Psychosomatic Disorders

Chapter 15
Stress-Induced Cardiomyopathy: Mechanism and Clinical Aspects

Jun-Won Lee and Byung-il William Choi

15.1 Introduction

The heart has been used as a classic symbol to represent emotion from ancient times. For example, heartbreak or heartache is an informal expression used when we feel pain due to emotional events eliciting sorrow, grief, sense of loss, anger, anxiety, and panic. In Korea, the word "hwabyung" means "anger" or "fire" disease [1]. The most common symptoms are chest tightness, dyspnea, and heat sensation, and patients with this culture-related anger syndrome often pound their chest with fists to relieve the symptoms. Predisposing factors of hwabyung are known to be related to psychological stressors. Psychological stressors need to be considered an important issue, especially in cardiovascular diseases [2]. Depression is an established risk factor for coronary heart diseases [3]. Stress-induced cardiomyopathy (SICM) is currently regarded as a suitable model of cardiovascular psychophysiology. This chapter discusses the mechanism and clinical aspects of SICM.

15.2 Typical Scenario of Stress-Induced Cardiomyopathy

The typical features of SICM are summarized as follows: (a) SICM mimics ST-segment elevation myocardial infarction (STEMI) which demands immediate action to revascularize the infarcted coronary artery. (b) Coronary angiography

J.-W. Lee, M.D. (✉)
Division of Cardiology, Department of Internal Medicine, Yonsei University Wonju College of Medicine, 162 Ilsan-dong Wonju, Gangwon Province 220-701, Korea
e-mail: ljwcardio@yonsei.ac.kr

B.-i.W. Choi, M.D., FACC, FAHA
Division of Cardiology, Medical College of Wisconsin, Milwaukee, WI 53226, USA
e-mail: bchoi@mcw.edu

K.B. Koh (ed.), *Somatization and Psychosomatic Symptoms*,
DOI 10.1007/978-1-4614-7119-6_15, © Springer Science+Business Media New York 2013

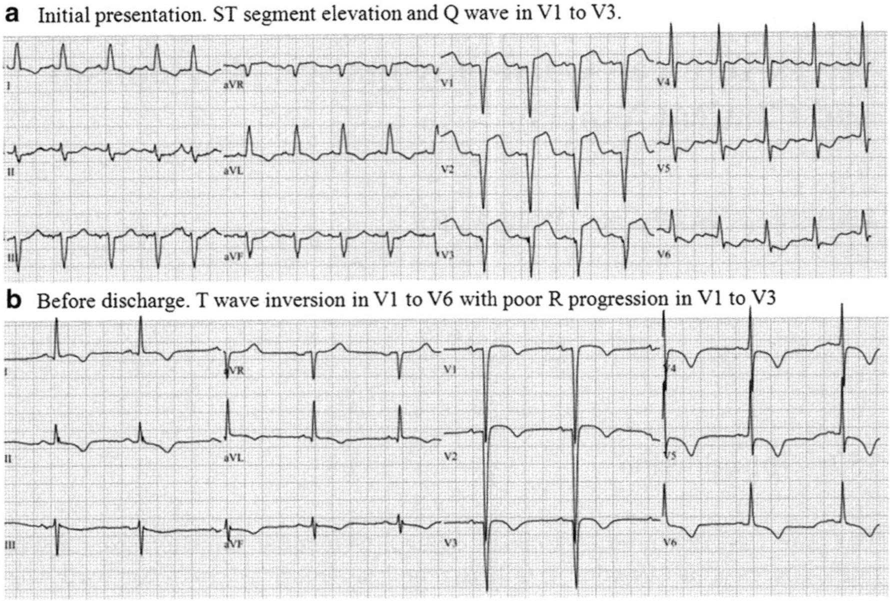

Fig. 15.1 Electrocardiogram at initial presentation (**a**) and before discharge (**b**)

shows no significant stenosis, but global systolic dysfunction of the left ventricle causes acute heart failure. (c) The prognosis is generally favorable, and left ventricular function recovers fully within 1–2 weeks.

The following is an illustrative case. A 59-year-old postmenopausal woman visited the emergency department with acute chest pain. She had no medical history but suffered from heavy psychological burden as debts were to be paid within 1 week. Her blood pressure was 152/94 mmHg, and pulse rate was 98 beats/min. Electrocardiography showed sinus rhythm and ST-segment elevation with Q wave in leads V1 through V3 (Fig. 15.1a). Echocardiography showed reduced left ventricular systolic function (35 %) and global akinesia of mid to apex of the left ventricle. Emergent coronary angiography was performed to rule out STEMI and showed no significant stenotic lesion. Left ventriculography revealed apical ballooning of the ventricle. Cardiac biomarkers were slightly elevated (creatinine kinase MB 7.4 ng/mL, troponin I 1.56 ng/mL), and the level of B-type natriuretic peptide (BNP) was relatively high (649 pg/mL). On the 2nd hospital day, she started to complain of exacerbation of dyspnea, and chest X-ray showed pulmonary congestion. She was intubated and ventilated due to worsening tachypnea and decreased oxygen saturation. Her blood pressure fell to 80/50 mmHg. Continuous IV inotropic agent was infused into the jugular vein, and she was moved to the medical intensive care unit (ICU). After 3 days of heart failure management with diuretics, she was successfully extubated. On the 9th hospital day before discharge, follow-up transthoracic echocardiography revealed normal left ventricular ejection fraction (LVEF) (57 %) and complete recovery of the global wall motion abnormality. However, giant T wave inversion was still observed in precordial leads (Fig. 15.1b) and persisted for 2 months. She was discharged on the 10th day without any complications.

15.3 Historical Background

In 1980, Cebelin and Hirsch [4] reported an important pathologic finding suggesting "stress cardiomyopathy" in victims of homicidal assaults. Fifteen victims died of physical assault with no direct internal injuries, and 11 of them showed degenerative changes in cardiac myofibrils. The authors suggested the relationship between stress and its effect on the heart via a catecholamine-mediated response. A case of pulmonary edema due to severe psychological stress in a 44-year-old woman was reported in 1986 [5]. Her chest pain developed just half an hour after she heard of her son's suicide. Her cardiac systolic function was seriously depressed, and left ventricular cineangiogram showed global akinesis and ballooning of the left ventricle.

Physical conditions (such as subarachnoid hemorrhage or pheochromocytoma) which result in high levels of plasma catecholamine are known to induce myocardial dysfunction similar to psychological stress [6, 7]. SICM became more well known after the term "takotsubo-like left ventricular dysfunction" was first described by Sato et al. [8] in 1990. Takotsubo means Japanese octopus trap, and the feature of apical ballooning of the left ventricle in SICM resembles takotsubo. From this point, many physicians became interested in this phenomenon, and stress cardiomyopathy was reused by Pavin et al. [9] in 1997. Nowadays, the number of publications on this syndrome is significantly increasing, and the field of investigation is expanding from basic science to neurocardiology [10–17].

15.4 Definition

In 2008, the Mayo Clinic suggested criteria for the diagnosis of SICM [18], but these criteria are ambiguous and need further revision due to advanced understanding of this syndrome. These criteria consist of four requisites: (a) transient hypokinesis, akinesis, or dyskinesis in the left ventricular mid-segments with or without apical involvement; abnormalities in regional wall motion extending beyond a single epicardial vascular distribution; and the presence (often, but not always) of stressors as a trigger; (b) the absence of obstructive coronary disease or angiographic evidence of acute rupture of plaques that could be responsible for the observed wall motion abnormalities; (c) new electrocardiographic abnormalities (ST-segment elevation and/or inverted T wave) or modest elevation of serum levels of cardiac troponin; and (d) the absence of pheochromocytoma or myocarditis.

15.5 Demographics and Clinical Features

15.5.1 Age and Sex Predominance

Postmenopausal women account for over 80 % of cases, and the mean age of patients is over 60 years [19]. However, the proportion of males to females differs markedly in reported cases. Park et al. [20] reported that 71 % of diagnosed cases in the medical ICU were men. Our data showed that 69 % of cases were female [21]. A recent case report demonstrated that SICM can occur even in a newborn after fetal distress [22]. This discrepancy may be due to selection bias or depend on different situations. SICM may develop at any age and in either sex.

15.5.2 Precipitating Triggers

Triggers of SICM are psychological stressors, physical stressors, or a combination of both. Situations causing tension, sense of loss, grief, anxiety (fear, panic), and anger can be psychological stressors [18, 23]. Physical stressors include severe illnesses such as asthma, chronic obstructive pulmonary disease, acute cholecystitis, diabetic ketoacidosis, buccal cavity abscess, cancer, intracranial hemorrhage, and thyrotoxicosis [21, 23]. Multiple contusions or procedure-related events may share both triggers.

Madhavan et al. [24] suggested that the underlying comorbid conditions of SICM were significantly associated with physical stressors. The duration and intensity of stressors may determine the diverse clinical presentations and outcomes.

15.5.3 Clinical Presentation

Chest pain and dyspnea are the most common symptoms. Gianni et al. [25] reported that chest pain was the cardinal symptom (68 %) followed by dyspnea (18 %). However, Madhavan et al. [24] demonstrated that almost half of patients had dyspnea (45 %) and developed heart failure. Lee et al. [21] found that dyspnea was the most frequent presentation at initial admission. There seems to be a close relationship between the types of stressors and symptoms. If trigger factors are emotional and/or acute in onset, there is a tendency to have more chest pain. In contrast, physical stressor and/or sustained stimulus appears to be related to dyspnea [26]. In addition, mental change, syncope, cardiogenic shock, heart block, and ventricular fibrillation were also reported [19, 21, 23, 25].

15.5.4 *Laboratory Findings and Electrocardiography*

BNP and cardiac biomarkers (CK-MB fraction and troponin) are usually elevated [19, 25]. BNP is a popular marker representing heart failure, and cardiac biomarkers determine the degree of myocardial damage. BNP elevation is higher in patients with heart failure [24] and those with SICM who suffer from events (combination of any death or cardiogenic shock) [21], but a statistical significance was not found. BNP levels were higher in SICM patients compared with STEMI patients, while systolic function of the left ventricle and hemodynamic parameters were similar in the two disorders [27]. Ahmed et al. [28] demonstrated that BNP was universally elevated in SICM and a significantly elevated ratio of BNP to troponin T was a biological indicator of SICM. The levels of the inflammatory biomarker such as C-reactive protein (CRP) were elevated in SICM patients and correlated with baseline LVEF [29]. In addition, the correlation between CRP and BNP levels was significant [29], and the magnitude of elevated CRP was as high as that found in acute myocardial infarction [27].

ST-segment elevation is seen in about 70 % of cases. Other findings consist of T wave inversion (64 %) and Q wave (32 %) [25]. The QTc interval is usually prolonged in the acute phase, and elevated ST-segment can evolve into giant T wave inversion [30, 31]. Takashio et al. [32] showed that high heart rate and the sum of ST-segment elevation were independent predictors of inhospital complications of SICM.

15.6 Imaging Findings

SICM shows various clinical and pathophysiologic aspects in different imaging studies including echocardiography, coronary angiography with left ventriculography, cardiac magnetic resonance (CMR) imaging, and nuclear imaging.

Echocardiography is the most useful imaging modality for diagnosis, management, and prediction of adverse outcome, providing both anatomical and physiologic information. In addition, echocardiography is a noninvasive bedside approach, without the use of contrast, and has the advantages of real-time monitoring and repeatability [33].

The typical findings of SICM are ballooning of the apex and decreased systolic function, with relatively preserved basal function (Fig. 15.2). A reported range of mean LVEF is 20–49 %, and the systolic function is improved within days to weeks [31]. However, some patients fail to recover systolic function [34], and delayed recovery of systolic function within 1 week was an independent risk factor of mortality [26]. Although it is believed that the basal area of the left ventricle is preserved, a quantitative method to assess myocardial function (strain echocardiography) revealed that the value of longitudinal strain in several segments (basal anterior and

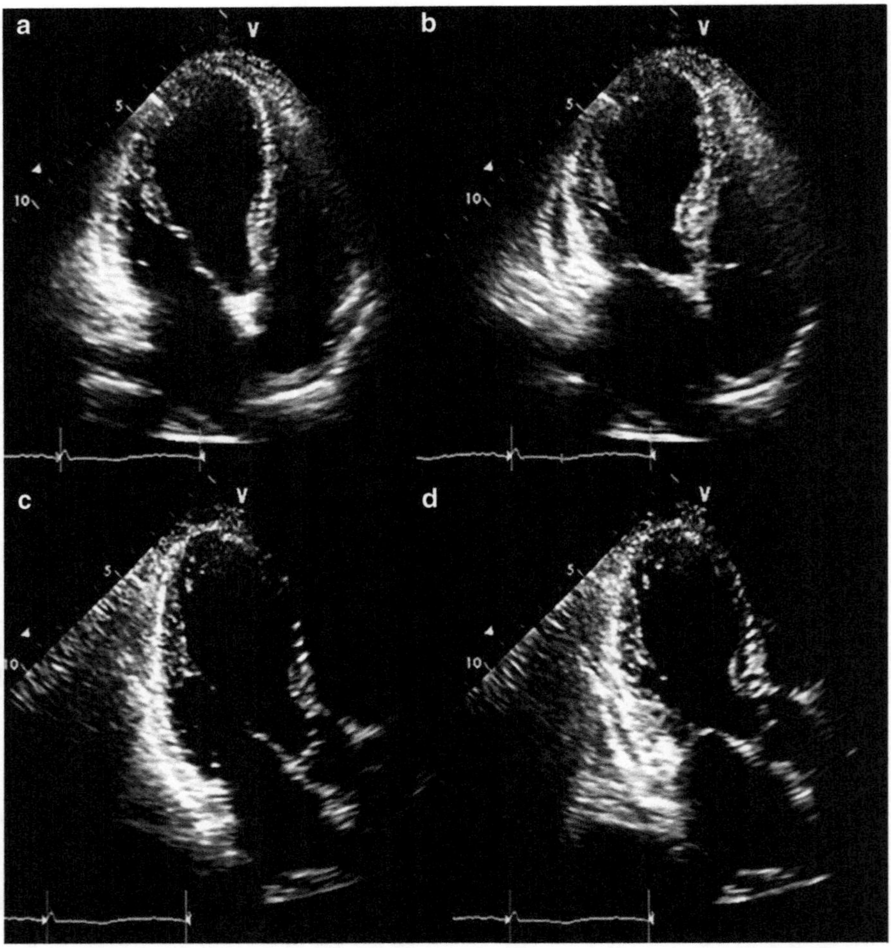

Fig. 15.2 Echocardiography shows apical ballooning and reduced global left ventricular systolic function (**a** end-diastole, **b** end-systole in apical four-chamber view, **c** end-diastole, **d** end-systole in apical three-chamber view)

anteroseptal segments) was also diminished [35]. In the variant type, the value was lowest at the mid-level of the left ventricle.

The presence of dynamic left ventricular outflow tract (LVOT) obstruction is important in determining the management strategy in SICM. Hypertrophy of the basal septum can induce the Venturi effect which is observed when blood flows through a narrower LVOT, pressure is decreased, and velocity is increased. This effect results in drawing of the anterior mitral leaflet toward the interventricular septum during the systolic period. Earlier closure of the LVOT and reduced stroke volume leads to low cardiac output and cardiogenic shock. Cardiogenic shock may be exacerbated by inotropic agents (dopamine, dobutamine). One in four patients

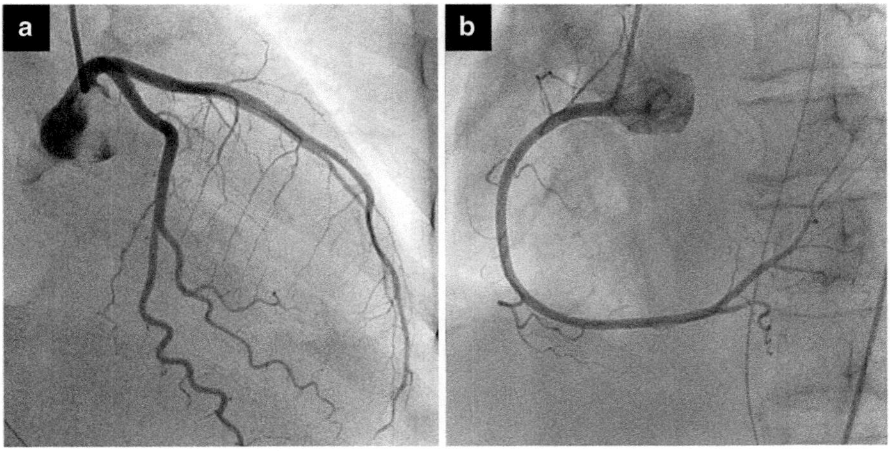

Fig. 15.3 Coronary angiography shows nearly normal coronary artery (**a**: left coronary artery, **b**: right coronary artery)

with SICM has septal thickening and mitral regurgitation [36]. Merli et al. [37] reported the association between septal thickening and LVOT obstruction, especially in elderly women. The development of mitral regurgitation is related to LVOT obstruction or a secondary change due to left ventricular enlargement (tethering) [38, 39].

It is known that the right ventricle may also be involved in SICM. The coincidence of right and left ventricular dysfunction is not rare and is associated with longer hospitalization, severe heart failure, the need for intra-aortic balloon pump, and even cardiopulmonary resuscitation [40].

Thrombus formation in the apical segment may lead to multiple systemic emboli such as cerebrovascular ischemic accident, renal infarction, or bowel infarction in the recovery phase [41]. The overall incidence of thrombus formation is about 2.5 % [42]. Immediate administration of heparin and short-term use of warfarin are essential to prevent thromboembolic events. Contrast echocardiography helps to exclude thrombus in the case of a poor echo window of the apical endocardial border [33].

Coronary angiography is performed mainly to rule out obstruction of the coronary artery. However, significant flow-limiting stenosis of the coronary artery is not regarded as a prerequisite (Fig. 15.3). Although several cases have shown the coexistence of coronary artery disease and takotsubo cardiomyopathy [43–46], Gianni et al. [25] excluded the possibility of vasoconstriction in multivessels because provocation tests with acetylcholine or ergonovine induced multivessel spasm in only one third of patients. Therefore, vasospasm is not the main precipitating factor of SICM. Left ventriculography is often used to determine left ventricular function and wall motion abnormality (Fig. 15.4).

CMR imaging is considered the gold standard modality for tissue characterization of the myocardium, wall motion abnormality, quantitative measurement of volume,

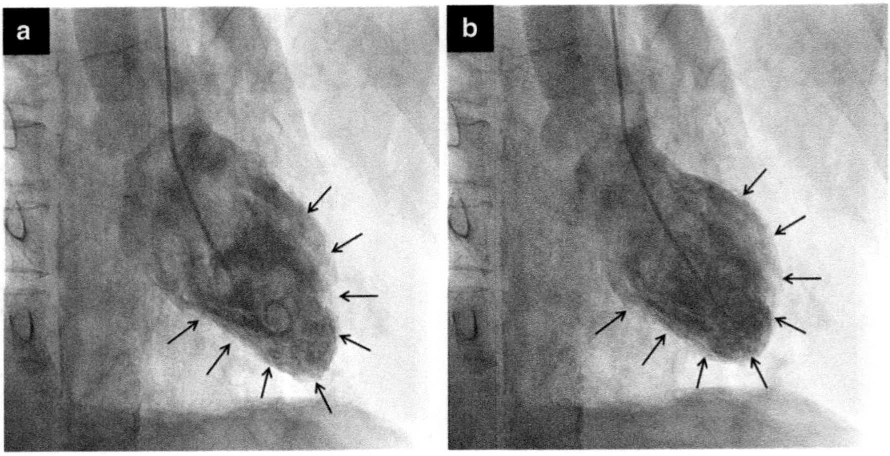

Fig. 15.4 Left ventriculogram shows ballooning from the apex to mid-level (*arrows* in figure) with relatively preserved systolic motion of basal level in the left ventricle (**a**: end-diastolic phase, **b**: end-systolic phase)

and systolic function. Recent efforts by Avegliano et al. [47] demonstrated, for the first time, the morphologic pattern of mild late gadolinium enhancement (LGE) in SICM. The pattern of late gadolinium uptake corresponded to localized inflammation and edema in the area of abnormal wall motion. This may be evidence of diffuse microcirculatory damage rather than epicardial pathology. Naruse et al. [48] determined the clinical impact of LGE. They showed that LGE patients in the subacute phase had more cardiogenic shock and needed a longer time to restore normal electrocardiographic findings and wall motion.

Fluorine-18 fluorodeoxyglucose positron emission tomography (^{18}F-FDG PET) is an established imaging modality to assess glucose metabolism in the heart, lungs, and the brain. Glucose uptake in the left ventricle in the acute phase was reduced, but not absent, and at 3-month follow-up, an even distribution of glucose uptake was observed, suggesting reversible viability [49].

^{123}Iodine-metaiodobenzylguanidine (MIBG) is useful to evaluate the cardiac sympathetic function. MIBG is a neurotransmitter analogue of norepinephrine and shares the same processes of uptake, storage, and release in the presynaptic sympathetic nerve endings. But MIBG is not metabolized and does not interact with the postsynaptic receptors. The localized and retained ^{123}iodine-MIBG can be imaged by single-photon emission computed tomography (SPECT) [50, 51]. The heart-to-mediastinum ratio (HM ratio) and the myocardial washout rate are commonly used as quantitative indices. Akashi et al. [52] demonstrated that HM ratio at 3–4 h after MIBG injection was decreased and washout rate was increased in acute phase of SICM. Decreased HM ratio suggests reduced cardiac MIBG uptake and impaired adrenergic nervous function which improved gradually at 3-month follow-up. Increased washout rate implies myocardial injuries with a resultant sympathetic hyperactivity, suggesting norepinephrine spillover from the presynaptic sympathetic nerve endings or increased extraneuronal clearance of excessive MIBG [52].

15.7 Treatment and Prognosis

There are no specific treatments for SICM. Diuretics can be used to improve pulmonary congestion and symptoms of heart failure. Inotropes should be used cautiously and avoided in patients who have a risk of LVOT obstruction [25]. Beta-blockers are thought to protect the heart against excess catecholamines. However, a recent retrospective study by Palla et al. [53] failed to prove the protective effect of beta-blocker pretreatment. Clinical parameters and severity of presentation were not different in patients treated and not treated with low-dose beta-blocker. One of the limitations in this study was that the pretreatment drugs used were selective beta-1 blockers (metoprolol and atenolol). Combined alpha and beta-blockers (carvedilol) would have a beneficial effect. However, this needs further investigation. In addition, a higher dose of beta-blocker would be advantageous in SICM [53].

The prognosis of SICM is known to be favorable, but fatal outcomes are often reported. The incidence of inhospital mortality is different in published articles and ranges from 1.1 % [25] to 15 % [34]. Adverse outcomes include acute heart failure, cardiogenic shock, arrhythmia, cardiac thrombus, ventricular rupture, and even death [19, 25, 31]. Delayed recovery of left ventricular function (within 1 week), dynamic LVOT obstruction, RV dysfunction, and the presence of cardiac thrombi are potential prognostic indicators for negative outcome.

15.8 Stress and Catecholamines: The Link between Brain and Heart

15.8.1 Evidence Suggesting a Connection Between Brain and Heart

Akashi et al. [54] reported an elevated level of plasma norepinephrine in four of 7 cases of SICM. Plasma catecholamines were 2–3 times higher in patients with SICM than in those with myocardial infarction [55] and were 7–34 times higher than normal controls. Status epilepticus also elevates plasma catecholamine levels [56, 57]. Cases of coincidence of SICM and seizures were investigated by Le Ven et al. [15]. All seizures were generalized (grand mal) with long duration and severe characteristics. This implies that the severity of seizures could impact the heart and induce SICM. Seizure-associated SICM was found to be more common in younger male patients, and SICM patients with seizure had less chest pain but more cardiogenic shock and frequent recurrence of SICM than those without seizure [16]. Summers et al. [17] retrospectively reviewed 224 patients diagnosed with SICM and posterior reversible encephalopathy syndrome. This series of case reports supported the evidence of a close connection between brain and heart.

15.8.2 Stress and the Stress System

Our body is constantly stimulated by numerous psychological and/or physical stressors. These stressors are perceived and integrated in the brain with cumulated stimuli which command the body to respond appropriately with neuroendocrine hormones via neuronal pathways and the bloodstream. The "stress system" is related to a series of protective adaptations to maintain body homeostasis. If the response is inappropriate or excessive, deleterious physiologic consequences may develop [58, 59].

Dr. John Hunter (1728–1793), an English cardiologist, was quoted saying, "My life is in the hands of any rascal who chooses to annoy me" [60]. In fact, during a strenuous argument in a board meeting at St. George in 1793, he died from a sudden heart attack. This anecdote illustrates the link between brain and heart.

15.8.3 Neuroanatomical and Functional Pathways of the Stress System

The stress system is highly coordinated by the central nervous system and peripheral targets. The primary biological systems are the hypothalamic-pituitary-adrenocortical (HPA) axis and the sympatho-adrenomedullary axis.

Initiation of cognitive appraisal occurs in the prefrontal and frontal cortices. The lateral prefrontal cortices receive input from the visual, auditory, and motor areas, as well as from the areas of memory and emotion, such as the hippocampus, cingulate gyrus, amygdala, and temporal regions (limbic system). The hypothalamus is interconnected with the higher frontal cortical regions and the lower pituitary gland [30]. Following stressful stimuli, the hypothalamus synthesizes and secretes corticotrophin-releasing hormone (CRH), which induces the release of adrenocorticotropic hormone (ACTH) from the anterior pituitary gland. ACTH stimulates the adrenal cortex and causes the adrenal gland to secrete cortisol. This sequential process is known as the HPA axis [30, 61].

The locus ceruleus (major source of norepinephrine-producing neurons) is located in the lateral floor of the 4th ventricle and is associated with the autonomic nervous system. The locus ceruleus forms complex networks with the prefrontal cortex, amygdala, hypothalamus, medullary reticular formation, and paraventricular nucleus [30, 62]. Concentrated norepinephrine in the locus ceruleus spreads throughout the brain [63]. This release of norepinephrine triggers the sympathetic nervous system in the thoracolumbar spinal cord which has synapses at the target organ, especially the chromaffin cells of the adrenal medulla [64]. Finally, the adrenal medulla releases catecholamines (norepinephrine and epinephrine) into the systemic circulation, which increases cardiovascular tone and respiration [56]. The locus ceruleus-norepinephrine circuit enables our body to respond rapidly to physiologic demand. Walter Cannon named this phenomenon the "fight-or-flight response" [65].

15.8.4 Catecholamine Spillover and Cardiovascular Responses

Recurrent and sustained stimulus due to psychological or physical stressors can result in catecholamine spillover through a feedback loop between the brain and peripheral neurohormonal system. This feedback system can result in SICM. The concurrence of a catecholamine surge and cardiac dysfunction-associated subarachnoid hemorrhage or pheochromocytoma has previously been reported [6, 66]. The effect of catecholamine spillover on the cardiovascular system is summarized into three components: (a) direct toxicity of catecholamines, (b) microvascular spasm, and (c) signal trafficking of ß-adrenoreceptors.

Firstly, the direct cardiac toxicity of catecholamines was proven in the 1970s. Rona et al. and Boutet el al. [67, 68] demonstrated that the sarcolemma (plasma membrane of cardiomyocytes) was damaged directly by an intravenous injection of catecholamines. The sarcolemma compromises accumulated intracellular calcium and subsequent cellular death of the cardiomyocyte [69, 70]. Secondly, imaging studies have shown that catecholamines cause microvascular dysfunction of the coronary artery [28, 47, 49, 52]. Recently, Uchida et al. [71] demonstrated that catecholamine-induced coronary microvascular spasm was followed by endothelial cell apoptosis shown by myocardial biopsy and suggested that apoptosis following microvascular spasm may be the missing link between stress and SICM. Finally, excessive stimulation of catecholamines switches the signaling cascades of ß-adrenoreceptors. These ß-adrenoreceptors are coupled with G proteins which consist of three subtypes: G-α, G-β, and G-γ. Ligand-receptor binding results in conformational changes in the ß-adrenoreceptors (dissociation of G-α and G-$\beta\gamma$), following downstream signal transduction. $ß_1$-adrenoreceptor stimulates only the G-α_s protein, but $ß_2$-adrenoreceptor combines with both G-α_s and G-α_i (opposite action of G-α_s) [72]. G-α_s-associated signaling results in inotropic (increased contractility), lusitropic (accelerated relaxation), and chronotropic (increased heart rate) effects. In contrast, the G-α_i protein has negative effects. During catecholamine spillover, the binding of epinephrine to $ß_2$-adrenoreceptor activates G-α_i and switches signal transduction. Cardiac function then deteriorates until the switched signal trafficking of ß-adrenoreceptor recovers [73].

15.9 Estrogen Effects

The predominance of SICM in postmenopausal women demonstrates that estrogen has crucial effects on the cardiovascular system. Indeed, 17-ß-estradiol increased cardiac output and improved arterial flow velocity with a reduction in vascular resistance [74]. The expression of endothelial nitric oxide synthase (eNOS) is significantly affected by estrogen. Estrogen also induces the expression of important genes for cardioprotection [75]. This evidence provides insight into why postmenopausal women are vulnerable to stress-related events.

15.10 Conclusions

Psychological and/or physical stressors threaten body homeostasis, and the stress system is activated to allow adaptation to the changing circumstances. The central nervous system is highly coordinated and interconnected with the peripheral system via the HPA and sympatho-adrenomedullary axes. Myocardial function may be adversely affected by inappropriate spillover or sustained release of catecholamines. These harmful effects include direct cardiotoxicity, microvascular spasm followed by endothelial cell apoptosis, and signal trafficking of ß-adrenoreceptors. Estrogen deficiency partly contributes to the development of stress-induced cardiomyopathy (SICM).

SICM may be a severe form of catecholamine-mediated cardiac response. A variety of stressors have been reported to be potent trigger factors, and cardiac profiles may be different according to the intensity and exposure duration of stressors. Several imaging modalities have revealed the characteristics of SICM. In particular, echocardiography plays a leading role in evaluating and managing SICM. There is no proven therapeutic strategy to treat and protect against SICM, other than empirical use of beta-blockers. Collaboration between cardiologists, psychiatrists, and neuroscientists is needed to elucidate the mechanism of SICM and therapeutic as well as preventive measure for SICM.

References

1. Min, S. K. (2008). Clinical correlates of hwa-byung and a proposal for a new anger disorder. *Psychiatry Investigation, 5*, 125–141.
2. Hjemdahl, P., Rosengren, A., & Steptoe, A. (2011). *Stress and cardiovascular disease*. New York: Springer.
3. Kent, L. K., & Shapiro, P. A. (2009). Depression and related psychological factors in heart disease. *Harvard Review of Psychiatry, 17*, 377–388.
4. Cebelin, M. S., & Hirsch, C. S. (1980). Human stress cardiomyopathy. Myocardial lesions in victims of homicidal assaults without internal injuries. *Human Pathology, 11*, 123–132.
5. Ryan, T. J., & Fallon, J. T. (1986). Case reports of the Massachusetts general hospital. Weekly clinicopathological exercises. Case 18–1986. A 44-year-old woman with substernal pain and pulmonary edema after severe emotional stress. *The New England Journal of Medicine, 314*, 1240–1247.
6. Pollick, C., Cujec, B., Parker, S., et al. (1988). Left ventricular wall motion abnormalities in subarachnoid hemorrhage: An echocardiographic study. *Journal of the American College of Cardiology, 12*, 600–605.
7. Iga, K., Gen, H., Tomonaga, G., et al. (1989). Reversible left ventricular wall motion impairment caused by pheochromocytoma-a case report. *Japanese Circulation Journal, 53*, 813–818.
8. Sato, H., Tateishi, H., & Uchida, T. (1990). Takotsubo-type cardiomyopathy due to multivessel spasm. In K. Kodama, K. Haze, & M. Hon (Eds.), *Clinical aspect of myocardial injury from ischemia to heart failure*. Tokyo: Kagaku Hyoronsha.
9. Pavin, D., Le Breton, H., & Daubert, C. (1997). Human stress cardiomyopathy mimicking acute myocardial syndrome. *Heart, 78*, 509–511.

10. Rockman, H. A., Koch, W. J., & Lefkowitz, R. J. (1997). Cardiac function in genetically engineered mice with altered adrenergic receptor signaling. *American Journal of Physiology, 272*, H1553–H1559.
11. Sharkey, S. W., Maron, B. J., Nelson, P., et al. (2009). Adrenergic receptor polymorphisms in patients with stress (tako-tsubo) cardiomyopathy. *Journal of Cardiology, 53*, 53–57.
12. Izumi, Y. (2010). New model of Takotsubo-like left ventricular dysfunction in cynomolgus monkey. *Nihon Yakurigaku Zasshi, 136*, 103–106.
13. Vriz, O., Minisini, R., Citro, R., et al. (2011). Analysis of beta1 and beta2-adrenergic receptors polymorphism in patients with apical ballooning cardiomyopathy. *Acta Cardiologica, 66*, 787–790.
14. Ueyama, T., Yamamoto, Y., Ueda, K., et al. (2011). Cardiac and vascular gene profiles in an animal model of takotsubo cardiomyopathy. *Heart and Vessels, 26*, 321–327.
15. Le Ven, F., Pennec, P. Y., Timsit, S., et al. (2011). Takotsubo syndrome associated with seizures: An underestimated cause of sudden death in epilepsy? *International Journal of Cardiology, 146*, 475–479.
16. Stöllberger, C., Wegner, C., & Finsterer, J. (2011). Seizure-associated Takotsubo cardiomyopathy. *Epilepsia, 52*, e160–e167.
17. Sommers, M. R., Madhavan, M., Chokka, R. G., et al. (2012). Coincidence of apical ballooning syndrome (tako-tsubo/stress cardiomyopathy) and posterior reversible encephalopathy syndrome: Potential common substrate and pathophysiology? *Journal of Cardiac Failure, 18*, 120–125.
18. Prasad, A., Lerman, A., & Rihal, C. S. (2008). Apical ballooning syndrome (Tako-Tsubo or stress cardiomyopathy): A mimic of acute myocardial infarction. *American Heart Journal, 155*, 408–417.
19. Bybee, K. A., Kara, T., Prasad, A., et al. (2004). Systematic review: Transient left ventricular apical ballooning: A syndrome that mimics ST-segment elevation myocardial infarction. *Annals of Internal Medicine, 141*, 858–865.
20. Park, J. H., Kang, S. J., Song, J. K., et al. (2005). Left ventricular apical ballooning due to severe physical stress in patients admitted to the medical ICU. *Chest, 128*, 296–302.
21. Lee, J. W., Kim, J. Y., Youn, Y. J., et al. (2010). Clinical characteristics and prognostic factors of stress-induced cardiomyopathy. *Korean Circulation Journal, 40*, 277–282.
22. Greco, C. A., De Rito, V., Petracca, M., et al. (2011). Takotsubo syndrome in a newborn. *Journal of the American Society of Echocardiography, 24*(471), e5–e7.
23. Akashi, Y. J., Nef, H. M., Möllmann, H., et al. (2010). Stress cardiomyopathy. *Annual Review of Medicine, 61*, 271–286.
24. Madhavan, M., Rihal, C. S., Lerman, A., et al. (2011). Acute heart failure in apical ballooning syndrome (Takotsubo/stress cardiomyopathy): Clinical correlates and Mayo clinic risk score. *Journal of the American College of Cardiology, 57*, 1400–1401.
25. Gianni, M., Dentali, F., Grandi, A. M., et al. (2006). Apical ballooning syndrome or takotsubo cardiomyopathy: A systematic review. *European Heart Journal, 27*, 1523–1529.
26. Lee, P. H., Song, J. K., Sun, B. J., et al. (2010). Outcomes of patients with stress-induced cardiomyopathy diagnosed by echocardiography in a tertiary referral hospital. *Journal of the American Society of Echocardiography, 23*, 766–771.
27. Madhavan, M., Borlaug, B. A., Lerman, A., et al. (2009). Stress hormone and circulating biomarker profile of apical ballooning syndrome (Takotsubo cardiomyopathy): Insights into the clinical significance of B-type natriuretic peptide and troponin levels. *Heart, 95*, 1436–1441.
28. Ahmed, K. A., Madhavan, M., & Prasad, A. (2012). Brain natriuretic peptide in apical ballooning syndrome (Takotsubo/stress cardiomyopathy): comparison with acute myocardial infarction. *Coronary Artery Disease, 23*, 259–264.
29. Morel, O., Sauer, F., Imperiale, A., et al. (2009). Importance of inflammation and neurohumoral activation in Takotsubo cardiomyopathy. *Journal of Cardiac Failure, 15*, 206–213.
30. Balkin, D. M., & Cohen, L. S. (2011). Takotsubo syndrome. *Coronary Artery Disease, 22*, 206–214.
31. Zeb, M., Sambu, N., Scott, P., et al. (2011). Takotsubo cardiomyopathy: A diagnostic challenge. *Postgraduate Medical Journal, 87*, 51–59.

32. Takashio, S., Yamamuro, M., Kojima, S., et al. (2012). Usefulness of sum of ST-segment elevation on electrocardiograms (limb leads) for predicting in-hospital complications in patients with stress (Takotsubo) cardiomyopathy. *American Journal of Cardiology, 109*, 1651–1656.
33. Lee, J. W., & Kim, J. Y. (2011). Stress-induced cardiomyopathy: The role of echocardiography. *Journal of Cardiovascular Ultrasound, 19*, 7–12.
34. Sharkey, S. W., Winderburg, D. C., Lesser, J. R., et al. (2010). Natural history and expansive clinical profile of stress (tako-tsubo) cardiomyopathy. *Journal of the American College of Cardiology, 55*, 333–341.
35. Heggemann, F., Weiss, C., Hamm, K., et al. (2009). Global and regional myocardial function quantification by two-dimensional strain in Takotsubo cardiomyopathy. *European Journal of Echocardiography, 10*, 760–764.
36. El Mahnoud, R., Mansencal, N., Pilliere, R., et al. (2008). Prevalence and characteristics of left ventricular outflow tract obstruction in Tako-Tsubo syndrome. *American Heart Journal, 156*, 543–548.
37. Merli, E., Sutcliffe, S., Gori, M., et al. (2006). Tako-Tsubo cardiomyopathy: New insights into the possible underlying pathophysiology. *European Journal of Echocardiography, 7*, 53–61.
38. Parodi, G., Del Pace, S., Salvadori, C., et al. (2007). Left ventricular apical ballooning syndrome as a novel cause of acute mitral regurgitation. *Journal of the American College of Cardiology, 50*, 647–649.
39. Haghi, D., Rohm, S., Suselbeck, T., et al. (2010). Incidence and clinical significance of mitral regurgitation in Takotsubo cardiomyopathy. *Clinical Research in Cardiology, 99*, 93–98.
40. Elesber, A. A., Prasad, A., Bybee, K. A., et al. (2006). Transient cardiac apical ballooning syndrome: Prevalence and clinical implications of right ventricular involvement. *Journal of the American College of Cardiology, 47*, 1082–1083.
41. Haghi, D., Papavassiliu, T., Heggemann, F., et al. (2008). Incidence and clinical significance of left ventricular thrombus in tako-tsubo cardiomyopathy assessed with echocardiography. *QJM, 101*, 381–386.
42. de Gregorio, C., Grimaldi, P., & Lentini, C. (2008). Left ventricular thrombus formation and cardioembolic complications in patients with Takotsubo-like syndrome: A systematic review. *International Journal of Cardiology, 131*, 18–24.
43. Winchester, D. E., Ragosta, M., & Taylor, A. M. (2008). Concurrence of angiographic coronary artery disease in patients with apical ballooning syndrome (tako-tsubo cardiomyopathy). *Catheterization and Cardiovascular Interventions, 72*, 612–616.
44. Bandorski, D., Braun, O., Kramer, W., et al. (2008). Coincidence of coronary artery disease and takotsubo cardiomyopathy in a 72-year-old female patient. *Medizinische Klinik (Munich, Germany), 103*, 665–669.
45. Gaibazzi, N., Ugo, F., Vignali, L., et al. (2009). Tako-Tsubo cardiomyopathy with coronary artery stenosis: A case-series challenging the original definition. *International Journal of Cardiology, 133*, 205–212.
46. Parker, J. A., Amerini, A. L., Autschbach, R., et al. (2012). Takotsubo cardiomyopathy with concurrent multivessel obstructive coronary artery disease: Proposition for a new clinical entity and first case surgical experience. *Interactive Cardiovascular and Thoracic Surgery, 14*, 108–109.
47. Avegliano, G., Huguet, M., Costabel, J. P., et al. (2011). Morphologic pattern of late gadolinium enhancement in Takotsubo cardiomyopathy detected by early cardiovascular magnetic resonance. *Clinical Cardiology, 34*, 178–182.
48. Naruse, Y., Sato, A., Kasahara, K., et al. (2011). The clinical impact of late gadolinium enhancement in Takotsubo cardiomyopathy: Serial analysis of cardiovascular magnetic resonance images. *Journal of Cardiovascular Magnetic Resonance, 13*, 67.
49. Skovgaard, D., Holmvang, L., Bang, L. E., et al. (2010). Imaging of Takotsubo cardiomyopathy. *Clinical Nuclear Medicine, 35*, 967–971.

50. Perrone-Filardi, P., Paolillo, S., Dellegrottaglie, S., et al. (2011). Assessment of cardiac sympathetic activity by MIBG imaging in patients with heart failure: a clinical appraisal. *Heart, 97*, 1828–1833.
51. Carrió, I., Cowie, M. R., Yamazaki, J., et al. (2010). Cardiac sympathetic imaging with mIBG in heart failure. *JACC. Cardiovascular Imaging, 3*, 92–100.
52. Akashi, Y. J., Nakazawa, K., Sakakibara, M., et al. (2004). 123I-MIBG myocardial scintigraphy in patients with "takotsubo" cardiomyopathy. *Journal of Nuclear Medicine, 45*, 1121–1127.
53. Palla, A. R., Dande, A. S., Petrini, J., et al. (2012). Pretreatment with low-dose scintigraphy in patients with y does not affect severity of Takotsubo cardiomyopathy. *Clinical Cardiology*. doi:10.1002/clc.21983.
54. Akashi, Y. J., Nakazawa, K., Sakakibara, M., et al. (2003). The clinical features of takotsubo cardiomyopathy. *QJM, 96*, 563–573.
55. Wittstein, I. S., Thiemann, D. R., Lima, J. A., et al. (2005). Neurohumoral features of myocardial stunning due to sudden emotional stress. *The New England Journal of Medicine, 352*, 539–548.
56. Meierkord, H., Shorvon, S., & Lightman, S. L. (1994). Plasma concentrations of prolactin, noradrenaline, vasopressin and oxytocin during and after a prolonged epileptic seizure. *Acta Neurologica Scandinavica, 90*, 73–77.
57. Simon, R. P., Aminoff, M. J., & Benowitz, N. L. (1984). Changes in plasma catecholamines after tonic-clonic seizures. *Neurology, 34*, 255–257.
58. Chrousos, G. P. (2009). Stress and disorders of the stress system. *Nature Reviews. Endocrinology, 5*, 374–381.
59. Chrousos, G. P., & Gold, P. W. (1992). The concepts of stress and stress system disorders: Overview of physical and behavioral homeostasis. *The Journal of the American Medical Association, 267*, 1244–1252.
60. Castiglioni, A. (1947). Chapter 18. In E. B. Krumbhaar (Ed.), *A history of medicine*. New York: Knopf.
61. Dunn, A. J., & Berridge, C. W. (1990). Is corticotrophin-releasing factor a mediator of stress responses? *Annals of the New York Academy of Sciences, 579*, 183–191.
62. Sara, S. J. (2009). The locus coeruleus and noradrenergic modulation of cognition. *Nature Reviews Neuroscience, 10*, 211–223.
63. Amaral, D. G., & Sinnamon, H. M. (1977). The locus coeruleus: Neurobiology of a central noradrenergic nucleus. *Progress in Neurobiology, 9*, 147–196.
64. Ulrich-Lai, Y. M., & Herman, J. P. (2009). Neural regulation of endocrine and autonomic stress responses. *Nature Reviews Neuroscience, 10*, 397–409.
65. Cannon, W. B. (1915). *Bodily changes in pain, hunger, fear and rage*. New York: D. Appleton & Co.
66. Scott, I. U., & Gutterman, D. D. (1995). Pheochromocytoma with reversible focal cardiac dysfunction. *American Heart Journal, 130*, 909–911.
67. Rona, G., Boutet, M., & Huttner, I. (1975). Membrane permeability alterations as manifestation of early cardiac muscle cell injury. *Recent Advances in Studies on Cardiac Structure and Metabolism, 6*, 439–451.
68. Boutet, M., Hüttner, I., & Rona, G. (1976). Permeability alteration of sarcolemmal membrane in catecholamine-induced cardiac muscle cell injury. In vivo studies with fine structural diffusion tracer horse radish peroxidase. *Laboratory Investigation, 34*, 482–488.
69. Kassim, T. A., Clarke, D. D., Mai, V. Q., et al. (2008). Catecholamine-induced cardiomyopathy. *Endocrine Practice, 14*, 1137–1149.
70. Bloom, S., & David, D. L. (1972). Calcium as mediator of isoproterenol-induced myocardial necrosis. *The American Journal of Pathology, 69*, 459–470.
71. Uchida, Y., Egami, H., Uchida, Y., et al. (2010). Possible participation of endothelial cell apoptosis of coronary microvessels in the genesis of Takotsubo cardiomyopathy. *Clinical Cardiology, 33*, 371–377.

72. Rosenbaum, D. M., Rasmussen, S. G., & Kobika, B. K. (2009). The structure and function of G-protein-coupled receptors. *Nature, 459*, 356–363.
73. Lyon, A. R., Rees, P. S., Prasad, S., et al. (2008). Stress (Takotsubo) cardiomyopathy-a novel pathophysiological hypothesis to explain catecholamine-induced acute myocardial stunning. *Nature Clinical Practice. Cardiovascular Medicine, 5*, 22–29.
74. Collins, P., Rosano, G. M., Jiang, C., et al. (1993). Cardiovascular protection by oestrogen: A calcium antagonist effect? *Lancet, 341*, 1264–1265.
75. Murphy, E., & Steenbergen, C. (2007). Cardioprotection in females: A role for nitric oxide and altered gene expression. *Heart Failure Reviews, 12*, 293–300.

Chapter 16
Poststroke Depression: Mechanisms and Management

Kyung Bong Koh

16.1 Introduction

Stroke, defined as a sudden loss of blood supply to the brain leading to permanent damage caused by thrombotic, embolic, or hemorrhagic events, ranks as the leading cause of death in patients aged 50 years and older [1]. Poststroke depression is defined as depression occurring in the context of a clinically apparent stroke [2].

Stroke often results in major changes in a person's life; a stroke survivor can suffer loss of health, occupation, social roles, and independence [2]. Depression such as adjustment disorder with depressed mood might occur after a patient was paralyzed from a stroke. Grief and demoralization would be expected as normal, but withdrawal associated with hopelessness and refusal to participate in potentially effective rehabilitation efforts would be considered maladaptive [3].

Aside from its clinical importance, poststroke depression may provide a unique opportunity to investigate the neurobiology of depression. Some studies have suggested that stroke survivors have a higher rate of major depressive disorder compared with physically ill patients with similar levels of disability [4]. This possible difference has been interpreted as evidence that poststroke depression is directly caused by the ischemic brain lesions that disrupt aminergic pathways or neural circuits involved in mood regulation [5–7]. Stroke is one of the few conditions in the Diagnostic and Statistical Manual (DSM)-IV [8] as listed "directly" causing depression. Thus, poststroke depression is diagnosed differently from depression following a myocardial infarction or a hip fracture. Yet, the literature does not necessarily support this conceptualization [2].

K.B. Koh, M.D., Ph.D. (✉)
Department of Psychiatry, Yonsei University College of Medicine,
50 Yonsei-ro, Seodaemun-gu, Seoul 120-752, Korea
e-mail: kbkoh@yuhs.ac

K.B. Koh (ed.), *Somatization and Psychosomatic Symptoms*,
DOI 10.1007/978-1-4614-7119-6_16,

In addition to the emotional well-being of the stroke survivor, the recognition and treatment of depression is important as depression is associated with increased disability [9], increased cognitive impairment [10, 11], poor rehabilitation outcome [12, 13], morbidity [14–16], and increased suicidality and mortality [17].

A key problem, which may lead to the undertreatment of poststroke depression, is that both the patient and the physician often do not accept this condition as a treatable illness [18]. A more worrying problem is that when evaluating an older patient, the physician concentrates on other aspects of the patient and dismisses depressive symptoms. Unfortunately, it has been estimated that 80 % of poststroke depression patients may not be diagnosed by nonpsychiatric clinicians [19].

The purpose of this chapter is to review the scope of problems, prevalence, mechanisms of poststroke depression, and the current knowledge base relevant to the management of poststroke depression. This section will focus on the mechanisms and management options available for poststroke depression.

16.2 Scope of Problems

The physical and psychological sequelae caused by stroke can be devastating [20]. Poststroke depression is an unresolved issue in the recovery and rehabilitation of stroke patients. It has been considered the most common neuropsychiatric condition after stroke [21]. Poststroke depression is associated with deficits in activities of daily living, as well as functional, cognitive, and social deficits that potentially limit the rehabilitation outcomes [22]. Stroke can also damage the patient's self-esteem [23]. Other consequences of poststroke depression include higher health costs, diminished social abilities, increased risk of vascular-related events, and increased suicidality and mortality [17, 24, 25].

16.3 Prevalence of Poststroke Depression

Depression is a common consequence of stroke up to 2–3 years after stroke onset [26]. The prevalence rates of poststroke depression vary from 6 % to 79 % [27, 28]. In a study using the Beck Suicidal Ideation Scale, 35 % of Korean inpatients with acute stroke showed severe suicidal ideation [29]. These rates reflect the considerable variation between studies and among different populations. Poststroke depression rates depend on the settings in which patients are examined, with greater rates among hospital inpatient-based locations (general hospital wards or rehabilitation centers) than community-based settings [20, 30]. Based on pooled data, the overall prevalence of major depression is 21.7 % and minor depression is 19.5 % [1]. Therefore, depression occurs in about 40 % of acute stroke patients [1].

16.4 Mechanisms of Poststroke Depression

It has been proposed that the primary biological mechanism most likely underlying poststroke depression is the direct effect of ischemic insults on neural circuits involved in mood regulation [31, 32]. An injury to the brain's catecholamine pathway reduces the release of neurotransmitters with depression as a likely result. Depletion of cortical biogenic amines is found after a disruption of frontal-subcortical circuits after stroke [33]. Some researchers have reported that specific ischemic lesions (i.e., left anterior and left basal ganglia lesions, lesions close to the frontal pole) are associated with the occurrence of poststroke depression [6, 7, 34, 35]. These data suggest a direct biological link between stroke and depression [2].

In addition to this anatomical basis of depression, there is growing evidence that abnormalities in proinflammatory protein release provoked by brain injury or regional dysfunction may play a crucial role in the physiological and neurochemical dysfunctions that may underlie the pathophysiology of depression. There is a great deal of human and animal experiments documenting the fact that cerebral ischemia leads to the perturbation of proinflammatory cytokine levels such as interleukin (IL)-1 beta, IL-6, and IL-18, and tumor necrosis factor-alpha [36]. These cytokines have also been shown to result in the widespread activation of indolamine 2,3-dioxygenase, which metabolizes tryptophan to kynurenine, thus depleting serotonin [36]. Further, antidepressant drugs have an anti-inflammatory effect [37].

Other mechanisms of poststroke depression have also been proposed. For example, Kohen et al. [38] recently demonstrated that people with the serotonin transporter gene polymorphism s/s genotype are three times more likely to have poststroke depression than patients with the l/l or l/xl genotype polymorphisms. Further, patients with the serotonin transporter gene polymorphism STin2 9/12 or 12/12 genotype are four times more likely to be depressed than patients with the STin2 10/10 genotype polymorphism. However, the mechanisms by which these genes increase or decrease the probability of developing depression are not known [1].

The primary psychosocial mechanisms proposed to be the cause of poststroke depression are psychosocial stressors associated with a stroke affecting mood [39, 40]. Several reasons support a psychosocial mechanism. First, some of the evidence supporting a biological mechanism for poststroke depression has not been consistently replicated. A recent meta-analysis of all relevant published studies failed to identify any association between poststroke depression and left anterior lesions or left hemispheric lesions [41]. Second, the similarities between poststroke depression and "functional" depression in terms of symptoms and treatment response profiles have also been interpreted as evidence that poststroke depression is an expected psychological reaction to a devastating event and not a unique biological consequence of stroke [42–44]. Third, the identification of several risk factors for poststroke depression that are not specific to stroke has also been interpreted as evidence supporting a psychosocial mechanism.

According to a recent systematic review by Hackett and Anderson [45], several factors have been consistently and positively associated with depression following stroke, such as stroke severity, physical disability, and cognitive impairment. In particular, severity of disability is more predictive of depression than lesion location [46] and is also one of the strongest and most consistent risk factors of poststroke depression [47].

Other predictors of poststroke depression are female gender [48], family or personal history of mood disorder [49, 50], neuroticism [14], impaired social support [51], and negative life events [51]. Additionally, social isolation and living alone have been identified as predictive risk factors for poststroke depression [52–54]. Although the evidence supporting cognitive impairment [46, 50, 55, 56] or aphasia [57, 58] as risk factors is less robust, their potential association with poststroke depression can be understood as a form of disability that can overwhelm coping skills [2].

However, most poststroke depression appears to be multifactorial in origin, although some stroke survivors may have poststroke depression purely biological in origin and some purely psychological [59]. Ultimately, a better delineation of the risk factors for poststroke psychopathology and understanding of their relative importance will contribute to the development of a systematic approach to identify stroke survivors at risk for significant poststroke psychopathology. Similarly, understanding the influence of various factors on treatment response variability could lead to the design of better treatment algorithms [2].

16.5 Clinical Manifestations of Poststroke Depression

Poststroke depression occurring within the first 3 months of stroke is classified as "early" [60]. Early poststroke depression patients have more somatic signs compared with psychological symptoms [61]. Peak incidence and greater severity of depression commonly occur between 6 months and 2 years after stroke [62]. Robinson et al. [62] found major depression in assessments immediately after a stroke in almost one-third of patients and noted that 60 % of those patients still were depressed 1 year later [63–65].

Clinically, there are differences between depressed younger and older people. Among depressed younger adults, symptoms of fatigue, sleep disturbance, psychomotor retardation, and hopelessness about the future are more commonly reported, whereas subjective complaints of poor memory and lack of concentration are more commonly reported among depressed older adults [66].

16.6 Screening and Evaluation of Poststroke Depression

In a systematic review, Hackett and Anderson [45] recommended that the gold standard method for diagnosing poststroke depression is using a semistructured psychiatric interview that meets all the standards needed for a specific diagnostic criterion (e.g., DSM criteria or International Classification of Diseases for major depressive disorder, adjustment disorder, or dysthymic disorder).

The Geriatric Depression Scale (GDS) has been considered reliable for use in elderly patients [67]. The GDS is most useful in the diagnosis of depression among patients with higher levels of function and only mild cognitive impairment [68]. Additionally, the Brief Assessment Schedule Depression Cards (BASDEC) was developed to evaluate depression in elderly patients in a hospital ward environment [69].

16.7 Diagnosis of Poststroke Depression

Diagnosis of poststroke depression is limited by comorbid factors such as (1) aphasia, (2) cognitive impairment, and (3) overlap between symptoms of depression and symptoms of stroke. For example, symptoms of depression, such as loss of energy, decreased appetite, and insomnia, may also be found among nondepressed stroke patients secondary to the hospital environment, use of medications, other medical conditions, and the physical sequelae of stroke [59]. Fedoroff et al. [43] found that, with the exception of early morning awakening, all neurovegetative and psychological symptoms of depression are significantly more frequent among patients with depressed mood as compared to those without depressed mood.

On the other hand, many methods of diagnosing depression rely on somatic symptoms that, in turn, may complicate the diagnosis of poststroke depression [70]. When depression and somatic diseases are present concomitantly, the diagnosis and treatment of poststroke depression are even more complicated and can have an adverse impact on clinical presentation and the prognosis of the underlying disease [70].

In addition, the following factors contribute to the difficulty in diagnosing poststroke depression: (1) lack of proper training of mental health-care professionals to recognize which symptoms are more related to stroke than depression and (2) medical care providers usually have limited knowledge about the differences between depression and typical signs of aging and stroke [71]. Therefore, clinicians should define a set of valid criteria for diagnosing poststroke depression [72].

16.8 Management of Poststroke Depression

Early and aggressive treatment of poststroke depression is required to minimize the cognitive and performance deficits that depression inflicts on the patient during the recovery period [23]. The biopsychosocial approach to the treatment of depression is highly recommended because poststroke depression may result from a combination of biological, psychological, and social factors [2].

All treatments must be modified according to the patient's needs, including the cost, accessibility, and availability [45]. Effective treatment will generally include the participation of the family and other support networks [45]. Under all circumstances, the treating clinician should monitor a patient presenting with depression at least weekly for the first 6 weeks to evaluate mood changes, suicidal thinking, physical safety, social life, and adverse effects of any drugs that have been prescribed [45].

Major goals of such a treatment regimen include reducing depressive symptoms, improving mood and quality of life, using health-care resources appropriately, and reducing the risks of medical complications [73]. The management of poststroke depression includes pharmacotherapy, psychotherapy, electroconvulsive therapy (ECT), and physical exercise.

16.8.1 Psychopharmacotherapy

Overall, studies demonstrate that antidepressants are well tolerated in stroke patients and that over 60 % of patients with poststroke depression respond to medication [2]. However, psychopharmacotherapy may be particularly complicated in elderly poststroke depression patients, who often have high rates of medical comorbidity and polypharmacy and are more vulnerable to the adverse effects of antidepressants [59]. It is important that the antidepressants used be effective in controlling mood disorders and also lack adverse effects on cognitive function since patients who have had strokes often experience cognitive impairment [70]. There are many variables involved in the psychopharmacotherapy of elderly patients, including pharmacokinetic changes associated with aging, drug interactions with other medications, preexisting illnesses, and adverse effects of the drugs on the elderly due to their increased vulnerability [59].

16.8.1.1 Antidepressants

Antidepressants can be effective in treating most moderate and severe depressive disorders such as major depressive disorder, but antidepressants are generally not indicated for mild forms because the balance of benefit and risk is not satisfactory for elderly stroke patients [59]. Evidence suggests that about 65 % of patients with poststroke depression improve with psychoactive drugs as compared to 44 % of patients treated with placebo [74]. Selective serotonin receptor inhibitors (SSRIs) are better tolerated than tricyclics, and significant antidepressant efficacy has been demonstrated for sertraline and citalopram [22]. Therefore, it is advisable to treat poststroke depression with SSRIs of proven efficacy and switch to nortriptyline if there is no significant improvement after an adequate trial and there are no contraindications for the use of tricyclics [22].

Further, SSRIs are the first choice for poststroke depression treatment in elderly patients due to their lower potential for drug interaction and side effects [59]. There is a beneficial effect of medication on response rates, as well as a significant reduction in depression scores as compared to placebo treatment [22]. However, there is no consistent evidence of the benefit of psychopharmacotherapy in treating poststroke depression based on remission [22].

An important finding in a meta-analysis [74] is that the benefit of psychoactive agents in reducing depressive symptoms is significant after 3 or 4 weeks of treatment and increases with continued treatment. Maintenance treatment may also be recommended in order to achieve optimal outcomes and prevent relapse [22]. Thus, antidepressants should be continued at least for 4 months after initial recovery and should be changed if no response is seen after 6 weeks [75]. Antidepressant treatment also should be continued for a minimum of 6 months in those patients who respond to psychopharmacotherapy. Antidepressant treatment can then be slowly withdrawn, or in case of relapse, it can be continued for a longer duration [76, 77].

In summary, there is converging evidence of good antidepressant response with SSRIs and tricyclic antidepressants [22]. Antidepressants should be continued for at least 4–6 weeks and maintained to achieve optimal outcomes and prevent relapse [45].

16.8.1.2 Psychostimulants

Methylphenidate is a safe and efficient therapy for elderly patients with poststroke depression. Fast onset of action (usually within 3–10 days) and relatively few adverse effects of methylphenidate may offer significant benefits over tricyclic antidepressants, which require 2–4 weeks for the onset of action [78]. In addition to few side effects, methylphenidate therapy has many benefits including mood elevation, better motor function, and the ability to perform regular daily activities [59]. Therefore, this drug may be particularly important for enhancing active participation in rehabilitation programs for patients who have had recent strokes [22].

16.8.2 Nonpsychopharmacological Management

Nonpsychopharmacological interventions in poststroke depression include psychotherapy, electroconvulsive therapy (ECT), and transcranial magnetic stimulation. Psychological interventions are the preferred method of treatment for mild mood disorders [45] and are reserved for those in whom antidepressants are either inappropriate or not tolerated [79]. Psychological treatments include behavioral therapy, cognitive behavioral therapy (CBT), problem-solving therapy, and life review therapy [80]. Additionally, Watkins et al. [81] recently showed that motivational interviewing may be effective in improving patients' mood 3 months after stroke.

Treatment of adjustment disorder after a stroke is primarily psychosocial. The focus should be on nonspecific support, education, and psychotherapeutic clarification of the individual's conflicts in the context of the physical illness [3]. In particular, emphasis should be placed on maintaining the person's self-esteem in psychotherapy [23]. Support from family and friends is also essential in treatment. Unfortunately, there are some drawbacks to these interventions, including the costs in terms of staff time and expertise and patients' slow and delayed response in comparison to psychopharmacotherapy. Psychological interventions often require several weeks before showing any clinical improvements [59].

16.8.2.1 Cognitive Behavioral Therapy (CBT)

CBT has a very strong and positive effect on patients because it not only improves and builds confidence but also enhances their daily lifestyle through a range of activities. CBT is designed to challenge dysfunctional thoughts or beliefs that are associated with low mood and to collaboratively establish more functional thoughts or beliefs [72]. CBT is based on providing insight using psychoeducation, collaborative empiricism, active problem solving, assessing the nature and quality of support, and improving the patient's adaptation to a new lifestyle after a stroke [82]. Patients examine how their thoughts may contribute to affective symptoms and feelings and how they can transform them [83]. The treatment requires qualified health professionals to constantly evaluate participants, making it easier to satisfy the diverse needs of individuals. However, patients with cognitive impairment and/or aphasia are not suited to this treatment form [59].

For individuals diagnosed with a range of chronic and disabling physical conditions, such as stroke and poststroke depression, a 12-week course of CBT may be effective [84]. In general, approximately six to eight regular sessions should be provided to patients over a period of 10–12 weeks, with most people experiencing improvements in mood and/or a reduction in symptoms after 2 months of therapy. Responses to therapy should be reviewed after eight sessions. A therapy extension period of 6 months is considered necessary for a person who has multiple issues or severe comorbidity [45].

However, in a randomized controlled trial, Lincoln et al. [85] demonstrated that CBT was not effective in the treatment of poststroke depression. Additionally, a Cochrane review of depression interventions after stroke found that psychotherapeutic intervention for poststroke depression including CBT failed to provide evidence of effectiveness [86].

Given these contradictory results, psychotherapy should be combined with antidepressants to reduce residual symptoms and the risk of relapse in patients with severe depression and in those with moderate or severe depression who refuse antidepressants [87].

16.8.2.2 Physical Exercise, Activity, and Physical and Speech Therapy

Physical exercise during the subacute recovery phase of stroke has a beneficial effect on depressive symptoms [88]. In most psychological treatments, a behavioral activation component is often involved, which addresses the problem of limitations in activity. Some of these approaches primarily focus on the meaningfulness of the activity during the treatment, which may help to intensify and maintain cognition and target depression [89]. Additionally, physical therapy and speech therapy may also be helpful for poststroke depression patients in regaining a sense of sound body and self-esteem.

16.8.2.3 Care Management (Activate-Initiate-Monitor Intervention)

Williams and colleagues [90] conducted a randomized trial of a care management intervention (Activate-Initiate-Monitor intervention) versus usual care for the treatment of poststroke depression. The Activate-Initiate-Monitor intervention was carried out by nurse care managers under the supervision of physicians and consisted of three main steps: (1) "activate" stroke survivors and their families to understand and accept the diagnosis of depression and the need for treatment, (2) initiate antidepressant medication, and (3) monitor treatment effectiveness. Stroke survivors randomized to usual care received an identical number of baseline and telephone sessions as a control treatment. Results indicated that care management of depression in patients with recent ischemic stroke produces greater remission of depression and reduction in depressive symptoms than usual care alone. The remission rate of 39 % in the intervention group was comparable or superior to that reported in most antidepressant trials in non-stroke-related depression patients [90].

16.8.2.4 Integrated Care Pathway

The integrated care pathway (ICP) may be a suitable model for a systematic approach to managing poststroke depression patients [76, 91]. This system includes screening for depression and assessing the severity of depression using psychological instruments, such as the Hamilton Rating Depression Scale, Beck Depression Inventory II (BDI-II) [92], and a clinical interview. The ICP model also suggests selecting a treatment such as psychopharmacotherapy and the use of a formal psychiatric consultation. Sometimes other instruments such as the Structured Assessment for Depression in Brain Damaged (SADBD) [93] individuals and the Stroke Aphasic Depression Questionnaire (SAD) [94] may be required to assess depression in those with severe language or communication deficits.

However, a multidisciplinary approach needs to be included in this program to facilitate more effective management of these patients. Thus, treatment of depression after stroke should include psychiatrists or psychologists, neurologists or neurosurgeons, rehabilitation medicine specialists, nurses, physical therapists, and speech therapists.

16.8.2.5 Electroconvulsive Therapy

Electroconvulsive therapy (ECT) has been reported to be effective in treating poststroke depression, causing few side effects and no neurological deterioration [95]. Its primary indication is severe depressive illness or when a disorder (or its symptoms) is considered potentially life-threatening [45]. However, ECT is not a recommended therapy for poststroke depression patients, and adverse events such as cardiac complications, memory loss, and delirium suggest caution in the use of ECT for older, poststroke depression patients [45] because of the risk of depression relapse [95] and the development of medical complications [96].

Case 1

A 49-year-old female patient was admitted to the department of neurosurgery via the emergency room with a sudden onset of headache and loss of consciousness. She underwent surgery with the diagnosis of aneurysmal rupture at the middle cerebral artery. However, she suffered from its sequelae, including right hemiparesis, aphasia, impaired orientation to time, memory disturbance, and diminished intellectual functioning. She was then transferred to the department of rehabilitation medicine, where she underwent physical therapy and speech therapy. She was referred to the department of psychiatry after being discharged from the hospital.

On her first visit to the outpatient psychiatry department, a mental status examination revealed signs of an organic mental disorder and of adjustment disorder with depression: weeping spells, loss of self-esteem caused by loss of bodily functions, impaired memory, and slurred speech. She received supportive psychotherapy and medication including haloperidol and fluoxetine biweekly for 3 months and then monthly for 2 years. Additionally, she underwent physical therapy and speech therapy at the department of rehabilitation medicine. Despite her many disabilities, she continued to practice writing and speaking briefly.

Physical therapy helped her lift her right hand to some degree, but not completely. It was possible for the patient to communicate with her family members and friends with the help of the speech therapist, but it was still difficult for her to form sentences. She was sometimes frustrated by her limited ability to speak and lift her arm, but she looked joyful as her slurred speech improved. She continued to exercise outside her house and to receive physical therapy at home everyday.

About 5 months later, she reported feeling thankful for her husband's warm and encouraging attitude. Her speech had drastically improved, and she was able to talk with her friends on the phone, albeit fast. She was surprised that she was again able to say numbers in German as she had forgotten how to immediately after her illness. Her memory also improved. However, she still exhibited bouts of sudden tearfulness, particularly when recalling her survival from her near-death experience. She began to write letters to her friends and her two sons who had been studying abroad. She was able to recall the names of her friends completely. Her stuttering also notably improved. Her friends encouraged her by saying, "Now you can talk better than 1 month ago" and "You do not stutter at all," although she did not notice those changes.

She continued to exercise at the fitness center. She was able to go outside without being accompanied by her husband. She began to understand the Chinese characters she had forgotten after her illness. Additionally, her vocabulary use and understanding increased. She was also able to speak in a low tone and was surprised that she was still able to completely lift her right arm.

Case 2

A 70-year-old male patient with stroke was admitted to the department of neurology. His brain lesion was found to have multiple diffuse embolisms, the prognosis of which was judged to be irreversible and hopeless by the neurologist. The patient was transferred to the department of rehabilitation medicine for supportive care of the stroke sequelae, including hemiparesis and aphasia. He required physical therapy and speech therapy but declined treatment and refused to eat.

He was referred to the department of psychiatry for consultation. He was severely depressed because he could no longer live as an independent person and instead had to be absolutely dependent on his wife. He was diagnosed with major depressive disorder, and an antidepressant, sertraline (Zoloft), was administered. His wife, who had devoted most of her time to taking care of him, was also tearful and appeared tired because of her husband's pessimistic and uncooperative attitude. After 4 weeks of treatment with the antidepressant, his depression was greatly improved. Thereafter, he began to participate in physical therapy and speech therapy. Even after being discharged from the hospital, he continued to exercise and to receive physical therapy and speech therapy. They moved to Canada where their daughter was living. After 7 years, he returned to Korea with his wife and was assessed at the hospital. He was observed to be able to put on his shoes, stand up and walk with the help of his wife, and even talk, which was very surprising given his status at the last visit.

These two cases suggest the impact that stroke sequelae have on patients' and their partners' emotions and self-esteem. This suggests that a multidisciplinary approach could be effective in assessing and treating poststroke depression. In particular, treatment of poststroke depression should be integrative, including biological treatment such as antidepressants, psychotherapy, physical exercise, and physical and speech therapy.

16.9 Prevention of Poststroke Depression

Given the adverse effects of poststroke depression on recovery of activities of daily living and cognitive functioning, as well as the increased mortality rate, prevention of poststroke depression using antidepressant medications may play an increasingly prominent role in the management of patients following acute stroke [1]. A double-blind, placebo-controlled study performed by Robinson et al. [97] showed that escitalopram as a preventive drug, compared with placebo over the first year after stroke, decreases the frequency of poststroke depression. However, in a systematic review of trials on psychopharmacological therapy in poststroke depression, Hackett et al. [98] reported that although antidepressants are able to reduce mood disorder symptoms, they have no clear effect on the prevention of depressive illness after stroke.

In a Cochrane review, Anderson et al. [99] found that there is no consistent evidence for a significant effect of psychoactive treatment to prevent depression, although the overall rate of depression is lower among patients treated with antidepressants. Additionally, there is a significant but small improvement in psychological distress after active psychotherapy, but there is no significant difference between active and control treatments when the outcome is depression as diagnosed with a structured interview [99]. Therefore, the overall benefit with consideration for potential side effects and complications of active treatment is still unclear. Psychological treatment is better tolerated than psychoactive drugs, but the evidence is so far negative. Therefore, preventive treatment for poststroke depression cannot be recommended at this stage [22].

16.10 Future Directions

It is crucial that future studies on the prevention and treatment of poststroke depression use adequate methods for randomized controlled trials. It should be possible to identify a subgroup of patients that will selectively respond to a given treatment modality (e.g., patients with dysthymia or adjustment disorder may show a better response to psychotherapy than patients with major depressive disorder). A better approach to designing prevention studies is to compare different treatment modalities. Future studies should also aim to investigate the putative neuroprotective role of antidepressants on cellular damage after stroke. Phenomenological differences between late-life depression and poststroke depression can then be better characterized. Further, pharmacogenetics may help to predict which of the available psychoactive agents has the highest efficacy and tolerability ratio for a given patient [22].

16.11 Conclusions

Stroke severity, physical disability, cognitive impairment, and increased mortality are positively associated with depression following stroke. Most poststroke depression appears to be multifactorial. The diagnosis of poststroke depression is limited by comorbid factors, such as aphasia, cognitive impairment, and overlap between symptoms of depression and symptoms of stroke. Poststroke depression may result from a combination of biological, psychological, and social factors. Therefore, poststroke depression is a good candidate for an integrative or biopsychosocial approach.

Antidepressants can be effective in most moderate and severe depressive disorders (e.g., major depressive disorder). There is converging evidence of good antidepressant response with SSRIs and tricyclic antidepressants. An adequate duration of antidepressant treatment should be considered in order to produce and maintain significant effects. Additionally, psychotherapy including cognitive behavioral therapy may help patients with milder depression (e.g., adjustment disorder with depressed mood or dysthymic disorder) and those with side effects or contraindications for antidepressants.

Multidisciplinary and integrative approaches can help in the assessment and treatment of poststroke depression patients. Care management interventions such as Activate-Initiate-Monitor intervention and the integrated care pathway may be suitable models for a systematic approach to managing poststroke depression patients. However, more organized and systematic approaches or programs need to be developed to manage such patients more effectively.

References

1. Robinson, R. G., & Spalletta, G. (2010). Poststroke depression: A review. *Canadian Journal of Psychiatry, 55*, 341–349.
2. Whyte, E. M., & Mulsant, B. H. (2002). Post-stroke depression: Epidemiology, pathophysiology, and biological treatment. *Biological Psychiatry, 52*, 253–264.
3. Cohen-Cole, S. A., & Harpe, C. (1987). Assessment of depression in the medically ill. In A. Stoudemire & B. S. Fogel (Eds.), *Principles of medical psychiatry* (pp. 23–36). Orlando, FL: Grune & Stratton.
4. Folstein, M., Maiberger, R., & McHugh, P. (1977). Mood disorder as a specific complication of stroke. *Journal of Neurology, Neurosurgery & Psychiatry, 40*, 1018–1020.
5. Robinson, R., Shoemaker, W., Schlumpf, M., et al. (1975). Effect of experimental cerebral infarction in rat brain on catecholamines and behavior. *Nature, 255*, 332–334.
6. Robinson, R., Kubos, K., Starr, L., et al. (1984a). Mood disorders in stroke patients: Importance of location of lesion. *Brain, 107*, 81–93.
7. Starkstein, S. E., Robinson, R. G., Berthier, M. L., et al. (1988). Differential mood changes following basal ganglia versus thalamic lesions. *Archives of Neurology, 45*, 725–730.
8. American Psychiatric Association. (1994). *Diagnostic and statistical manual of mental disorders* (4th ed.). Washington, DC: American Psychiatric Association.
9. Lenze, E., Rogers, J., Martire, L., et al. (2001). The association of late-life depression and anxiety with physical disability: A review of the literature and prospectus for future research. *The American Journal of Geriatric Psychiatry, 9*, 113–135.
10. Austin, M., Mitchell, P., & Goodwin, G. (2001). Cognitive deficits in depression: Possible implications for functional neuropathology. *The British Journal of Psychiatry, 178*, 200–206.
11. Butters, M., Becker, J., Nebes, R., et al. (2000). Changes in cognitive functioning following treatment of late-life depression. *The American Journal of Psychiatry, 157*, 1949–1954.
12. Gillen, R. T. H., McKee, T. E., Gernert-Dott, P., et al. (2001). Depressive symptoms and history of depression predict rehabilitation efficiency in stroke patients. *Archives of Physical Medicine and Rehabilitation, 82*, 1645–1649.
13. Paolucci, S., Antonucci, G., Grasso, M., et al. (2001). Poststroke depression, antidepressant treatment and rehabilitation results: A case-controlled study. *Cerebrovascular Diseases, 12*, 264–271.
14. Morris, P., Raphael, B., & Robinson, R. (1992). Clinical depression is associated with impaired recovery from stroke. *The Medical Journal of Australia, 157*, 239–242.
15. Parikh, R., Robinson, R., Lipsey, J., et al. (1990). The impact of poststroke depression on recovery in activities of daily living over a 2-year follow-up. *Archives of Neurology, 47*, 785–789.
16. Robinson, R., Lipsey, J., Rao, K., et al. (1986). Two-year longitudinal study of post-stroke mood disorders: Comparison of acute-onset with delayed-onset depression. *The American Journal of Psychiatry, 143*, 1238–1244.
17. Schulz, R., Beach, S., Ives, D., et al. (2000). Association between depression and mortality in older adults: The Cardiovascular Health Study. *Archives of Internal Medicine, 160*, 1761–1768.
18. Rabins, P. (1996). Barriers to diagnosis and treatment of depression in elderly patients. *The American Journal of Geriatric Psychiatry, 4*, 79–83.

19. Schubert, D., Taylor, C., Lee, S., et al. (1992). Detection of depression in the stroke patient. *Psychosomatics, 33*, 290–294.
20. Poynter, B., Schuman, M., Diaz-Granados, N., et al. (2009). Sex differences in the prevalence of post-stroke depression: A systematic review. *Psychosomatics, 50*, 563–569.
21. Robinson, R. G. (1997). Neuropsychiatric consequences of stroke. *Annual Review of Medicine, 48*, 217–229.
22. Starkstein, S. E., Mizrahi, R., & Power, B. D. (2008). Antidepressant therapy in post-stroke depression. *Expert Opinion on Pharmacotherapy, 9*, 1291–1298.
23. Cassem, N. H. (1991). Depression. In N. H. Cassem (Ed.), *MGH handbook of general hospital psychiatry* (pp. 237–268). St. Louis, MO: Mosby-Year Book.
24. Ensinck, K., Schuurman, A., van den Akker, M., et al. (2002). Is there an increased risk of dying after depression? *American Journal of Epidemiology, 156*, 1043–1048.
25. Glassman, A., & Shapiro, P. (1998). Depression and the course of coronary artery disease. *The American Journal of Psychiatry, 155*, 4–11.
26. Berg, A., Palomaki, H., Lehtihalmes, M., et al. (2003). Poststroke depression: An 18-month follow-up. *Stroke, 34*, 138–143.
27. Whyte, E., Mulsant, B., Vanderbuilt, J., et al. (2004). Depression after stroke: A prospective epidemiological study. *The Journal of the American Society for Geriatric Dentistry, 52*, 774–778.
28. Provinciali, L., & Coccia, M. (2002). Post-stroke and vascular depression: A critical review. *Neurological Science, 22*, 417–428.
29. Kim, S., Kim, Y., Choi, N., et al. (2001). Suicidal ideation of patients in the acute stage of stroke. *Journal of Korean Neuropsychiatric Association, 40*, 243–252.
30. Gaete, J., & Bogousslavsky, J. (2008). Post-stroke depression. *Expert Review of Neurotherapeutics, 8*, 75–92.
31. Robinson, R. (2005). Vascular depression and poststroke depression: Where do we go from here? *The American Journal of Geriatric Psychiatry, 13*, 85–87.
32. Robinson, R., Starr, L., Lipsey, J., et al. (1984). A two-year longitudinal study of post-stroke mood disorders: Dynamic changes in associated variables over the first six months of follow-up. *Stroke, 15*, 510–517.
33. Dieguez, S., Staub, F., Bruggimann, L., et al. (2004). Is poststroke depression a vascular depression? *Journal of Neurological Sciences, 226*, 53–58.
34. Robinson, R., & Szetela, B. (1981). Mood change following left hemisphere brain injury. *Annals of Neurology, 9*, 447–453.
35. Starkstein, S., Robinson, R., & Price, T. (1987). Comparison of cortical and subcortical lesions in the production of poststroke mood disorders. *Brain, 110*, 1045–1059.
36. Spalletta, G., Bossu, P., Ciaramella, A., et al. (2006). The etiology of poststroke depression: A review of the literature and a new hypothesis involving inflammatory cytokines. *Molecular Psychiatry, 11*, 984–991.
37. O'Brien, S. M., Scott, L. V., & Dinan, T. G. (2006). Antidepressant therapy and C-reactive protein levels. *The British Journal of Psychiatry, 188*, 449–452.
38. Kohen, R., Cain, K. C., Mitchell, P. H., et al. (2008). Association of serotonin transporter gene polymorphisms with poststroke depression. *Archives of General Psychiatry, 65*, 1296–1302.
39. Gainotti, G., Azzoni, A., & Marra, C. (1999). Frequency, phenomenology and anatomical-clinical correlates of major post-stroke depression. *The British Journal of Psychiatry, 175*, 163–167.
40. House, A. (1996). Depression associated with stroke. *Journal of Neurology and Psychiatry, 8*, 453–457.
41. Carson, A., MacHale, S., Allen, K., et al. (2000). Depression after stroke and lesion location: A systematic review. *Lancet, 356*, 122–126.
42. Paradiso, S., Ohkubo, T., & Robinson, R. (1997). Vegetative and psychological symptoms associated with depressed mood over the first two years after stroke. *International Journal of Psychiatry in Medicine, 27*, 137–157.
43. Fedoroff, J., Starkstein, S., Parikh, R., et al. (1991). Are depressive symptoms nonspecific in patients with acute stroke? *The American Journal of Psychiatry, 148*, 1172–1176.

44. Lipsey, J., Spencer, W., Rabins, P., et al. (1986). Phenomenological comparison of poststroke depression and functional depression. *The American Journal of Psychiatry, 143*, 527–529.
45. Hackett, M., & Anderson, C. (2005). Treatment options for post-stroke depression in the elderly. *Aging Health, 1*, 95–105.
46. Singh, A., Black, S., Herrmann, N., et al. (2000). Functional and neuroanatomic correlations in post-stroke depression: The sunnybrook stroke study. *Stroke, 31*, 637–644.
47. Murphy, E. (1982). Social origins of depression in old age. *The British Journal of Psychiatry, 141*, 134–142.
48. Angeleri, F., Angeleri, V. A., Foschi, N., et al. (1993). The influence of depression, social activity, and family stress on functional outcome after stroke. *Stroke, 24*, 1478–1483.
49. Starkstein, S. E., & Robinson, R. G. (1989). Affective disorders and cerebral vascular disease. *The British Journal of Psychiatry, 154*, 170–182.
50. Starkstein, S. E., Robinson, R. G., Honig, M. A., et al. (1989). Mood changes after right-hemisphere lesions. *The British Journal of Psychiatry, 155*, 79–85.
51. Robinson, R. G. (2003). Poststroke depression: Prevalence, diagnosis, treatment, and disease progression. *Biological Psychiatry, 54*, 376–387.
52. Aben, I., Verhey, F., Honig, A., et al. (2001). Research into the specificity of depression after stroke: A review on an unresolved issue. *Progress in Neuro-Psychopharmacology & Biological Psychiatry, 25*, 671–690.
53. Ouimet, M. A., Primeau, F., & Cole, M. G. (2001). Psychosocial risk factors in poststroke depression: A systematic review. *Canadian Journal of Psychiatry, 46*, 819–828.
54. Hackett, M., & Anderson, C. (2005). Predictors of depression after stroke: A systematic review of observational studies. *Stroke, 36*, 2296–2301.
55. Andersen, G., Vestergaard, K., Ingemann-Nielsen, M., et al. (1995). Risk factors for post-stroke depression. *Acta Psychiatrica Scandinavica, 92*, 193–198.
56. Robinson, R., Starr, L. B., Kubos, K., et al. (1983). A two-year longitudinal study of post-stroke mood disorders: Findings during the initial evaluation. *Stroke, 14*, 736–741.
57. Berg, A., Palomaki, H., Lehtihalmes, M., et al. (2001). Poststroke depression in acute phase after stroke. *Cerebrovascular Diseases, 12*, 14–20.
58. Starkstein, S., Robinson, R., & Price, T. (1988). Comparison of patients with and without poststroke major depression matched for size and location of lesion. *Archives of General Psychiatry, 45*, 247–252.
59. Lokk, J., & Delbari, A. (2010). Management of depression in elderly stroke patients. *Neuropsychiatric Disease and Treatment, 6*, 539–549.
60. Carod-Artal, F. (2007). Are mood disorder a stroke risk factor? *Stroke, 38*, 1–3.
61. Beblo, T., & Driessen, M. (2002). No melancholia in poststroke depression? A phenomenologic comparison of primary and poststroke depression. *Journal of Geriatric Psychiatry and Neurology, 15*, 44–49.
62. Robinson, R., Bolduc, P., & Price, T. (1987). Two-year longitudinal study of poststroke mood disorders: Diagnosis and outcome at one and two years. *Stroke, 18*, 837–843.
63. Wilkinson, P., Wolfe, C., Warburton, F., et al. (1997). A long-term follow-up of stroke patients. *Stroke, 28*, 507–512.
64. Sharpe, M., Hawton, K., House, A., et al. (2009). Mood disorders in long-term survivors of stroke: Associations with brain lesion location and volume. *Psychological Medicine, 20*, 815–828.
65. Astrom, M., Adolfsson, R., & Asplund, K. (1993). Major depression in stroke patients. A 3-year longitudinal study. *Stroke, 24*, 976–982.
66. Christensen, H., Jorm, A., Mackinnon, A., et al. (1999). Age differences in depression and anxiety symptoms: A structural equation modeling analysis of data from a general population sample. *Psychological Medicine, 29*, 325–339.
67. Agrell, B., & Dehlin, O. (1989). Comparison of six depression rating scales in geriatric stroke patients. *Stroke, 20*, 1190–1194.
68. Carod-Artal, F., Ferreira Coral, L., Trizotto, D., et al. (2009). Poststroke depression: Prevalence and determinants in Brazilian stroke patients. *Cerebrovascular Diseases, 28*, 157–165.

69. Adshead, F., Cody, D., & Pitt, B. (1992). BASDEC: A novel screening instrument for depression in elderly medical inpatients. *British Medical Journal, 305*, 397.
70. Gusev, E., & Bogolepova, A. (2009). Depressive disorders in stroke patients. *Neuroscience and Behavioral Physiology, 39*, 639–643.
71. Strober, L. B., & Arnett, P. A. (2009). Assessment of depression in three medically ill, elderly populations: Alzheimer's disease, Parkinson's disease, and stroke. *Clinical Neuropsychology, 23*, 205–230.
72. Laidlaw, K. (2007). Poststroke depression and CBT with older people. In G.-T. Dolores, M. S. Ann, & W. T. Lary (Eds.), *Handbook of behavioral and cognitive therapies with older adults* (pp. 233–248). New York: Springer.
73. Alexopoulos, G., Buckwalter, K., Olin, J., et al. (2002). Comorbidity of late life depression: An opportunity for research on mechanisms and treatment. *Biological Psychiatry, 52*, 543–558.
74. Chen, Y., Guo, J. J., Zhan, S., et al. (2006). Treatment effects of antidepressants in patients with post-stroke depression: A meta-analysis. *The Annals of Pharmacotherapy, 40*, 2115–2122.
75. Snow, V., Lascher, S., & Mottur-Pilson, C. (2000). Pharmacologic treatment of acute major depression and dysthymia: Clinical guideline, part 1. *Annals of Internal Medicine, 132*, 738–742.
76. Turner-stokes, L., & Hassan, N. (2002). Depression after stroke: A review of the evidence base to inform the development of an integrated pathway. Part 1: Diagnosis, frequency and impact. *Clinical Rehabilitation, 16*, 231–247.
77. Williams, L. S. (2005). Depression and stroke: Cause or consequence? *Seminars in Neurology, 25*, 396–409.
78. Lazarus, L., Winemiller, D., Lingam, V., et al. (1992). Efficacy and side effects of methylphenidate for poststroke depression. *The Journal of Clinical Psychiatry, 53*, 447–449.
79. Paolucci, S. (2008). Epidemiology and treatment of post-stroke depression. *Neuropsychiatric Disease and Treatment, 4*, 145–154.
80. Scogin, F., Welsh, D., Hanson, A., et al. (2006). Evidence-based psychotherapies for depression in older adults. *Clinical Psychology: Science and Practice, 12*, 222–237.
81. Watkins, C., Auton, M., Deans, C., et al. (2007). Motivational interviewing early after acute stroke: A randomized, controlled trial. *Stroke, 38*, 1004–1009.
82. Gallagher-Thompson, D., Steffen, A., Thompson, L., et al. (2008). *Handbook of behavioral and cognitive therapies with older adults*. New York: Springer.
83. Gebretsadik, M., Jayaprabhu, S., & Grossberg, G. (2006). Mood disorders in the elderly. *The Medical Clinics of North America, 90*, 789–805.
84. Kemp, B., Corgiat, M., & Gill, C. (1992). Effects of brief cognitive-behavioral group psychotherapy on older persons with and without disabling illness. *Behavior, Health, & Aging, 2*, 21–28.
85. Lincoln, N., & Flannaghan, T. (2003). Cognitive behavioral psychotherapy for depression following stroke: A randomized controlled trial. *Stroke, 34*, 111–115.
86. Hackett, M., Anderson, C., & House, A. (2009). Interventions for treating depression after stroke. *Stroke, 40*, e487–e488.
87. Australian, R. (2004). Australian and new Zealand clinical practice guidelines for the treatment of depression. *The Australian and New Zealand Journal of Psychiatry, 38*, 389–407.
88. Lai, S. M., Studenski, S., Richards, L., et al. (2006). Therapeutic exercise and depressive symptoms after stroke. *Journal of American Geriatrics Society, 54*, 240–247.
89. Fiske, A., Wetherell, J., & Gatz, M. (2009). Depression in older adults. *Annual Review of Clinical Psychology, 5*, 363–389.
90. Williams, L. S., Kroenke, K., Bakas, T., et al. (2007). Care management of post-stroke depression: A randomized, controlled trial. *Stroke, 38*, 998–1003.
91. Turner-Stokes, L., Hassan, N., Pierce, K., et al. (2002). Managing depression in brain injury rehabilitation: The use of an integrated care pathway and preliminary report of response to sertraline. *Clinical Rehabilitation, 16*, 261–268.
92. Beck, A. T., Ward, C. H., Mendelssohn, M. J., et al. (1961). An inventory for measuring depression. *Archives of General Psychiatry, 4*, 561–571.

93. Gordon, W. A., Hibbard, M. R., Egelko, S., et al. (1991). Issues in the diagnosis of post-stroke depression. *Rehabilitation Psychology, 36*, 71–87.
94. Sutcliffe, L. M., & Lincoln, N. B. (1998). The assessment of depression in aphasic stroke patients: The development of the Stroke Aphasic Depression Questionnaire. *Clinical Rehabilitation, 12*, 506–513.
95. Murray, G. B., Shea, V., & Conn, D. K. (1986). Electroconvulsive therapy for poststroke depression. *The Journal of Clinical Psychiatry, 47*, 258–260.
96. Currier, M., Murray, G., & Welch, C. (1992). Electroconvulsive therapy for poststroke depressed geriatric patients. *The Journal of Neuropsychiatry and Clinical Neurosciences, 4*, 140–144.
97. Robinson, R., Jorge, R., Moser, D., et al. (2008). Escitalopram and problem-solving therapy for prevention of poststroke depression: A randomized controlled trial. *Journal of the American Medical Association, 299*, 2391–2400.
98. Hackett, M., Anderson, C., & House, A. (2005). Management of depression after stroke: A systematic review of pharmacological therapies. *Stroke, 36*, 1092–1097.
99. Anderson, C. S., Hackett, M. L., & House, A. (2004). Interventions for preventing depression after stroke. *Cochrane Database of Systematic Reviews, 2*, 1–55.

Chapter 17
Cancer in a Psychosomatic Perspective

Adriaan Visser

17.1 Introduction

Cancer as a life-threatening disease brings *intense* feeling of anxiety and insecurity to patients and their family members. Improvements by early detection and its treatment, the increase of survival, and the aging populations make cancer more chronic and require attention to long-term adjustment and coping [1]. These are reasons to take serious the psychosocial problems of cancer patients and to apply appropriate interventions to these patients. They hold true for their family members and proxies too, e.g., partner, children, siblings, grandparents, and friends whose lives are also affected by this disease. So, on the average one new cancer case may often directly affect 10 persons. This suggests that cancer needs to be seen in a psychosomatic perspective. Efforts to study the influence of psychological factors on the development of cancer and its progress were still so far not so successful [2]. However, psychosocial problems of cancer patients are mainly related to mind-body relationship, although the cause of cancer is in the body. Therefore, we gain insight into cancer from the knowledge of psychosomatic medicine.

This chapter will focus on the psychosocial problems and effective interventions in breast and prostate cancer patients, the two most common types of cancer. Based on the available knowledge on these topics, the author will mainly describe results of studies in the United States, the United Kingdom, Australia, and the Netherlands. Given the emphasis on the mind-body model, the use of rehabilitation programs and the challenges of complementary approaches will also be addressed.

A. Visser, Ph.D. (✉)
Knowledge Center Innovations in Care, Rotterdam University of Applied Sciences, 3001 HA, P.O. Box 25035, Rotterdam, The Netherlands
e-mail: adriaan.visser@planet.nl

K.B. Koh (ed.), *Somatization and Psychosomatic Symptoms*,
DOI 10.1007/978-1-4614-7119-6_17, © Springer Science+Business Media New York 2013

17.2 Incidence and Mortality of Cancer

Cancer is a leading cause of death in the world. WHO data [3] indicate 7.6 million people died of cancer worldwide in 2008. Incidence is anticipated to increase up to 50 million in 2020 [1]. In the United States, approximately 1.2 million new cancers are diagnosed annually, and one-fifth of all deaths are from cancer. In the United Kingdom, approximately 273,000 new cancer cases are diagnosed each year, and 160,000 people die from it [3]. In Australia, cancer is the leading cause of death, accounting for approximately one-quarter of all deaths [4].

17.2.1 Breast Cancer

Breast cancer is the most common cancer in females in Europe. It is estimated that in the year 2000, there were 350,000 new breast cancer cases in Europe, while the number of deaths from breast cancer was estimated at 130,000. Breast cancer is responsible for 26.5 % of all new cancer cases among women in Europe, and 17.5 % of cancer deaths [5]. The estimates of new breast cancer cases for individual European countries for the year 2000 are the highest for the Netherlands, Denmark, France, Belgium, and Sweden [5]. The total number of Dutch women with breast cancer is approximately 9.3 per 1,000 women (in total 76,000) [6]. The incidence of breast cancer among women increased in 1990, which was due to the introduction of a general health program to screen women between the age of 50 and 70 years. In 1999, women of 70–75 years of age could also participate in the breast cancer screening program, resulting in increased incidence up to 123 per 100,000 women. In 2007, the incidence was 130 per 100,000 women. This figure is an increase of 30 % compared to 1989. In 2009, 13,177 women were diagnosed with breast cancer [7]. Therefore, these results suggest that the incidence of breast cancer is likely to be increased in the future.

17.2.2 Prostate Cancer

It is estimated that worldwide, the incidence of prostate cancer is 536,279 new cases in 2000 [3]. In 2009, over 9,000 new cases have been diagnosed in the Netherlands [7]. Prostate cancer patients are frequently diagnosed in later disease stages because prostate cancer progresses slowly. Symptoms such as urinary problems become manifest in an advanced disease phase and are attributed to age rather than to cancer, so often leading to seek delayed treatment [8, 9].

17.3 Psychosocial Problems in Cancer Patients

Physical and psychosocial difficulties associated with cancer diagnoses and its treatments are well documented in the literature [10]. The general problems are anxiety, social problems, meaning of life, and spirituality. In many breast cancer patients, anxiety and feelings of uncertainty about the future occur as well as feelings of guilt [11, 12], depression [13, 14], and posttraumatic stress disorder [15, 16]. The most common psychopathological syndromes are depressive, anxious, and cognitive problems (e.g., lack of concentration).

Depression and anxiety can be considered as related to the disease itself or situational, and they are mostly of subclinical intensity [17]. So, it is important to note that cancer is not necessarily associated with psychiatric disorders. Anxiety and depression are normal reactions in case of cancer. A Dutch study shows that only 5 % of the cancer patients can be indicated as having psychiatric disorders [18]. However, subclinical psychological problems and symptoms may be common too. Many survivors experience high levels of stress and anxiety associated with fear that the cancer may recur. Survivors of cancer may also experience a number of other psychological problems, including impaired body image, sexual dysfunction, and loss of fertility. Uncertainty about how to interpret and appropriately handle symptoms often leads to excessive worry, avoidance of symptom complaints, or somatic vigilance. Social problems such as stigmatization, vocational discrimination, and financial difficulties have also been reported [19].

17.3.1 Psychosocial Problems of Breast Cancer Patients

Despite increases in incidence, mortality rates of breast cancer patients have fallen. Due to the increasing survival rates, researchers and clinicians have turned to investigating the psychosocial issues facing breast cancer survivors [19]. Psychosocial morbidity in cancer patients has been estimated by the assessment of quality of life, satisfaction with care, and, more recently, patient's needs. Research on quality of life has indicated that the diagnoses and subsequent treatment of cancer impair patients' work and social activities, home management, relationships with family and others, sleep patterns, and sexual activity. In addition, studies exploring the psychological sequelae of cancer have suggested that cancer patients experience clinically significant levels of anxiety and depression [4]. Patients with cancer experience considerable burden, unmet psychosocial needs, and psychiatric morbidity, but few receive appropriate psychosocial support [20].

In general, women with breast cancer are recognized as a group of patients who report problems and high levels of need for psychosocial care across the illness trajectory. Some studies have demonstrated that female breast cancer survivors experience significantly higher levels of psychological morbidity than healthy women [19]. Based on the available literature, the most prudent conclusion is that due to cancer, only a small subset of breast cancer survivors experience severe psychological distress. The majority of breast cancer survivors will not be diagnosed with psychiatric disorders but may experience psychological symptoms and problems of living with cancer which disrupt the quality of life [19].

17.3.2 Psychosocial Problems of Prostate Cancer Patients

Although there is an increasing number on studies on the psychosocial impact of prostate cancer, most knowledge of psycho-oncology is still based on research on young women with breast cancer. During the last decade, the amount of studies has been growing; it probably has been recognized that men with prostate cancer has been a neglected area in psycho-oncology for decades [21].

Prostate cancer is unique for several reasons. It affects only males and more specifically older males. Before the age of 40, prostate cancer is rare, but the incidence rises with age with a peak around the age of 70 [7]. Contrary to other types of cancer, prostate cancer is growing slowly and thus makes it possible to consider what to do or even the choice to do nothing but monitor closely (watchful waiting). As a result of treatment, prostate cancer patients often will experience specific problems such as micturition disturbance, incontinence, erectile disorders, and bowel problems, apart from problems that accompany cancer in general such as fatigue, anxiety, and pain [22]. Although there is a growing attention to cancer in the media, it is still a disease with a taboo. Prostate cancer can bear an extra stigma since it manifests itself in the sexual, urination, and defecation areas which are shameful to most people. For instance, a substantial number (26 %) of men feel shame during digital rectal examinations [23] or would not undergo a digital rectal examination at all because of shame [24].

Due to their uncertainty about prognosis and treatment-related side effects, prostate cancer patients experience physical, emotional, and social problems, which may develop feelings of distress in almost 35 % of all cases [8]. Besides general cancer-related problems (e.g., pain, fatigue), a lot of prostate cancer patients report specific problems such as erectile dysfunction, incontinence, and urinary and intestinal disturbances during the first years after treatment [4, 25–27], which may lead to daily distress [25, 27–29]. Voerman et al. [22] found posttraumatic stress reactions in one-third of the patients. Disease stage, treatment, and socioeconomic status cohere with these posttraumatic stress reactions [25]. Studies distinguished psychological, social, and physical dimensions in relation to stress. According to Sanson-Fisher et al. [4], prostate cancer patients experience needs for support in the psychological, informational, and daily living domains.

The health-related quality of life (HRQOL) in prostate cancer patients needs to be seen in relationship with different treatment modalities and time since diagnosis. That is because treatments not only provide a good survival rate but also adverse side effects which seriously impact on the quality of life. The concept of HRQOL is multidimensional. There is a wide consensus that HRQOL includes the following four domains: (1) physical health, such as continence or absence of pain; (2) functional health, such as self-care, mobility, and role activities; (3) social health, indicating the quality of interpersonal relationships; and (4) psychological health, indicating cognitive function, psychiatric morbidity, and psychological distress [29]. There are a lot of studies about the quality of life of prostate cancer patients. However, these results are often only circulating in the medical field and often not applied to analyses of the psychosocial conditions of the patients.

17.4 Needs for Psychosocial Support

The step from the psychosocial problems of cancer patients to the use of supportive facilities requires attention to the need for psychosocial support. Having psychosocial problems does not automatically lead to the use of services. Needs can be defined as the requirement of some action or resource that is necessary, desirable, or useful to attain optimal well-being in cancer patients. Soothill et al. [30] defined significant unmet needs as those needs that patients identify as both important and unsatisfied. Until this moment, there is very little information about the unmet needs of cancer patients [21].

Research on the need is hampered by a number of methodological limitations, including conceptual uncertainties of defining "need" as "problems"; focusing on a specific type or stage of cancer or a particular treatment modality, or on specific domains of need rather than a range of patient needs; and recruiting study samples from only one treatment center. Several of these problems are solved by the development of Supportive Care Needs Survey (SCNS) [4]. The purpose of the SCNS instrument was to provide a direct and comprehensive assessment of the multidimensional impact of cancer on the lives of cancer patients and the specific issues where patients require the most help. Sanson-Fisher et al. [4] reported that the highest levels of the need for breast cancer patients were found to be in the psychological domain, which accounted for half of the top ten. The five items on the psychological domain are fears about the cancer spreading, fears about the cancer recurring, concerns and the worries about those close to the patient, uncertainty about the future, and feelings about death and dying. The three items on health system and information domain are to be informed about the things he/she can do to help himself/herself get well, to be informed about cancer that is under control or diminishing, and to be informed about his/her results as soon as possible. The two items on psychological and daily living domain are lack of energy and tiredness and not being able to do the things he/she used to do [4].

Some survivors of breast cancer have continued needs for information about health insurance, preventative treatments, genetic counseling, diet and exercise, and complementary therapies which may persist for many months or years after the end of the treatment as presented by Thewes et al. [19]. The results of this study show that women with breast cancer have psychological, support, and information needs.

These needs concern the informal support, support from treatment team, support groups, professional counseling, as well as psychological and support needs of the family. The information needs reported are written information during the treatment, information needs of the family, and ongoing information needs [19]. The majority of the respondents expressed the opinion that information and good relationships with health-care professionals were important, and few expressed dissatisfaction with these aspects of needs. Items of significant unmet needs cluster around aspects of managing daily life, emotions, and social identity. The needs are more likely to be experienced by patients who are younger, have a long-standing illness or disability, do not own and/or use a car, and/or have no religious faith. Furthermore, significant unmet needs relate to the patients' ability to talk freely to a caregiver about the cancer, the degree to which the cancer interferes with social activities, and whether financial difficulties are experienced [30].

Visser et al. [31] reported in a study on 20 Dutch health-care professionals that 45 % stated that there is a lack of an institute that provides information for cancer patient in their region. The most important issues are a meeting place, providing patients and their proxies with information, special hours, and linking people to special psychosocial care professionals. Patients were asked similar questions at a website, and 60 % stated they missed a care center as well. A recent study in Friesland shows that 47 % of the respondents (patients) stated that there is need for psychosocial support during or after the treatment. Still the question on why they have those needs remains unanswered [31]. Focusing on the significant unmet needs of cancer patients in relation to their psychosocial concerns fits with recent policy initiatives to streamline cancer services [30].

In a recent study on needs among 122 Dutch women with breast cancer, the need for and use of psychosocial care was questioned [32]. The need for psychological issues is found to be the highest, e.g., they need psychosocial care to help them with their fear that the cancer is spreading, their uncertainty about the future, and their worries about the people who are close to them. They also need help with their feelings of sadness, anxiety, and depression. Younger women need more psychosocial care in this domain than older women. On the physical side, a lot of women need help as well, because they are not able to do the things they used to do, feeling tired and lacking energy. The Dutch women also have moderate to high needs for psychosocial care in the sexuality area. They need help in the change of sexual feelings and change in their sexual relationship. In addition, they need information about the relationship between sexuality and their illness. Especially so do younger women and who do not have a long-lasting intimate relationship. Overall the authors conclude that women who have a low quality of life and low health status have more needs in all the domains. Psychosocial care team and medical staff should give more attention to the psychological, physical, and sexual needs of this group of patients [32]. A study among Dutch men with prostate cancer found that their supportive needs were especially concerning psychological, health-care system, sexual, and physical issues [33].

17.5 Psychosocial Interventions for Cancer Patients

Psychosocial care can be defined as concerned with the psychological and emotional well-being of the patient and their family/caregivers, including issues of self-esteem, insight into the adaptation to the illness and its consequences, communication, social functioning, and relationships [32]. Psychosocial care is the active support for cancer patients and their partners during the period of time of the illness as well as the period after their illness. This care consists of basic care provided by medical specialists, such as information and emotional support, and professional care provided by psychological specialists. Among others, professional care consists of psychoeducation, psychotherapy, individual counseling, group therapy, and revalidation [34].

There is evidence that interventions aimed at improving patient outcomes do benefit patients with cancer [4], although this view has been critically discussed in the literature as well. Lepore and Coyn [35] have their doubts about the effect of psychological treatments, but they believe that the evidence is insufficient to conclude that psychological treatments for cancer patient are ineffective and unaccepted [35]. In a Dutch study, Schrameijer and Brunenberg [18] investigated the psychosocial problems of cancer patients, the use of support facilities, and the unmet needs for psychosocial support. This cross-sectional study showed that the majority of cancer patients were confronted with psychosocial problems, but only one-third had looked for supportive care, and about 10 % of the patients had actually found professional psychosocial help. The rate of participation in psychosocial care studies is often not so high (about 50–60 %); one-third show dropout, and only about 50 % are followed up [35]. Besides the highest participation by women, the higher educated, younger patients and those with an autochthon background tend to participate in the studies.

However, in recent years there have been important changes with respect to care for cancer patients:

- More supportive care facilities are available for cancer patients in the form of psychosocial departments in hospitals and specialized psycho-oncology institutes [36].
- Nurses are more widely involved in patient education and in provider-patient communication in oncological settings [37].
- The social climate with respect to cancer has become increasingly open, as stimulated by the Dutch Cancer Society (KWF) and also by patient organizations [38].

In the Netherlands, there is a large variety of psychosocial care facilities for cancer patients and their proxies. Psycho-oncological centers offer help by professionally trained psychologists. The patients may be referred to the centers by general practitioners, oncologist, or by self-reference. The therapy is nearly totally reimbursed [36].

There is growing attention to cancer patients and their proxies by foundations functioning as open walking-in houses (hospitality centers), emphasizing the importance of support by trained volunteers. Activities are meeting fellow patients, creative activities, walking, meditation, fashion shows, and groups for children with a parent with cancer. These walking-in houses are appreciated very well and seem to enhance the quality of life of the visitors. However, despite the increased attention, very little is known about the needs of the visiting patients and their proxies, their background characteristics, evaluation of experiences, and possible effects of walking-in houses on their well-being [31].

Some professionals suppose that every cancer patient needs care, because of the crisis they will experience once they are confronted with cancer. Others think that patients are capable of managing this crisis on their own, with help from their environment [36]. Now there is more attention to psychosocial care in medical protocols; this care is given by medical professionals. There is a priority to screen those patients who need specialized psychosocial care [36].

Recently the stress management training applying mindfulness is growing, showing positive effects on the quality of life, release of tension and relief of physical suffering, vigor and lowering depression and feelings of anger, and increasing meaning of life. The patients are very satisfied with this intervention, although they sometimes not only like to be trained in silence but also to have attention to the topic of cancer and the possibilities to exchange experiences. It is one of the most popular interventions with a lot of positive evidence that it works [39].

17.5.1 Interventions for Breast Cancer Patients

There are a lot of studies on the psychosocial interventions for breast cancer patients. Among them there are the following modalities: individual and group therapy, social support groups, existential and experiential group therapy, meditation, and mindfulness training. Effects of these interventions are measured concerning better emotional adjustment, improvement of mood and quality of life, less distress, anxiety and depression, and less disease- and treatment-related complaints (e.g., nausea, vomiting, pain, and sleep disturbance) [40].

It has been found that support given to women with breast cancer has a positive effect on their reactions to the illness [32] and may even prolong their survival [41], although the latter is critically discussed and controversial due to methodological flaws. There is also no sufficient evidence that psychosocial interventions may affect life expectancy.

The methodology of intervention studies has been criticized for the following reasons: no randomization, no comparison between different interventions, dropout, and no standardization of measurements. However, there is a need among women for psychosocial support. So if they participate, they are very satisfied, with an average score of 8 on a 10-point scale [35].

In summary, research has shown that there are increasing numbers of breast cancer survivors, and while the majority of women adjust well to breast cancer, among survivors, negative psychosocial consequences and/or need for information may persist for many years after the end of treatment [19].

17.5.2 Supportive Care for Prostate Cancer Patients

Studies indicate that in order to cope with their problems, prostate cancer patients look for supportive care. Voerman et al. [42] argue in their study on determinants of group participation that the a*ttitude*, s*ocial support*, and *efficacy* factors influence the supportive care-seeking behavior. Corboy et al. [43] also concluded that attitudes toward different kinds of support services, instead of the experienced problems, are predictive for actual care use. Other studies [44, 45] emphasize the importance of an individualized approach to help men address thoughts and feelings after the diagnosis or a more gender-adapted approach. Daeter et al. [33] concluded that men experience *priority needs*, which means they search information and support in order to be able to do the things important to them. This is consistent with conclusions of Sanson-Fisher's et al. [4] and Bisson's et al. [46] that standard care should consist of adequate support and information. A Dutch study found a significant predictable value of psychological and physical needs and depression for the use of future care among prostate cancer patients. These needs were more important than attitude in relation to care-seeking behavior.

In spite of the problems of prostate cancer patients, men make limited use of supportive care interventions that are often not widely available as shown in a 2002 review by Voerman et al.[22]. Dutch centers for psychosocial supportive care also observe this phenomenon [46, 47]. Voerman et al. [22] describe seven intervention studies. Emotional support seems to be of minor importance to men. In general, men prefer information about the disease and treatment in a formal setting with expert speakers focusing on information and education. Information packages, telephone interventions, and interventions alternating recreation activities with discussion sessions were well accepted by the patients. Further, the effect of interventions on anxiety and distress was limited, and studies were small sized and had other design limitations [22]. Twelve new intervention studies were published since 2002. Their impact is still rather limited. Ineffective interventions, due to organizational problems as well as contradictory study results, have been reported [48–51]. Patient's information seeking is found to be successful at improving their knowledge, quality of life, and satisfaction with care, especially when combined with a group discussion [51–53]. On the other hand, studies found that much of the educational material used for prostate cancer patients omitted important information or was incorrect [54]. The lack of supportive care interventions, the increasing incidence of prostate cancer, and the related psychosocial problems underline the need for development of intervention, which addresses the patient's problems.

17.6 Rehabilitation Programs

The interventions in psycho-oncology are mainly based on psychological approaches, using a mind-body model, as shown in the above studies. The rehabilitation programs start from the body, applying sport activities, fitness training, muscular training, and cardiac activities. It is easy to be referred to a rehabilitation center by general practitioners and oncologists due to the fact that rehabilitation is an existing medical treatment and reimbursed by the health insurance companies. The number of participants rose to more than 3000 patients in the Netherlands since it started in 1996. Follow-up evaluation of rehabilitation is well accepted by the patients, especially by men who are not so attracted by interventions based on talking only; these men like something to do. Studies and reviews showed positive effects on the quality of life, fitness, physical functioning, cardiopulmonary indicators, exhaustive grades, muscle strength, and improvement of symptoms (e.g., fatigue) [55–59]. These physical approaches are often combined with psychoeducation and cognitive behavioral therapy. Interesting is that in a few studies, additional cognitive behavioral therapy did not enhance the effects, which suggests that patients with cancer favor the pure rehabilitation approach [58, 59]. This seems contrary to the psychosomatic medicine approaches stressing the value of psychological and psychiatric interventions. However, more comparative studies are needed to solve the effects of different approaches.

17.7 Complementary Interventions

To enhance their quality of life, cancer patients often turn to the use of complementary and alternative medicine. Worldwide, 29–70 % of the general population and 42–50 % of cancer patients and palliative care patients use yearly at least one form of complementary and alternative medicine [60]. Massage and relaxation techniques are the forms of care most commonly used [61]. From massage and touches, patients learn to connect their illness with their feelings, with themselves, and with the world around them, leading to reduction in symptoms and improvement in quality of life. This approach is a part of the mind-body medicine, defined as focusing on the interaction among the brain, mind, body, and behavior, and the powerful ways in which psychological, social, spiritual, and behavioral factors can directly affect health. [60]

It has been observed that massage decreases anxiety, depression, anger, pain, nausea, dyspnea, fatigue, and sleep disturbance and improves the quality of life and neuroendocrine-immune functions. Massages often are combined with the use of aromas and essential oils, which may enhance the effects of massages. Studies on the effects of relaxation therapies show reduced emotional suppression and improvement in the quality of life of in- and outpatients and relief of symptoms such as depression, anxiety, improvement in distress, sleep disturbance, fatigue, pain, and nausea and vomiting. Besides these mind-body approaches, art and music therapy are very beneficial for cancer patients, because they are nonverbally oriented. Participation in groups using art therapy may lead to an increased meaning of life and spirituality, less complaints, and less use of professional care [60–62].

17.8 Conclusions

Cancer is a somatic disease which leads to a lot of psychosocial problems. This disease not only concerns the patients but also their family members. Cancer often confronts people with existential questions: why me, why now, and what is the meaning of it in my life? What can be learned from psycho-oncology concerns the openness of all the health-care providers at any moment for all physical, psychological, social, and spiritual problems. This too requires the attention to the needs for supportive care facilities. Based on these needs, the psycho-oncology can offer a lot of interventions. Although the effects of interventions are often not well documented, the patients value this therapeutic help very much. The interventions include not only psychological help but also rehabilitations programs, giving more attention to the body which may be related to the experience of cancer patients with their bodily complaints. From this perspective, complementary approaches, also more based on a mind-body orientation, such as massage and relaxation, may be very helpful and beneficial for these patients.

Acknowledgments I would like to thank Bert Voerman, Dorine Schoustra, and Laura Daeter for citing their excellent reviews and studies.

References

1. Holland, J. C. (1998). *Psycho-oncology*. New York: Oxford University Press.
2. Garssen, B. (2004). Psychological factors and cancer development: Evidence after 30 years of research. *Clinical Psychology Review, 24*, 315–338.
3. World Health Organization. (2011). Accessed November 2011, www.who.int
4. Sanson-Fisher, R., Girgis, A., Boyes, A., et al. (2000). The unmet supportive care needs of patients with cancer. *Cancer, 88*, 226–237.
5. Tyczynski, J. E., Bray, F., & Parkin, D. M. (2002). Breast cancer in Europe. *European Network of Cancer Registries (ENCR), 2*. www.encr.com.fr
6. Nationaal Kompas Volksgezondheid. (2011, October). *RIVM*. Den Haag: Ministerie van Welzijn Gezondheid en Sport. www.nationaalkompas.nl
7. Facts and Figures of the Integraal Kankercentrum Nederland. (2011). November 1. www.cijfersoverkanker.nl/selecties
8. Muilekom, H. A. M., & Spil, J. A. (2006). *Handboek prostaatcarcinoom*. Maarssen: Elsevier Gezondheidszorg.
9. McDowell, M., Occhipinti, S., Ferguson, M., et al. (2010). Prospective predictors of psychosocial support service use after cancer. *Psycho-Oncology, 20*, 788–791.
10. Adler, N. E., & Page, A. E. K. (2008). *Cancer for the whole patient*. Washington, DC: The National Academies Press.
11. Dunkel-Schetter, C., Feinstein, L. G., Taylor, S. E., et al. (1992). Patterns of coping with cancer. *Health Psychology, 11*, 79–87.
12. Fallowfield, L. J., Hall, A., Maguire, G. P., et al. (1990). Psychological outcomes of different treatment policies in women with early breast cancer outside a clinical trial. *British Medical Journal, 301*, 575–580.

13. Massie, M. J., & Popkin, M. K. (1998). Depressive disorders. In J. C. Holland (Ed.), *Psycho-oncology*. New York: Oxford University Press.
14. van't Spijker, A., Trijsburg, R. W., & Duivenvoorden, H. J. (1997). Psychological sequelae of cancer diagnosis: A meta-analytical review of 58 studies after 1980. *Psychosomatic Medicine, 59*, 280–293.
15. Passik, S. D., & Grummon, K. L. (2003). Posttraumatic stress disorder. In J. C. Holland (Ed.), *Psycho-oncology*. New York: Oxford University Press.
16. Mehnert, A., Lehmann, C., Graefen, M., et al. (2009). Depression, anxiety, post-traumatic stress disorder and health-related quality of life and its association with social support in ambulatory prostate cancer patients. *European Journal of Cancer Care, 19*, 736–745.
17. Bastecky, J., Tondlova, H., Veselá, J., et al. (1996). Prevalence of psychopathology in patients suffering from breast and gastrointestinal cancer. *Patient Education and Counseling, 28*, 75–78.
18. Schrameijer, F., & Brunenberg, W. (1992). *Psychosociale zorg bij kanker. Patiënten en hulpverleners over problemen en hulpaanbod*. Utrecht: Nederlands centrum Geestelijke Volksgezondheid.
19. Thewes, B., Butow, P., Girgis, A., et al. (2004). The psychosocial needs of breast cancer survivors; a qualitative study of the shared and unique needs of younger versus older survivors. *Psycho-Oncology, 13*, 177–189.
20. Girgis, A., Breen, S., Stacey, F., et al. (2009). Impact of two supportive care interventions on anxiety, depression, quality of life, and unmet needs in patients with nonlocalized breast and colorectal cancers. *Journal of Clinical Oncology, 27*, 6180–6190.
21. Visser, A., & van Andel, G. (2003). Psychosocial and educational aspects in prostate cancer patients. *Patient Education and Counseling, 49*, 203–206.
22. Voerman, B., Fischer, M., Visser, A., et al. (2004). Prostate cancer: A review of the literature on psychosocial problems and psychosocial interventions. *Gedrag en Gezondh: Tijdschr Psychol Gezondh, 32*, 251–270.
23. Naccarato, A. M., Reis, L. O., Matheus, W. E., et al. (2011). Barriers to prostate cancer screening: Psychological aspects and descriptive variables: Is there a correlation? *The Aging Male, 14*, 66–71.
24. Romero, F. R., Romero, K. R., Brenny, F. T., et al. (2008). Reasons why patients reject digital rectal examination when screening for prostate cancer. *Archivos Españoles de Urología, 61*, 759–765.
25. Voerman, B., Visser, A., Fischer, M., et al. (2012). Elderly male patients: Traumatic stress and need for support in prostate cancer patients. Abstract of 4th European Congress on Older Persons: the Future of Care. Free University, Amsterdam, 4–7 October, 2010.
26. Huang, G. J., Sadetsky, N., & Penson, D. F. (2010). Health-related quality of life for men treated for localized prostate cancer with long-term follow-up. *Journal of Urology, 183*, 2206–2212.
27. Dale, W., Bilir, P., Han, M., Meltzer, D., et al. (2005). The role of anxiety in prostate carcinoma: A structured review of the literature. *Cancer, 104*, 467–478.
28. Pirl, W. F., & Mello, J. (2002). Psychological complications of prostate cancer including commentary by Dineen, K., Eton, D. T., Von Gunten, C. F., et al. *Oncology, 11*, 1448
29. Van Andel, G., Bottomley, A., Fossa, S. D., et al. (2008). An international field study of the EORTC QLQ-PR25: A questionnaire for assessing the health-related quality of life of patients with prostate cancer. *European Journal of Cancer, 44*, 2418–2424.
30. Soothill, K., Morris, S. M., Harman, J., et al. (2001). The significant unmet needs of cancer patients: Probing psychosocial concerns. *Supportive Care in Cancer, 9*, 597–605.
31. Visser, A., Breed, W., Geluk, W., et al. (2009). The value of open walking-in houses for cancer patients and their proxies: History, use, needs and evaluation. *Nederlands Tijdschrift Oncologie, 6*, 248–255.
32. Schoustra, D., & Visser, A. P. (2012). *The unmet psychosocial care needs in breast cancer patients in the Netherlands*. Master thesis, Report De Vruchtenburg, Rotterdam.

33. Daeter, L., Visser, A., & Van der Hooft-Lemans, T. (2012). *Determinants of seeking psychosocial care in Dutch men with prostate cancer*. Master thesis, Report De Vruchtenburg, Rotterdam.
34. Facts and Figures of the Integraal Kankercentrum Zuid. (2011). November 1. www.ikz.nl
35. Lepore, S. J., & Coyne, J. C. (2006). Psychological interventions for distress in cancer patients: A review of reviews. *Annals of Behavioral Medicine, 32*, 85–92.
36. De Haes, H., Gualthérie van Weezel, L., & Sanderman, R. (2009). Psychologische patiëntenzorg in de oncologie. *Handboek voor de professional* (2e druk). Assen: Van Gorcum BV.
37. Kruijver, J. (2001). *Communication between nurses and admitted cancer patients*. Thesis, Utrecht University, Utrecht.
38. Boerrigter, G. H., Honing, C., Leer, E. M., et al. (1999). De balans van een halve eeuw kankerbestrijding. Uitgave Nederlandse Kankerbestrijding/Koningin Wilhelmina Fonds, bij gelegenheid van het vijfjarig jubileum. Bohn Stafleu van Loghum, Houten.
39. Kieviet-Stijnen, A., Visser, A., Garssen, B., et al. (2008). Mindfulness-based stress reduction training for oncology patients: Patients' appraisal and changes in well-being. *Patient Education and Counseling, 72*, 436–442.
40. Lindop, E., & Canon, S. (2001). Evaluating the self-assessed support needs of women with breast cancer. *Journal of Advanced Nursing, 34*, 760–771.
41. Spiegel, D. (1992). Effects of psychosocial support on patients with metastatic breast cancer. *Journal of Psychosocial Oncology, 10*, 113–120.
42. Voerman, B., Visser, A., Fischer, M., et al. (2007). Determinants of participation in social support groups for prostate cancer patients. *Psycho-Oncology, 16*, 1092–1099.
43. Corboy, D., McLaren, S., & McDonald, J. (2011). Predictors of support service use by rural and regional men with cancer. *The Australian Journal of Rural Health, 19*, 185–190.
44. Halbert, C. H., Wrenn, G., Weathers, B., et al. (2001). Sociocultural determinants of men's reactions to prostate cancer diagnosis. *Psycho-Oncology, 19*, 553–560.
45. Helgason, A. R., Dickman, P. W., Adolfsson, J., et al. (2001). Emotional isolation: Prevalence and the effect on well-being among 50-80-year-old prostate cancer patients. *Scandinavian Journal of Urology and Nephrology, 35*, 97–101.
46. Bisson, J. I., Chubb, H. L., Bennett, S., et al. (2002). The prevalence and predictors of psychological distress in patients with early localized prostate cancer. *BJU International, 90*, 56–61.
47. Stichting De Vruchtenburg (2010). *Annual report 2009*, Rotterdam.
48. Oliffe, J. L., Halpin, M., Bottorff, J. L., et al. (2008). How prostate cancer support groups do and do not survive: British Columbian perspectives. *American Journal of Men's Health, 2*, 143–155.
49. Helgeson, V. S., Lepore, S. J., & Eton, D. T. (2006). Moderators of the benefits of psychoeducational interventions for men with prostate cancer. *Health Psychology, 25*, 348–354.
50. Berglund, G., Petersson, L. M., Eriksson, K. C., et al. (2007). "Between Men": a psychosocial rehabilitation programme for men with prostate cancer. *Acta Oncologica, 46*, 83–89.
51. Lepore, S. J., Helgeson, V. S., Eton, D. T., et al. (2003). Improving quality of life in men with prostate cancer: A randomized controlled trial of group education interventions. *Health Psychology, 22*, 443–452.
52. Templeton, H., & Coates, V. (2004). Evaluation of an evidence-based education package for men with prostate cancer on hormonal manipulation therapy. *Patient Education and Counseling, 55*, 55–61.
53. Tarnhuvud, M., Wandel, C., & Willman, A. (2007). Nursing interventions to improve the health of men with prostate cancer undergoing radiotherapy: A review. *European Journal of Oncology Nursing, 11*, 328–339.
54. Walling, A. M., Maliski, S., Bogorad, A., et al. (2004). Assessment of content completeness and accuracy of prostate cancer patient education materials. *Patient Education and Counseling, 54*, 337–343.
55. van der Peet, E. (2005). *Systematische literatuur search naar revalidatieprogramma's [Systematic literature search on revalidation programs]*. Maastricht: Integraal Kankercentrum Limburg.
56. Knols, R., Aaronson, N. K., Uebelhart, D., et al. (2005). Physical exercise in cancer patients during and after treatment. *Journal of Clinical Oncology, 23*, 3830–3842.

57. McNeely, M. L., Campbell, K. L., Row, B. H., et al. (2006). Effects of exercises on breast cancer patients and survivors. *Canadian Medical Association Journal, 175*, 34–41.
58. Korstjens, I. (2008). *Cancer rehabilitation*. Thesis, Maastricht University, Maastricht.
59. May de Groot, A. M. (2008). *Rehabilitation in cancer: Training and talking?*. Thesis, Maastricht University, Maastricht.
60. Visser, A., Schoolmeesters, A., van den Berg, M., et al. (2011). Methodological reflections on body-mind intervention studies with cancer patients. *Patient Education and Counseling, 82*, 325–334.
61. Busch, M. E. H., De Graeff, A., Hupkens, S. H. A., et al. (2010). *Richtlijn complementaire zorg (Guideline complementary care)*. Utrech: IKMN.
62. Visser, A., Wildenbeest, M., & Nieuwenhuizen, L. (2012). Evaluation of psychosocial support for people with cancer. *Medical Encounter, 26*, 19–21.

Chapter 18
Psychosocial Aspects of Breast Cancer: Focus on Interventions

Kyung Bong Koh

18.1 Introduction

The psychosocial aspects of breast cancer have received much attention due to the high prevalence and mortality of the disease, as well as the psychological effects of surgery on an organ with high accessory meaning (e.g., body image and self-image, sense of attractiveness, femininity, sexuality, nurturing capacity, and reproduction) [1].

The diagnosis, treatment, and treatment sequelae of breast cancer are major stressors for any woman; however, the psychological impact of the diagnosis and a woman's emotional response vary considerably depending on the medical parameters of the disease (i.e., stage at the time of diagnosis, treatment offered, and complications of treatment), the patient's psychological makeup (premorbid personality and prior personal experience with cancer), coping abilities, and the availability of emotional and financial support [2]. In addition, women who report more stressful life events have been shown to be at increased risk for cancer recurrence and at higher risk of death from breast cancer [3].

Loss is also an important concern for women with breast cancer. This was seen in a study of cognitive-existential group therapy in which many of the participants' concerns centered around a sense of profound loss: of the sense of a secure future, of good health, of bodily integrity, of self-esteem, of confidence, and of mastery over their lives [4]. The results from quality-of-life instruments showed that women were distressed by hair loss, change of body image, loss of a sense of attractiveness and femininity, and disturbed sexual functioning; these feelings of distress buttress the central role of loss [5] and are similar to findings among other cohorts [6–9].

Many women who have had a mastectomy report continued emotional discomfort when their partner touches their surgical site or reconstructed breast. Some

K.B. Koh, M.D., Ph.D. (✉)
Department of Psychiatry, Yonsei University College of Medicine,
50 Yonsei-ro, Seodaemun-gu, Seoul 120–752, Korea
e-mail: kbkoh@yuhs.ac

K.B. Koh (ed.), *Somatization and Psychosomatic Symptoms*,
DOI 10.1007/978-1-4614-7119-6_18, © Springer Science+Business Media New York 2013

report they are never again able to comfortably disrobe in public changing rooms, and many describe that some friends and colleagues never seem to stop scrutinizing their chests, always looking to see what is different [10].

Living with breast cancer imposes significant stress on the patients and requires well-developed coping skills. The patients' anxiety may depend on their coping style and age. For example, greater anxiety tends to be seen in women adopting a cognitive confrontational response (withstanding the illness) compared to other responses. Younger women appear likely to view breast cancer as a greater threat to their lives than older women [11], and they seem to show higher anxiety and greater worry when facing a potential diagnosis of malignancy [12]. To live with cancer is much more than adapting to the treatments and their various side effects. In addition to coping with the threat to life, many psychosocial issues must be addressed [13].

In particular, it is not only the above unique psychosocial and medical factors but also hormonal factors that may influence mood in breast cancer patients, so psychiatric diagnosis and treatment data on depression from other populations cannot be generalized to this population [14]. Therefore, in this chapter, the author reviews the research literature regarding psychological reactions to diagnosis, stage of treatment, and recurrence in patients with breast cancer, as well as psychiatric disorders and a variety of psychiatric treatment modalities available for them. Additionally, the author uses a case report to illustrate some therapeutic processes and reviews the biopsychosocial effects of psychological interventions.

18.2 Psychological Reactions to the Diagnosis, Treatment, and Recurrence of Breast Cancer

When a woman notices a suspicious symptom of breast cancer, her emotional reactions generally include terror, shock, or panic followed by emotional numbness, denial, or disbelief as she proceeds with the medical evaluation [15]. When a woman is told that she has breast cancer and that further diagnostic tests, surgery, chemotherapy, radiotherapy, or other treatments are necessary, her emotional reactions typically run from sorrow to despair and rage [10]. In particular, patients who suppress negative emotion tend to report more emotional distress, such as anxiety, depression and anger than did those who express negative emotion after being told the diagnosis of breast cancer and after surgery [16].

Many women who face mastectomy or limited resection fear dying while under anesthesia and also fear loss of autonomy. Most believe that preoperative waiting will be the most stressful time during the initial work-up and only later learn that waiting for the pathology report after surgery is much more stressful. A woman who has a choice between limited resection combined with irradiation or mastectomy is required to confront a different set of fears: how to adjust to the loss of the breast versus how to adjust to living with a breast that has become diseased. They may go into denial while they try to gather information [10].

A study of women who underwent mastectomy revealed five common stressors: hope for a cure, treatment effectiveness, fear of the unknown, progression of the disease, and pain [17]. Studies comparing the psychosocial outcome of mastectomy with lumpectomy and radiotherapy revealed some advantages to women treated with breast-conserving procedures in terms of body image, but there was very little difference in terms of psychiatric morbidity or sexual dysfunction [10].

Many women with breast cancer regard chemotherapy as the addition of yet more chemicals to a body that must have been so poisoned that the cancer developed in the first place. The anxiety that was present during the diagnostic work-up continues when some women with stage 1 breast cancer are asked to choose either chemotherapy or no further treatment. The experience of breast cancer leaves many women fearful for their future and worried that they may have made the wrong treatment decisions [10]. As the chemotherapy sessions continue, particularly if post-chemotherapy nausea or other side effects increase, women often come to face the chemotherapy sessions with dread [10]. It has also been reported that as compared to other treatments, chemotherapy is associated with higher levels of anxiety [18].

Aside from the transient side effects of fatigue, nausea, and vomiting, the most visible and detested side effect of chemotherapy is alopecia. After the loss of their breast, the loss of hair represents for many women yet one more assault on their femininity. These alterations in body image reinforce the view that many women hold that they have been mutilated and changed, which serves as a visible sign of their private conviction that they are emotionally scarred and forever vulnerable [10].

For women with estrogen receptor-positive tumors, the use of adjuvant antiestrogen therapy is usually considered. The presence of hot flashes, mood swings, and decreased libido resulting from low levels of estrogen further accentuate the "out of control" experience associated with breast cancer. For many women, the side effects of chemical menopause come as yet more in a series of "cruel surprises" following their diagnosis of breast cancer [10].

Given the wide range of uses of radiation therapy, women's responses vary greatly, as they do for chemotherapy. Feelings of claustrophobia are not uncommon as women wonder if they will be able to tolerate both the stimulation and the subsequent episodes of radiation therapy. Patients receiving radiation therapy also report intensified feelings of isolation and loneliness because they are separated from the radiation technician [10]. In addition, psychological distress (e.g., anxiety) prior to radiotherapy is known to be related to a distinct immunological (e.g., interleukin-6-soluble receptor) and behavioral response (e.g., fatigue) during radiotherapy [19].

For some women, time-intensive radiation therapy represents a daily reminder that they are fighting breast cancer. If women develop metastatic breast cancer, radiation therapy is used to reduce the metastases or to provide palliative relief from the side effects of the metastases. The heightened awareness of the severity of their illness understandably leads to increased anxiety and worry about death. Not uncommonly, women at this stage become increasingly claustrophobic during the radiation therapy process ("Being in the radiation therapy suite reminds me of being in a coffin.") [10].

As well, the diagnosis of recurrence of breast cancer is an emotionally catastrophic event. Women who experience rapid disease recurrence are frightened. The diagnosis of recurrence emotionally propels a woman back to the initial diagnosis. Such women describe having virtually the same emotional reactions (terror, shock, and disbelief) that they had when they were initially diagnosed [10]. Particularly breast cancer survivors who report high threat appraisal and low coping appraisal are known to have the highest fear of cancer recurrence [20].

The site of the recurrence significantly affects a woman's emotional burden. Adjusting to local recurrence as the only site of recurrence is emotionally much easier than adjusting to evidence of widespread disease. A woman who has radiographic evidence of bone metastases with no pain or physical limitation has a somewhat easier adjustment than does a woman who is told she has liver or brain metastases [10].

18.3 Psychiatric Disorders in Breast Cancer Patients

Psychiatric disorders are frequently comorbid with breast cancer. For example, in a cross-sectional study of 303 women with early-stage breast cancer, 45 % were diagnosed with a psychiatric disorder, among them, 42 % with depression and/or anxiety, 27.1 % with minor depression, 9.6 % with major depressive disorder (MDD), 8.6 % with anxiety disorder, and 6.9 % with phobic disorder [5]. In another study, 5–10 % of breast cancer patients met the DSM-IV criteria for posttraumatic stress disorder [21].

In particular, depression is a frequent but underrecognized and undertreated condition among breast cancer patients, which causes amplification of physical symptoms, increased functional impairment and poor treatment adherence [14]. In a Korean study, 14 % of breast cancer patients were reported to have depressive disorders [22]. One literature review found that about 10–25 % of breast cancer patients suffer from MDD [14]. The depression rate for breast cancer is considered to be higher than for most other cancers, with the exception of pancreatic and oropharyngeal cancer [23, 24]. One possible reason for the high prevalence of MDD in breast cancer patients is menopause and estrogen decline related to depression. The acute onset of premature menopause is a potential effect of chemotherapy. Additionally, endocrine therapy [e.g., ovarian suppression, selective estrogen receptor modulators (SERMs)] further depletes estrogen levels in both pre- and postmenopausal women. Estrogen is known to increase brain serotonin postsynaptic responsivity and is believed to cumulatively act as a serotonin agonist [25]. In certain brain regions, estrogen also acts as a cholinergic agonist and increases norepinephrine activity [26]. Therefore, estrogen may have an antidepressant-like effect by these multiple modulation.

There is also evidence that depression may independently lower plasma estrogen [27] and lead to an earlier perimenopause [28]. SERMs such as tamoxifen may modulate the central nervous system by estrogen antagonist actions, which, in turn, inhibit serotonergic mechanisms in the brain [29]. The effects of depression on estrogen and age of perimenopause may add to the adverse hormonal effects of chemotherapy and hormonal therapy in breast cancer patients [14].

Proinflammatory cytokines (e.g., interleukin [IL]-1, IL-6) released in response to the tissue damage that occurs during cancer treatment also may contribute to the high rates of depression in cancer patients [30–35].

18.4 Psychiatric Approaches for Patients with Breast Cancer

Therapeutic approaches generally used for cancer can be applied to treatment for patients with breast cancer, comprising a number of psychotherapeutic, behavioral, and psychopharmacologic techniques. Psychotherapeutic approaches include individual, family, and group therapy, as well as individual self-help treatment (e.g., patient-to-patient volunteers) and self-help groups. In particular, individual therapy that involves clear and open communication, expression of appropriate emotions, collaborative planning, and problem-solving has been shown to enhance adjustment and improve outcomes [36]. Behavioral interventions such as relaxation, biofeedback, systemic desensitization, hypnosis, and guided imagery are helpful for pain and anxiety during procedures and for nausea, vomiting, and cancer-related eating disorders. Psychopharmacologic management is effective for anxiety, depression, nausea, vomiting, and insomnia [37].

Individual therapy for patients with breast cancer can be divided into general treatment and specific treatment.

18.4.1 Individual Therapy

18.4.1.1 General Treatment

Crisis-Intervention Approach

Individual therapy utilizes a crisis-intervention approach in which the therapist (1) encourages the patient to express feelings, (2) offers support and optimism, (3) clarifies feelings, (4) interprets thoughts in psychodynamic terms, (5) encourages the patient to act on his or her circumstances, (6) explores the current situation in the context of the past, (7) focuses on specific relevant psychodynamic issues, and (8) limits the duration of therapy [38].

The therapeutic goal is not only to help the patient adjust to cancer but to utilize mobilized emotions and issues to resolve previously existing conflicts [39]. The psychotherapy of a cancer patient cannot occur in a vacuum which ignores the need for a direct attack on the primary illness and relies exclusively on a psychodynamic approach.

The educational component of this therapeutic system includes [39] (1) clarifying the state of the medical condition including diagnosis, prognosis, and therapeutic alternatives; (2) teaching about the effects of the cancer and its treatments; (3) teaching methods for relief of anxiety such as relaxation techniques, self-hypnosis, or biofeedback [40]; (4) providing an individualized method of utilizing visual imaging to combat the cancer; (5) supporting compliance with medical regimens; (6) teaching about lifestyle, diet, and exercise; (7) teaching about the common reactions of patients, relatives, and friends to cancer; and (8) self-help groups.

Clarification of the medical condition and related treatments is important. Informed patients have less fear and anxiety, lower levels of stress, and better functioning coping responses [41]. Relaxation techniques help patients feel that they can exercise control over their bodies as well as relieve pain and anxiety without extra medication [40]. In addition, lower stress level may be associated with enhanced cancer prognosis [40, 42]. This technique may also help prepare the patient for visual imaging [40].

These psychotherapeutic and educational approaches are all helpful in the management of cancer patients, although whether they favorably alter the prognosis of the cancer remains to be seen. However, they have been shown to lower psychological distress and improve treatment satisfaction and compliance [43]. The techniques of choice with each patient and family depend on individual needs and the modalities available. No single educational or psychological technique has been proven so successful that it should be imposed on every patient. An integrated approach selecting those techniques which are differentially helpful to each individual is strongly suggested [39].

Cognitive-Behavioral Therapy

Cognitive-behavioral treatment can be used effectively for patients with breast cancer. The overall aims of this treatment are to correct deficits in coping, to lower levels of distress, to reclaim personal control, to teach problem-solving methods, and to improve morale. More specifically, it is aimed to influence a patient's coping through educational means [13].

From several points of view, a cognitive-behavioral approach appears most useful for those patients identified as poor copers. First, it addresses a patient's coping deficits. Second, as a short-term device focused on the "here and now," educational intervention enables the clinician and the patient to collaborate in promoting the patient's self-control and responsibility for health. A third advantage of this treatment is cost-effectiveness. Increasing health-care costs makes it difficult to provide long-term psychosocial support to cancer patients, many of whom will return for multiple treatments and perhaps have several recurrences. Thus, a brief problem-solving intervention that is effective can multiply its effect over time. This kind of treatment offers patients an opportunity to learn a method for coping with problems while continuing to live with cancer [13].

The therapist must be knowledgeable of the medical aspects of the patient's disease, its prognosis, treatment, and common side effects. The therapist must also be flexible in approach; the focus of treatment shifts as the illness changes. Sometimes, psychotherapy is maintained by telephone for those patients too ill to come to the office [37].

Poorly coping patients can typically be identified as having two main deficits in their coping repertoire. First, they tend to overuse coping strategies that have been poorly effective in resolving problems, though they may have brought a temporary sense of relief, such as getting drunk. Second, and perhaps more important, a hallmark of poorly coping patients is that they are unable to generate a number of alternative coping strategies [13].

Good copers, conversely, are able to try a number of problem-solving approaches and to persevere until something effective is found and some degree of resolution is achieved. Also, these patients are able to evaluate and to rank order their approaches to problem-solving rather than giving each strategy equal weight. Therefore, they are able to face a perceived problem with hope and then imagine a range of consequences that might come about through the use of different strategies [13].

Treatments to improve coping begin by focusing on current issues. However, exploration of reactions to cancer often include situations unrelated to the illness [37]. Distressed cancer patients are encouraged to examine their situation, then to articulate their understanding of what might interfere with good coping and to explore options that are within reach in order to find a feasible, satisfactory solution [13].

In an approach that focuses on problem-solving, patients are taught to recognize, confront, and solve commonly encountered cancer problems [44, 45]. They are also taught a specific step-by-step procedure to problem-solving and then given the opportunity to practice with the therapist and apply it to personal problems related to the illness. In this way, the therapist attempts to teach and reinforce active coping skills [13].

In this intervention, problems are defined, approaches are evaluated, and consequences are cognitively considered in order to dissolve self-imposed blocks to behavioral action. The objectives are to strengthen internal controls and to reinforce flexibility about coping strategies, choice of goals, and personal resourcefulness [13].

The intervention follows the general principles of any short-term psychotherapy. In the first session, the patient is introduced to the program, its procedures, and rationale. A four-session contract is established, and the patient is informed that we will look at common problems faced by many cancer patients and the best and most practical ways to solve them. Ideas for problem-solving are taught, and patients are encouraged to practice these skills with their own problems. Relaxation is presented as a time-out procedure for managing stress and for identifying practical and successful means of problem-solving [46]. After explaining the rationale for "homework" as a way to promote self-management, the patient is given a "homework" assignment for the week which involves daily relaxation training.

In the second session, the therapist notes the patient's progress in relaxation training. The therapist works with the patient to generate possible problem-solving strategies for her particular issues and to develop ways to establish priorities among various possible approaches. Homework for the period between the second and third sessions involves more training in relaxation. This is tailored to the needs of individual patients on the basis of their skills and/or deficits in following the procedure. The third session places a heavy focus on problem-solving, and the process of problem-solving is reviewed. At this point, the therapist explores current personal problems with the patient and applies this approach to these problems [13].

The following step-by-step approach to problem-solving can be practically helpful for both the therapist and the patient as mentioned by Sobel and Worden [47]: "1) Clearly define the most important problem, 2) Recognize how you feel about the problem, 3) Relax and try not to think about a solution for a while, 4) Consider all possible solutions, even bad ones, 5) Try to ignore how other people might solve the problem, 6) Evaluate the pros and cons of each possible solution, 7) Arrange the various possible solutions into a list, starting with the least desirable or least practical one, 8) Make a choice, and 9) Briefly consider some favorable or positive aspects of the original problem. Can it be thought about differently?"

During the fourth session, the patient and therapist together evaluate the effectiveness of the approach for dealing with problems during the preceding week. The problem-solving steps are reviewed, and the patient is given written information about these steps. The need for further sessions is evaluated, and if appropriate, the therapist terminates the formal sessions. Many cancer patients who are distressed believe that change is impossible. However, the philosophy behind this cognitive intervention is that change is possible, that patients can be taught to take steps on their own, and that problems can be reorganized into manageable proportions [13].

Behavioral techniques include passive relaxation with visual imagery, progressive muscle relaxation, electromyographic (EMG) feedback, systematic desensitization, and cognitive distraction [48–50].

Visual imaging is sometimes recommended for cancer patients to counter the passivity of the disease and treatment process. This technique can be performed by utilizing visual images of their bodies actively fighting off the cancer. Patients are able to work with specific images devised by the therapist in order to meet individual needs. Although controversial, imaging techniques help patients feel more in control and less helpless. Patients who have used this technique were found to experience a sense of mastery, assertiveness, and competence [39].

These methods are useful as adjuvant treatments, combined with pharmacologic agents for pain and during chemotherapy infusions [37].

Psychopharmacotherapy

Mild or moderate depression often resolves spontaneously [51], with resolution of a precipitating stressor. However, severe depression, such as MDD, may significantly benefit from pharmacotherapy, psychotherapy, or a combination of both [14]. Moreover, the combination of antidepressant therapy and cognitive therapy may enhance long-term recovery from depression compared with cognitive therapy alone [52].

Selective serotonin reuptake inhibitors (SSRIs) (e.g., paroxetine) and serotonin-norepinephrine reuptake inhibitors (e.g., mirtazapine) may be effective in improving depression [53, 54] and decreasing menopausal symptoms in breast cancer survivors [55–61]. The mechanism for these effects is likely mediated by the serotonergic effects of these agents. In addition, the norepinephrine reuptake inhibitor reboxetine is known to be effective in breast cancer patients with MDD [62]. A study of bupropion in early-stage breast cancer patients on hormonal therapy following chemotherapy showed improvement in both sexual functioning and Beck Depression Inventory (BDI) depression scores [63].

Estrogen may also serve as an adjunct to the treatment of depression in postmenopausal women [14]. A few studies [64, 65] found that depressed postmenopausal women taking SSRIs had better improvement in depressive symptoms and quality of life if they received estrogen replacement therapy. Therefore, clinicians should be careful of the possibility that antidepressant efficacy will be lower in women taking an estrogen antagonist, such as tamoxifen [14].

Care of the Terminally Ill

In care of the terminally ill, the art and science of medicine and psychiatry are blended. Often the art is strongly influenced by the caregiver's personality, by the histories of the family and patient, and by their psychosocial values and issues [66]. Conflicts that arise regarding decisions about care may lead to requests for psychiatric consultation and intervention [37].

Terminally ill patients are those who have not responded to known curative measures, and their treatment is aimed at providing maximal comfort during their remaining life span. When the label "dying" is assigned to a patient, attitudes and behaviors of staff, family, and friends often assume a different character that tends to isolate or alienate patients from those they need most at that crucial time. We often forget that the person who is dying has not changed; only their life expectancy has changed, and their emotional needs may intensify [37].

During the terminal stage, support from those close to them and religion both appear to play critical roles in helping patients cope with the process of dying [67].

18.4.1.2 Specific Treatment

Psychosocial factors are becoming increasingly important components of the assessment and management of patients with breast cancer. Clearly, the development and evaluation of psychological interventions that ameliorate treatment side effects and enhance quality of life are needed [68].

Whatever the course of the disease, the treatment team should be alert to the ever-present possibility of psychological morbidity, which, if present, requires rigorous evaluation and judicious referral. This referral may not only help to reduce morbidity but, perhaps more importantly, may also prevent disease dominance over the lives of affected women [5].

In particular, at the stage of hospitalization and operation, the major problems which patients face include the risks of surgery, the loss of a breast (including a disturbed body image and reduced self-esteem), and the prognosis, which may induce fear of a painful death, followed by anger and acceptance. During this period, women are at increased vulnerability to a number of psychological problems as the series of physiological and psychosocial stressors generated by the illness is continuous. Thus, psychiatric care can be more intensely required than at any other stage. It is recommended in these circumstances to help patients gain support from those closest to them and to confront their situation with a fighting spirit [67].

The times of most frequent psychiatric referral of breast cancer patients are during initial treatment and during treatment of metastatic or recurrent disease at a radiation oncology clinic [69]. There is a high incidence of MDD in this outpatient breast cancer population, although oncologists frequently fail to recognize it. Because psychiatric management is an important part of overall treatment, breast care services need to include clinical staff whose job it is to provide supportive care [69].

Half of all cancer patients have a psychiatric disorder, usually adjustment disorder with depression. Effective psychotherapeutic treatment for depression has been found to affect the course of cancer. Psychotherapy also resulted in longer survival time for patients with breast cancer. Psychotherapeutic effects include changes in health maintenance behavior, health-care utilization, endocrine environment, and immune function. Specifically, effective treatment of depression in cancer patients results in better patient adjustment, reduced symptoms, and reduced cost of care and may influence the disease course. Thus, the treatment of depression in these patients may be considered part of medical as well as psychiatric treatment [70].

Active confrontation with a fighting spirit may help patients with breast cancer to live longer than if they were to surrender to helplessness and hopelessness [71]. Also, patients who actively confront their illness and the uncertainty that surrounds it have been shown to have better psychological health [12]. Among coping strategies of patients with cancer, confrontation was found to have a positive effect and externalization to have a negative effect on the resolution of patients' pending problems [72].

Billings and Moos [73] found that the use of active, problem-focused therapy and minimal use of avoidance were associated with fewer physical and psychological symptoms and that patients who coped via problem-solving and emotional regulation had less severe dysfunction. Consistent with this, Smith et al. [74] found that avoidance contributed significantly to psychological disturbance following stressful life events in elderly adults. These findings suggest that counseling and support aimed at promoting engagement, such as actively seeking information about the situation, accepting understanding from someone, and talking to someone about one's feelings, may reduce anxiety and depression in patients with a potentially life-threatening illness [12].

Early work by Greer and Morris [75] found suppression of anger to be associated with a higher risk of breast malignancy. Anger is found to be associated with anxiety and is frequently directed toward physicians, hospital staff, and families [76]. Anger as well as anxiety and depression should be appropriately managed, sometimes with the help of a psychiatrist.

With breast cancer, a symbol of femininity may be compromised, and a woman's loss of a breast may interfere with her identity. The psychological impact of breast cancer varies from one woman to another. It depends on the patient's age, personality, life experience, social and familial relationships, and psychological or psychiatric history. When a cancer is diagnosed, especially breast cancer in women, the overall psychological history should be taken into account [77]. The therapist should help the patient to adjust to surgery and disfigurement and should encourage a return to prior activities without fear of what others are thinking [13]. As later illustrated in a case report, concerns about loss of femininity can sometimes be overcome by the therapist's helping the patient to express her emotion and encouraging the husband to assist her without being confrontational.

Breast conservation surgery can be considered in patients with severe disturbance of body image [17], since, compared to mastectomy, this operation is associated with a less negative body image [5]. In readjusting to normal life, diversions from the illness and self-validation (or relativizing) seem to be helpful during periods of convalescence and chemoradiotherapy [67].

Among women with breast cancer, marital status and perceived social support are positively related to survival. Maunsell et al. [78] studied 224 women with newly diagnosed breast cancer and examined the relationship between social support and mortality. Married women had a relative death rate of 0.86 compared to unmarried women over a 7-year follow-up. The death rate was even lower among those who shared their feelings with more than one confidant. Thus, the availability of social support through marriage and friends proved to be a robust predictor of survival [79].

Social support from a spouse, another intimate, or a physician, as well as actively seeking social support, has been shown to be related to higher natural killer (NK) cell activity in patients with stages I and II breast cancer [80].

Patients with persistent concerns about body image, sexual desire, and sexual function should be referred to professionals who are trained in sexual rehabilitation. Treatment techniques include supportive psychotherapy, behavioral techniques such as relaxation, and gradual reeducation in sexual functioning [37].

Case

A woman in her late 30s with breast cancer who had undergone radical mastectomy became depressed, along with a perceived loss of femininity and loss of self-esteem caused by the mastectomy. After being discharged from the hospital, the patient was encouraged by her sister to see a psychiatrist. She said, "I can't tolerate living with only one breast" and complained of insomnia and a lack of interest in life. She also showed strong resentment and anger toward her husband, recalling that he had shown little concern about her situation and had returned home late at night a few times several months earlier. Accompanied by the patient, her husband said apprehensively, "My wife is trying to avoid sleeping in the same bed with me." During her sessions, the patient was allowed to vent her emotions, including anger toward her husband's negligence. Antidepressant (fluoxetine) and antianxiety (ethyl loflazepate) agents were administered twice daily. Her anger level was assessed using a hostility questionnaire. She recorded high scores on the anger subscale, saying "I seemed to get sick because I had a bad temper." Then, a variety of coping strategies were reviewed, including a few considered good for her situation. Through the application of the strategies, she began to introspectively search her inner self.

She found herself egotistic and self-centered, and she regretted getting into religion only externally but not internally. In addition, with her husband's understanding of the situation and his active assistance, the patient began to accept her own reality, to forgive her husband for mistreating her, and to regain her emotional stability and self-confidence. The issue relevant to her loss of femininity was not directly confronted by the psychiatrist. Rather, she was encouraged to vent her anger and do her limited daily activities, while she would deal with issues surrounding her illness. Also, the therapist encouraged her husband to actively participate in the therapeutic session. Such measures as the therapist's effort and the husband's assistance helped the patient to overcome her depression caused by loss of femininity and anger toward her spouse and to return to her routine activities.

18.4.2 Family Therapy

Family therapy is also an essential part of this therapeutic approach. The best technique for motivating the family to become involved in therapy is to point out the need all families have for help in communicating and coping when they must live with cancer [81]. The patient's spouse is helped to come to terms with the reality of the cancer while providing support and nurture. Often, the spouse may first need to vent his or her own fear, sadness, and anger. Family members of a cancer patient may altruistically deny their own need for help while focusing on the illness and the patient's needs. This can be overcome by educating family members to relax and cope with the cancer so that their lowered anxiety levels will, in turn, decrease the stress on the patient [39].

Work should be done with spouses and other family members to diminish negative expressions of hostility and criticism to the cancer patient and to provide supportive coping strategies. Reestablishment of the sexual relationship needs to be explored and encouraged [82, 83]. Couples and multifamily groups are particularly helpful with cancer patients and spouses as they permit the crisis to be shared with others, allowing for more cooperation in problem-solving [39].

18.4.3 Group Psychotherapy

Group psychotherapy may be advantageous for cancer patients, allowing them to receive support from others (patients or nonpatients) who have experienced and conquered similar problems of medical illness. The cancer patient in a group setting can easily learn that there are a range of normal reactions to illness and a range of healthy adaptive coping styles and strategies which others have employed to make the adjustment to illness easier. Group participation helps decrease the sense of isolation and alienation as the cancer patient and his family can see that they are not alone in adjusting to illness [37]. Spiegel et al. [84] have reported on their success in leading groups of patients with breast cancer at all stages of disease, ranging from recently diagnosed patients to the terminally ill. These types of groups, when directed by skilled leaders, can be highly rewarding for many patients. The principles of group therapy in general also apply to cancer patients [37].

A randomized trial of supportive-expressive group therapy was conducted for women with metastatic breast cancer [84]. Fifty of 86 women were randomly assigned to weekly support groups which emphasized building strong support bonds, expressing emotions, dealing directly with fears of dying and death, reordering life priorities, improving relationships with family and friends, enhancing communication and shared problem-solving with physicians, and learning self-hypnosis for pain control. Over a 10-year follow-up, there was a statistically significant survival advantage for women in the group therapy condition; they lived an average of 18 months longer.

18.4.4 Self-Help and Mutual Support Programs

Self-help and mutual support programs offer alternative support for patients and families. Life crises, such as bereavement, separation, divorce, drug addiction, and life-threatening illness, often provide the impetus for individuals to seek emotional support from others experiencing the same trauma. For example, Reach to Recovery was officially sponsored by the American Cancer Society in 1952 to meet the needs of women undergoing mastectomies [37].

Most self-help support networks for cancer patients work closely with professional medical services, thereby offering social support as an adjunct to medical care. The patient-to-patient program is one such program in which volunteers visit every newly admitted cancer patient. Such volunteers help decrease the sense of alienation and isolation of patients due to their unique knowledge and sensitivity, which comes from having undergone the same experience. In particular, veteran patient volunteers facilitate coping in the newly diagnosed patient [37].

Self-help programs staffed by cancer patients provide empathy and share common reactions experienced by cancer patients. These programs provide a great deal of support, information, and role models for successful adaptation and recovery [39].

18.5 Biopsychosocial Effects of Psychological Interventions

Psychological distress can influence tumor progression via many different pathways (e.g., genetic changes, immune surveillance, and pro-angiogenic processes). Psychological intervention has been shown to facilitate psychological adaptation to breast cancer [85]. Psychological interventions include strategies to reduce stress, improve mood, alter health behaviors, and maintain adherence to cancer treatment and care [86].

Psychological interventions were reported to have a number of favorable effects on biopsychosocial parameters in patients with breast cancer. For example, psychological interventions can attenuate emotional distress such as anxiety and depression manifested during radiotherapy treatment [87]. In addition, psychological interventions can influence neuroendocrine (e.g., cortisol) and immune function indicators, especially lymphocyte proliferation and Th1 cytokine production [85]. For example, those assigned to a 10-week group-based cognitive-behavioral stress management program evidenced better psychosocial adaptation (reduced anxiety symptoms) and physiological adaptation (lower cortisol and greater Th1 cytokine interleukin-2 (IL-2) and interferon-γ (IFN-γ) production) after adjuvant treatment compared to those in the control group [88]. In another study, immune responses paralleled psychological and behavioral improvements from psychological interventions. T-cell proliferation in response to PHA and Con A remained stable or increased for the intervention patients, whereas both responses declined for assessment-only patients [89]. Experiential-existential group psychotherapy reduced levels of plasma cortisol and prolactin compared to those in a waiting-list control group [90].

However, it was suggested that behavioral rather than immunity change was influential in achieving weaker symptoms and higher functional status. Therefore, distress reduction is highlighted as an important mechanism by which health can be improved in breast cancer patients [91]. Moreover, psychological adaptation in women with breast cancer can reduce anxiety and depressive mood and improve quality of life, which affects immune functions, such as increased production of the Th1 cytokine IL-2, IFN-γ, and tumor necrosis factor-α (TNF-α) [92].

Psychological interventions can also improve survival. Psychological intervention patients were found to have reduced risks of breast cancer recurrence and death from breast cancer compared with the assessment-only patients [86]. However, the relationship between supportive-expressive group therapy and longer survival was not replicated in another study [93].

18.6 Conclusions

Oncologists should be alert to each patient's emotional reactions and potential psychiatric problems, and if necessary, they should refer them to a psychiatrist or other mental health professionals. A number of psychotherapeutic, behavioral, and psychopharmacologic techniques are available for the care of patients with breast cancer. Psychotherapeutic modalities include individual, family, and group therapy, as well as self-help treatment, and involve general treatments that deal with crisis-intervention and use cognitive-behavioral approach, as well as specific treatments that address particular issues relevant to patients with breast cancer. Based on this review, it is apparent that proper and effective care for patients with breast cancer requires the combined use of a variety of therapeutic modalities as well as a multidisciplinary approach that includes psychiatric care. This chapter highlights the biopsychosocial effects of psychological interventions for distress reduction and psychological adaptation as an important mechanism by which health can be improved in breast cancer patients. The guidelines presented in this chapter are expected to contribute to the relief and prevention of emotional suffering stemming from experiences with the most common form of cancer in women.

References

1. Massie, M. J., & Holland, J. C. (1991). Psychological reactions to breast cancer in the pre- and post-surgical treatment period. *Seminars in Surgical Oncology, 7*, 320–325.
2. Rowland, J. H., & Massie, M. J. (1996). Patient rehabilitation and support. In J. R. Harris, M. E. Lippman, & M. Morrow (Eds.), *Disease of the breast*. Philadelphia: Lippincott-Raven.
3. Forsén, A. (1991). Psychosocial stress as a risk for breast cancer. *Psychotherapy and Psychosomatics, 55*, 176–185.
4. Kissane, D. W., Bloch, S., & Miach, P. (1997). Cognitive-existential group therapy for patients with primary breast cancer-techniques and themes. *Psycho-Oncology, 6*, 25–33.
5. Kissane, D. W., Clarke, D. M., Ikin, J., et al. (1998). Psychological morbidity and quality of life in Australian women with early-stage breast cancer: A cross-sectional survey. *The Medical Journal of Australia, 169*, 192–196.
6. Maguire, G. P., Lee, E. G., & Bevington, D. J. (1978). Psychiatric problems in the first year after mastectomy. *British Medical Journal, 279*, 963–965.
7. Fallowfield, L. J., Baum, M., & Maguire, G. P. (1986). Effects of breast conservation on psychological morbidity associated with diagnosis and treatment of early breast cancer. *British Medical Journal, 293*, 1331–1334.
8. Fallowfield, L. J., Hall, A., Maguire, G. P., et al. (1990). Psychological outcomes of different treatment policies in women with early breast cancer outside a clinical trial. *British Medical Journal, 301*, 575–580.
9. Sprangers, M. A. G., Groenvold, M., & Arraras, J. I. (1996). The European Organization for Research and Treatment of Cancer breast cancer specific quality-of-life questionnaire module. First results from a three country field study. *Journal of Clinical Oncology, 14*, 2756–2768.
10. Payne, D. K., Sullivan, M. D., & Massie, M. J. (1996). Women's psychological reactions to breast cancer. *Seminars in Oncology, 23*(Suppl. 2), 89–97.
11. Vinokur, A. D., Threatt, B. A., Vinokur-Kaplan, D., et al. (1990). The process of recovery from breast cancer for younger and older patients: Changes during the first year. *Cancer, 65*, 1242–1254.
12. Chen, C. C., David, A., Thompson, K., et al. (1996). Coping strategies and psychiatric morbidity in women attending breast assessment clinics. *Journal of Psychosomatic Research, 40*, 265–270.
13. Worden, J. W. (1987). Cognitive therapy with cancer patients. In A. Freeman & V. Greenwood (Eds.), *Cognitive therapy: Applications in psychiatric and medical settings*. New York: Human Science Press.
14. Fann, J. R., Thomas-rich, A. M., Katon, W. J., et al. (2008). Major depression after breast cancer: A review of epidemiology and treatment. *General Hospital Psychiatry, 30*, 112–126.
15. Massie, M. J., & Holland, J. (1989). Overview of normal reactions and prevalence of psychiatric disorders. In J. C. Holland & J. R. Rowland (Eds.), *Handbook of Psycho-oncology*. New York: Oxford University Press.

16. Iwamitsu, Y., Shimoda, K., Abe, H., et al. (2005). The relation between negative emotional suppression and emotional distress in breast cancer diagnosis and treatment. *Health Communication, 18*, 201–215.
17. Mamelock, A. E. (1995). Psychiatry and surgery. In H. I. Kaplan & B. J. Sadock (Eds.), *Comprehensive Textbook of Psychiatry*. Baltimore: Williams & Wilkins.
18. Lim, C. C., Devi, M. K., & Ang, E. (2011). Anxiety in women with breast cancer undergoing treatment: A systematic review. *International Journal of Evidence-Based Healthcare, 9*, 215–235.
19. Courtier, N., Gambling, T., Enright, S., et al. (2012). Psychological and immunological characteristics of fatigued women undergoing radiotherapy for early-stage breast cancer. *Supportive Care in Cancer*. doi:10.1007/s00520-012-1508-6.
20. McGinty, H. L., Goldenberg, J. L., & Jacobsen, P. B. (2012). Relationship of threat appraisal with coping appraisal to fear of cancer recurrence in breast cancer survivors. *Psycho-Oncology, 21*, 203–210.
21. Cordova, M. J., Andrykowski, M. A., Kenady, D. E., et al. (1995). Frequency and correlates of posttraumatic-stress-disorder-like symptoms after treatment for breast cancer. *Journal of Consulting and Clinical Psychology, 63*, 981–986.
22. Ha, E. H., Seo, J. E., Jeong, J., et al. (2008). Biopsychosocial predictors of depressive disorder in breast cancer patients. *Korean Journal of Clinical Psychology, 27*, 961–976.
23. Massie, M. J. (2004). Prevalence of depression in patients with cancer. *Journal of the National Cancer Institute Monographs, 32*, 57–71.
24. McDaniel, J. S., Musselman, D. L., Porter, M. R., et al. (1995). Depression in patients with cancer. Diagnosis, biology, and treatment. *Archives of General Psychiatry, 52*, 89–99.
25. Halbreich, U., Rojansky, N., Palter, S., et al. (1995). Estrogen auguments serotonergic activity in postmenopausal women. *Biological Psychiatry, 37*, 434–441.
26. Melzer, H. (1990). Role of serotonin in depression. *Annals of the New York Academy of Sciences, 600*, 486–495.
27. Young, E. A., Midgley, A. R., Carson, N. E., et al. (2000). Alteration in the hypothalamic-pituitary-ovarian axis in depressed women. *Archives of General Psychiatry, 57*, 1157–1162.
28. Harlow, B. L., Wise, L. A., Otto, M. W., et al. (2003). Depression and its influence on reproductive endocrine and menstrual cycle markers associated with perimenopause: The Harvard study of moods and cycles. *Archives of General Psychiatry, 60*, 29–36.
29. Sumner, B. E., Grant, K. E., Rosie, R., et al. (1999). Effects of tamoxifen on serotonin transporter and 5-hydroxytryptamine (2A) receptor binding sites and mRNA levels in the brain of ovariectomized rats with or without acute estradiol replacement. *Brain Research. Molecular Brain Research, 73*, 119–128.
30. Cleeland, C. S., Bennett, G. J., Dantzer, R., et al. (2003). Are the symptoms of cancer and cancer treatment due to shared biologic mechanism? A cytokine-immunologic model of cancer symptoms. *Cancer, 97*, 2919–2925.
31. Raison, C. L., & Miller, A. H. (2003). Depression in cancer: New developments regarding diagnosis and treatment. *Biological Psychiatry, 54*, 283–294.
32. Dantzer, R. (2001). Cytokine-induced sickness behavior: Where do we stand? *Brain, Behavior, and Immunity, 15*, 7–24.
33. Kronfol, Z., & Remick, D. G. (2000). Cytokines and the brain: Implications for clinical psychiatry. *The American Journal of Psychiatry, 157*, 683–694.
34. Capuron, L., & Dantzer, R. (2003). Cytokines and depression: The need for a new paradigm. *Brain, Behavior, and Immunity, 17*(suppl. 1), S119–S124.
35. Schiepers, O. J., Wichers, M. C., & Maes, M. (2005). Cytokines and major depression. *Progress in Neuro-Psychopharmacology & Biological Psychiatry, 29*, 201–217.
36. Spiegel, D. (1997). Psychosocial aspects of breast cancer treatment. *Seminars in Oncology, 24*, S1-36–S1-47.
37. Lesko, L. M., Massie, M. J., & Holland, J. C. (1987). Oncology. In A. Stoudemire & B. S. Fogel (Eds.), *Principles of medical psychiatry*. Orlando, FL: Grune & Stratton.

38. Marmor, J. (1979). Short-term dynamic psychotherapy. *The American Journal of Psychiatry, 136*, 149–155.
39. Kaufman, E., & Micha, V. G. (1987). A model for psychotherapy with the good-prognosis cancer patient. *Psychosomatics, 28*, 540–547.
40. Fiore, N. (1979). Fighting cancer: One patient's perspective. *The New England Journal of Medicine, 300*, 284–289.
41. Bloom, J. R., Ross, R. D., & Burnell, G. (1978). The effect of social support on patient adjustment after breast surgery. *Patient Counselling and Health Education, 1*, 50–59.
42. La Barba, R. C. (1970). Experimental and environmental factors in cancer. *Psychosomatic Medicine, 32*, 259–269.
43. Jerse, M. A., Whitman, H. H., & Gustafson, J. P. (1984). Cancer in adults. In H. B. Roback (Ed.), *Helping patients and their families cope with medical problems*. San Francisco: Jossey-Bass.
44. Janis, E., & Mann, L. (1997). *Decision-making*. New York: Free Press.
45. Spivack, G., Platt, J., & Schure, M. (1976). *The problem-solving approach to adjustment*. San Francisco: Jossey-Bass.
46. Benson, H. (1975). *The relaxation response*. New York: Morrow.
47. Sobel, H. J., & Worden, J. W. (1979). *Helping cancer patients cope: A problem solving intervention program for health care professionals*. New York: Guilford Press.
48. Burish, T. G., & Lyles, J. N. (1981). Effectiveness of relaxation training in reducing adverse reactions to cancer chemotherapy. *Journal of Behavioral Medicine, 4*, 65–78.
49. Morrow, G. R., & Morrell, B. S. (1982). Behavioral treatment for the anticipatory nausea and vomiting induced by cancer chemotheray. *The New England Journal of Medicine, 306*, 1476–1480.
50. Redd, W. H., Andresen, G. V., & Minagawa, Y. (1982). Hypnotic control of anticipatory emesis in patients receiving cancer chemotherapy. *Journal of Consulting and Clinical Psychology, 50*, 14–19.
51. Williams, J. W., Barrett, J., Oxman, T., et al. (2000). Treatment of dysthymia and minor depression in primary care: A randomized controlled trial in older adults. *Journal of the American Medical Association, 284*, 1519–1526.
52. Maguire, P., Hopwood, P., Tarrier, N., et al. (1985). Treatment of depression in cancer patients. *Acta Psychiatrica Scandinavica. Supplementum, 320*, 81–84.
53. Morrow, G. R., Hickok, J. T., Roscoe, J. A., et al. (2003). Differential effects of paroxetine on fatigue and depression: A randomized, double-blind trail from the University of Rochester Cancer Center Community Clinical Oncology Program. *Journal of Clinical Oncology, 21*, 4635–4641.
54. Thompson, D. S. (2000). Mirtazapine for the treatment of depression and nausea in breast and gynecological oncology. *Psychosomatics, 41*, 356–359.
55. Loprinzi, C. L., Kugler, J. W., Sloan, J. A., et al. (2000). Venlafaxine in management of hot flashes in survivors of breast cancer: A randomized controlled trial. *Lancet, 356*, 2059–2063.
56. Loprinzi, C. L., Sloan, J. A., Perez, E. A., et al. (2002). Phase III evaluation of fluoxetine for treatment of hot flashes. *Journal of Clinical Oncology, 20*, 1578–1583.
57. Stearns, V., Issacs, C., Rowland, J., et al. (2000). A pilot trial assessing the efficacy of paroxetine hydrochloride (Paxil) in controlling hot flashes in breast cancer survivors. *Annals of Oncology, 11*, 17–22.
58. Soares, C. N., Poitras, J. R., Prouty, J., et al. (2003). Efficacy of citalopram as a monotherapy or as an adjunctive treatment to estrogen therapy for perimenopausal and postmenopausal women with depression and vasomotor symptoms. *The Journal of Clinical Psychiatry, 64*, 473–479.
59. Kimmick, G. G., Lovato, J., McQuellon, R., et al. (2006). Randomized, double-blind, placebo-controlled, crossover study of sertraline (zoloft) for the treatment of hot flashes in women with early stage breast cancer taking tamoxifen. *The Breast Journal, 12*, 114–122.
60. Stearns, V., Beebe, K. L., Iyengar, M., et al. (2003). Paroxetine controlled release in the treatment of menopausal hot flashes: A randomized controlled trial. *Journal of the American Medical Association, 289*, 2827–2834.

61. Gordon, P. R., Kerwin, J. P., Boesen, K. G., et al. (2006). Sertraline to treat hot flashes: A randomized controlled, double-blind, crossover trial in a general population. *Menopause, 13*, 568–575.
62. Grassi, L., Biancosino, B., Marmai, L., et al. (2004). Effect of reboxetine on major depressive disorder in breast cancer patients: An open-label study. *The Journal of Clinical Psychiatry, 65*, 515–520.
63. Mathias, C., Cardeal Mendes, C. M., Ponde de Sena, E., et al. (2006). An open-label, fixed-dose study of bupropion effect on sexual function scores in women treated for breast cancer. *Annals of Oncology, 17*, 1792–1796.
64. Schneider, L. S., Small, G. W., & Clary, C. M. (2001). Estrogen replacement therapy and anti-depressant response to sertraline in older depressed women. *The American Journal of Geriatric Psychiatry, 9*, 393–399.
65. Schneider, L. S., Small, G. W., Hamilton, S. H., et al. (1997). Estrogen replacement and response to fluoxetine in a multicenter geriatric depression trial. Fluoxetine collaborative study group. *The American Journal of Geriatric Psychiatry, 5*, 97–106.
66. Holland, J. C. (1982). Psychological issues in the care of the terminally ill. In F. Flach (Ed.), *Directions in psychiatry*. New York: Hatherleigh.
67. Heim, E., Augustiny, K. F., Schaffner, L., et al. (1993). Coping with breast cancer over time and situation. *Journal of Psychosomatic Research, 37*, 523–542.
68. Walker, L. G., & Eremin, O. (1996). Psychological assessment and intervention: Future prospects for women with breast cancer. *Seminars in Surgical Oncology, 12*, 76–83.
69. Pendlebury, S. C., & Snars, J. (1996). Role of a psychiatry liaison clinic in the management of breast cancer. *Australasian Radiology, 40*, 283–286.
70. Spiegel, D. (1996). Cancer and depression. *The British Journal of Psychiatry, 30*(Suppl.), 109–116.
71. Greer, S., Morris, T., & Pettingale, K. W. (1979). Psychological response to breast cancer: Effect on outcome. *Lancet, 2*, 785–787.
72. Koh, K. B., & Kim, S. T. (1988). Coping strategy of cancer patients. *Journal of Korean Neuropsychiatric Association, 27*, 140–150.
73. Billings, A. G., & Moos, R. H. (1981). The role of coping responses in attenuating the stress of life events. *Journal of Behavioral Medicine, 4*, 139–157.
74. Smith, L. W., Patterson, T. L., & Grant, I. (1990). Avoidant coping predicts psychological disturbance in the elderly. *The Journal of Nervous and Mental Disease, 178*, 525–530.
75. Greer, S., & Morrs, T. (1975). Psychological attributes of women who develop breast cancer: A controlled study. *Journal of Psychosomatic Research, 19*, 147–153.
76. Peck, A. (1972). Emotional reactions to having cancer. *The American Journal of Roentgenology, Radium Therapy, and Nuclear Medicine, 114*, 591–599.
77. Daune, F. (1995). Psychological aspects of breast cancer. *Revue Médicale de Bruxelles, 16*, 245–247.
78. Maunsell, E., Jacques, B., & Deschenes, L. (1993). *Social support, a survival among women with breast cancer*. Presented at the annual Psycho-oncology meeting, Memorial Sloan-Kettering Cancer Center. New York.
79. Spiegel, D., & Kato, P. M. (1996). Psychosocial influences on cancer incidence and progression. *Harvard Review of Psychiatry, 4*, 10–26.
80. Levy, S. M., Herberman, R. B., Whiteside, T., et al. (1990). Perceived social support and tumor- estrogen/progesterone receptor status as predictors of natural killer cell activity in breast cancer patients. *Psychosomatic Medicine, 52*, 73–85.
81. Wellisch, D. (1980). Psychosocial problems of cancer. In C. M. Haskell (Ed.), *Cancer treatment*. Philadelphia: WB Saunders.
82. Pfeffenbaum, G., Pasnau, R., & Jamison, K. (1977). A comprehensive program of psychosocial care for mastectomy patients. *International Journal of Psychiatry in Medicine, 8*, 65–71.

83. Schain, W. S. (1982). Sexual problems of patients with cancer. In V. T. Devita, S. Hellman, & S. A. Rosenberg (Eds.), *Cancer: Principles and practices of oncology*. Philadelphia: JB Lippincott.
84. Spiegel, D., Bloom, J. R., & Yalom, I. D. (1981). Group support for patients with metastatic cancer: A randomized prospective outcome study. *Archives of General Psychiatry, 38*, 527–533.
85. McGregor, B. A., & Antoni, M. H. (2009). Psychological intervention and health outcomes among women treated for breast cancer: A review of stress pathways and biological mediators. *Brain, Behavior, and Immunity, 23*, 159–166.
86. Andersen, B. L., Yang, H. C., Farrar, W. B., et al. (2008). Psychologic intervention improves survival for breast cancer patients: A randomized clinical trial. *Cancer, 113*, 3450–3458.
87. Nunes, D. F., Rodriguez, A. L., da Silva, H. F., et al. (2007). Relaxation and guided imagery program in patients with breast cancer undergoing radiotherapy is not associated with neuroimmunomodulatory effects. *Journal of Psychosomatic Research, 63*, 647–655.
88. Antoni, M. H., Lechner, S., Diaz, A., et al. (2009). Cognitive behavioral stress management effects on psychosocial and physiological adaptation in women undergoing treatment for breast cancer. *Brain, Behavior, and Immunity, 23*, 580–591.
89. Andersen, B. L., Farrar, W. B., Golden-Kreutz, D. M., et al. (2004). Psychological, behavioral, and immune changes after a psychological intervention: A clinical trial. *Journal of Clinical Oncology, 22*, 3570–3580.
90. van der Pompe, G., Duivenvoorden, H. J., Antoni, M. H., et al. (1997). Effectiveness of a short-term group psychotherapy program on endocrine and immune function in breast cancer patients: An exploratory study. *Journal of Psychosomatic Research, 42*, 453–466.
91. Andersen, B. L., Golden-Kreutz, D., Emery, C. F., et al. (2007). Distress reduction from a psychological intervention contributes to improved health for cancer patients. *Brain, Behavior, and Immunity, 21*, 953–961.
92. Blomberg, B. B., Alvarez, J. P., Diaz, A., et al. (2009). Psychosocial adaptation and cellular immunity in breast cancer patients in the weeks after surgery: An exploratory study. *Journal of Psychosomatic Research, 67*, 369–376.
93. Spiegel, D., Butler, L. D., Giese-Davis, J., et al. (2007). Effects of supportive-expressive group therapy on survival of patients with metastatic breast cancer: A randomized prospective trial. *Cancer, 110*, 1130–1138.

Part VII
Specific Therapeutic Interventions and Biological Effects of Interventions

Chapter 19
Motivational Interviewing in Psychosomatic Medicine

Sung Hee Cho

19.1 Introduction

Motivational interviewing (MI) was developed by Miller in 1983 initially as a brief intervention for problem drinking to elicit motivation for change [1]. Since then, MI has been widely used in the treatment of various types of psychological problems and behavior problems. Psychological problems include anxiety, depression, post-traumatic stress disorder (PTSD), eating disorder, substance abuse and dependence, and pathological gambling, and behavior problems include medication adherence and health-related behaviors such as diet, smoking, exercise, and sexual behavior [2, 3]. MI also has been found to be effective in health-care settings such as dentistry, emergency department, mental health department, and rehabilitation center. A topical bibliography of research is found [4]; MI has been applied to a variety of physical diseases including asthma, head injury, cardiovascular disease (e.g., hypertension), diabetes, obesity, HIV/AIDS, and pain disorder. In addition, domestic violence, family relationships, and offenders are candidates for MI.

MI is a supportive style of communication and is defined as "a client-centered, directive method for enhancing intrinsic motivation to change by exploring and resolving ambivalence" [2]. MI is found to be effective in removing ambivalence and increasing an individual's confidence in his or her ability to make positive changes in his or her life.

MI is not a counseling but a communication style, developed to elicit a client's motivation for change and adherence to treatment. MI works when a clinician adheres to MI spirit, MI principles, and MI skills. Clients who are referred for consultation often look lacking in motivation to change; they seem to resist a change. Clinicians regard the clients as those who need a push to change and tend to use a

S.H. Cho, Ph.D. (✉)
Christian Studies Division, Baekseok University, 115 Anseo-dong, dongnam-gu, Cheonan, Chungnam Province 330-704, Korea
e-mail: cho@bu.ac.kr

K.B. Koh (ed.), *Somatization and Psychosomatic Symptoms*,
DOI 10.1007/978-1-4614-7119-6_19,

directive style of communication to tell those clients what to do and not to do. In fact, it is easier to tell them what to do or not to do, rather than to listen and reflect what they try to convey. On the other hand, MI involves listening as much as telling, guiding more than directing, and communicating more than coercing.

MI considers motivation as a state of readiness to change, rather than as a personality. Motivation is thought to fluctuate depending upon the relationship between the client and the clinician. Miller [2] states that motivation can be defined as the probability that a person will enter into, continue, and adhere to a specific change strategy. Direction of change is determined by the client and is supported as a goal of therapy by the clinician. Whether the client will follow a course of change depends on how much motivated he or she may be. Nevertheless, the clinician has a crucial role to play in helping the client enhance motivation for change.

19.2 The Clinical Population with Psychosomatic Symptoms

Psychosocial stressors play a role in influencing changes in psychosomatic symptoms. In explaining the relationship between stress and illness, Koh [5] stated that 71 % of medical (nonsurgical) inpatients experience psychosomatic disorders in Korea. They have stressors, most of which are chronic and ordinary daily stressors. Stressors affect their psychological state, causing depression and anxiety and leading to deterioration in physical symptoms.

When depression and anxiety lessen, psychosomatic symptoms become relieved. MI is found to be effective in reducing depression and in enhancing the effectiveness of approaches such as psychotherapy and drug therapy for depression [6, 7]. Arkowitz and Burke suggested that MI may be used as an integrative framework into which other therapies can be incorporated for the treatment of depression [6].

Domestic violence victims frequently experience psychosomatic symptoms that include chest pain, severe headache, digestion problems, body numbness, and arthritis [8, 9]. Violence victims go through a series of chronic stressors. The stressors include unanticipated, irregular violent acts of spouse, which induce chronic anxiety, fear, and depression [10, 11].

Women at shelters for domestic violence victims are usually in need of clinic visits for assessment and treatment due to various types of somatic symptoms during their stay. Women at shelters are brought to physical checkup on arrival, and most of them report chest pain, severe headache, body ache, indigestion, sleep disturbance, poor appetite, attention deficit, concentration problem, memory disturbance, and other cognitive problems. Depression, anger, frustration, fear, and helplessness are prominent among them. A variety of programs are provided for these women while they stay at shelters, including individual, couple, family, and group therapy. These programs are designed to help them empowered and to stand on their feet regardless of their further decisions.

Alleviating psychological distress helps reduce somatic discomforts. They are expected to change in self-efficacy, self-confidence, independent life style, and independent relationship; they need time for themselves in self-care, recovery, and job training.

Women at shelters know they should make a change in relationship with their spouses, their children, and their relatives, and about living conditions, but they feel afraid of making such changes. They feel helpless about doing something different from the way they are used to. They are so used to being told what to do or not to do; they are used to obeying what the spouses tell them to do and feeling little power and control about the surroundings. They are filled with frustration, depression, low self-esteem, fear, anxiety, anger, shame, social isolation, fear of financial burden, social pressure about divorce, and self-blame about spouse abuses. Severe guilty feeling, emptiness, and suicidal ideation are often reported. Some women suffer from insomnia and sometimes abuse alcohol or drugs. They isolate themselves from people and feel taken advantage of by others. During their stay at shelters, interpersonal conflicts occasionally occur and need staff intervention to solve the problems.

Women at shelters were given scales to measure depression and self-esteem, and 70–80 % of them scored within the range of high severity on depression scale [8, 9]. They had guilty feeling toward parents; shame, resentment, and guilt toward children; resentment toward in-laws; and fear and uncertainty about future.

Some studies found that the use of MI was effective in increasing self-efficacy of women at domestic violence shelters about ending violence and avoiding violent relationships [12, 13]. Hughes and Rasmussen [13] found MI to be effective in increasing self-esteem, self-concept, self-determination, self-strength, self-love, confidence, belief in capability of good life, decision-making, and responsibility for own growth; they found less anger, less fear, and less ambivalence.

19.3 Motivational Interviewing

MI is a communication style to enhance intrinsic motivation for change and to resolve ambivalence about change. It is defined as "client-centered, directive" style of communication founded on Roger's client-centered therapy [2]. MI focuses on ambivalence as a key to enhance motivation for change. Ambivalence may look like resistance and anger. However, when ambivalence is recognized by clients, it helps them make a decision and eventually enact change. MI is characterized as the overall "spirit," of which three components are collaboration, evocation, and autonomy [2].

19.3.1 MI Spirit

Collaboration refers to the clinician working in partnership with the client. A cooperative and collaborative partnership means equal power between the two. Involved in an active collaboration, the clinician does not direct the client in what to do, but they cooperate in the decision-making process. MI is an interview and conversation rather than a consultation or counseling [2]. The clinician does not teach but listen to and reflect what the client has in mind. There is respect for the client's past experience including achievement, trial and error, and attempts to make good changes in life. Client's goals become clear by collaborative endeavors.

Instead of giving the clients what they need or lack, for instance, medication, knowledge, information, insight, or skills, the clinician evokes from the clients what they already have or know and activate motivation for change. The resources inside their frame of reference are drawn out for the client to recognize them, and their self-efficacy is supported for the client utilize the resources and enact change. Each client has personal goals, values, concerns, and aspirations for future. MI evokes these elements the client has and helps the client be connected with them and motivated for change. It can be done only by evoking the client's own good reasons for change and arguments for change and understanding the client's own perspectives. During conversation, the clinician talks less than the client, elicits what the client has as resources and strengths for change, and reinforces the client to talk about these elements for himself.

Autonomy of the client is respected and honored. MI is based on the belief that the client can and do make choices, so a certain degree of detachment from the outcomes is required. There is acceptance that human nature resists being coerced and told what to do and not to do, and ultimately it is the client who decides and enacts what to do. On the other hand, there is acknowledgment that the client has right and freedom not to change, and ultimately it is the client who is responsible for the consequences. Information and advice, if needed from the clinician's point of view, may be given but only after finding out that the client wants to hear about it. When the autonomy to make a decision to hear about information and advice is respected, motivation for change is also elicited.

Miller and Rollnick [2] described four basic principles and fundamental skills of MI as expressing empathy, developing discrepancy, rolling with resistance, and supporting self-efficacy.

19.3.2 MI Principles

19.3.2.1 Express Empathy

MI employs the therapeutic skill of empathy throughout the course of conversation between the client and the clinician. It is possible only by listening to what the client says and by reflecting what it implies. There are the client's concerns, ambivalent feelings, ambition and aspiration, need, and desires, which can be drawn out by reflective listening. Empathic warmth is basically from acceptance of the client's feelings and perspectives without judging, criticizing, or blaming and acceptance of the ambivalence of the client as normal state of mind. Acceptance is not the same thing as agreement or approval of the client's perspective, that is, the clinician can have different opinion from that of the client. Important is that the clinician builds a working therapeutic relationship and supports the client's self-efficacy and responds to the client's point of view as understandable. Ambivalence and reluctance to change is accepted as normal.

19.3.2.2 Develop Discrepancy

Discrepancy is the ambivalence and dilemma between what the client is and does and what the client wants to be and what the client wants to do. MI involves helping the client more aware of the conflicts between the two. The awareness makes it possible for the client to become more objective about his or her present act and to make a commitment to change. Client's awareness of consequences, which conflict with his or her own goals in life, is important in a decision-making process. It is so-called contemplation stage of change [14] when the client faces the conflicts, and from this awareness the client is motivated to search alternatives to take in action for change [14]. Prochaska and DiClemente [14] suggested five stages of change: pre-contemplation, contemplation, preparation, action, and maintenance stage. In contemplation stage of change, the client both considers and rejects the ambivalence; when allowed to talk about it without interference, the client becomes empowered and motivated to make a decision and more likely to go forth without feeling pressured or coerced.

19.3.2.3 Roll with Resistance

MI considers resistance as a signal to change strategies [2]. Reflective listening to what the client feels under resistance is crucial to free from resistance and to keep motivated to change. Instead of confronting or arguing with the client's resistance, the clinician can turn or reframe client's statements slightly and create a new perspective toward change. Certainly, a new perspective is not imposed on the client; rather, the client is invited to perceive in a new perspective. Reflecting his ambivalence is another way to become free from resistance. Clients will gain insight into their fear and concerns about change and become motivated to change.

19.3.2.4 Support Self-Efficacy

MI considers self-efficacy as a key element in motivation for change, and the client's belief in the possibility of change is an important motivator. During the conversation the clinician helps the client talk about past achievements, future hope, desire, resources to utilize, and confidence to carry out personal change, which leads to self-efficacy. Affirming the client's past endeavors and current efforts is another way to support self-efficacy and to empower the client.

Rollnick et al. [4] related these four basic MI principles using the acronym RULE.

19.3.2.5 Resist the Righting Reflex (R)

Clinicians should resist "righting reflex" [4]; in other words, they have to refrain from correcting and giving advice without being requested to do so. Instead of correcting the client's present act, flaws, obstacles, and unmotivated state of mind, resisting such urge and listening to the client is more effective in keeping the client motivated to change. Resisting the urge to persuade or to fix the problem right is important to help the client not resist but go forth changing.

19.3.2.6 Understand the Client's Motivation (U)

The client needs to express his or her own good reasons or arguments to change or not to change. The client, not the clinician, is the one who must talk about his or her concerns, values, motivation, and what to expect from change or no change.

19.3.2.7 Listen to the Client (L)

The clinician's listening is essential to understand the client's motivation, and it involves an empathic interest in the client.

19.3.2.8 Empower the Client (E)

Engaging the client to explore how to make a change is more likely to create an action and make the change happen. It increases the client's self-efficacy.

19.3.3 MI Skills

MI suggests some fundamental skills which are consistent with the above principles: OARS in acronym.

19.3.3.1 Open-Ended Questions (O)

It is relatively easy to ask closed questions to obtain facts and opinions of the client, but MI utilizes open-ended questions to elicit the client to talk about what is in mind on his own. Active involvement can be induced by asking open-ended questions, which helps ambivalence to be elicited and expressed verbally.

19.3.3.2 Affirm (A)

Direct affirmation can help the client motivated and empowered to be engaged in the conversation. Appreciation and compliments are ways to affirm the client.

19.3.3.3 Reflective Listening (R)

Reflective listening is essential in MI. Reflective listening is an expression of empathy and makes the client feel accepted by the clinician. It is crucial in MI that empathy is directly related with motivation for change. Forms of reflection include simple reflection, amplified reflection, and double-sided reflection. Repeating the client's statement is a simple reflection; stating what it implies and reframing is an amplified reflection; stating ambivalence or underlying dilemma is a double-sided reflection. The clinician decides what to reflect, what to ignore, and what words to use in reflection. The client's statements which are related with change, such as concerns about change, reasons, needs, ability, and confidence about change, are called the client's change talk [2]. The client's change talk should be reflected back so that he or she can hear it again.

19.3.3.4 Summarize (S)

Summarizing on occasions during conversation as well as at the end of conversation is helpful for the client to feel empathized. The client hears in summary what has been said and realizes that the clinician has been attentively listening and feels respected. This motivates the client.

In addition to these skills, eliciting the client's change talk is crucial in helping the client make a commitment to take an action. The client's change talk is found to be the strongest predictor of behavior change [15]. The more change talk, the more possibility of change.

19.4 How MI Fits into Psychosomatic Population

The first principle of MI is expressing empathy. Empathy is a crucial element for therapeutic relationship and has a substantial effect on recovery from depression in clients [16, 17]. Therapeutic relationship is characterized by clinician's genuineness, unconditional positive regard, and acceptance. MI is a supportive style of communication, which generates less resistance than a more directive style does. Research findings show that when therapeutic suggestions are made in MI style, the suggestions are more likely to be carried out [18, 19].

Women at violence victim shelters who experience somatic symptoms tend to have PTSD, depression, ambivalence, low self-efficacy, and uncertainty about future. Due to these symptoms and psychological problems, their somatic symptoms tend to be prolonged. MI fits into their psychological problems and behavior change issues. Studies found that MI was also effective in reducing depression, anxiety, and fear, and resolving ambivalence [6, 7, 12, 13].

Women at shelters experience ambivalence while staying at the shelter; they feel guilty about their kids whom they have left for their husband to take care of. Some women enter the shelter alone saying they have made their mind not to contact anyone of family including kids till they feel stable emotionally and financially. As time flows and as they see other women living at the shelter with their kids, they start to miss more about connectedness and become more anxious about their future. Once they are safe at the shelter away from their abusive spouse and start receiving treatment for somatic symptoms, their determination fluctuates. Ambivalence becomes vivid, making them feel more depressed and emotionally unstable. Not all but some women experience more somatic symptoms.

It is noted that MI increases motivation for depressed people who are characterized as motivational deficit. In the middle of ambivalence, women at shelters seem to lose motivation to change and continue with somatic symptoms. Making determination to change helps them recover so that somatic symptoms will decrease. MI also helps express their anger toward others as well as themselves by reflective listening and affirming what they have tried to solve the problems in abusive situation even if not all effective. Affirming their inner power and strength to seek help is helpful for them to carry on and take their plans in action.

19.4.1 Engaging in Treatment

Engagement in treatment is predictive of change and of outcome. Clients differ in the level of motivation which is well explained by trans-theoretical model (TTM) of stages of change [14]. MI helps clients enhance their intrinsic motivation to engage in treatment as well as move from pre-contemplation stage to contemplation stage for change. As listed above, TTM illustrates five stages of change: pre-contemplation stage, contemplation stage, preparation stage, action stage, and maintenance stage. Women at shelters are noted with low level of motivation to engage in treatment by complaining of somatic pains, lack in energy, and want to skip attending sessions by excuses such as clinic visits, other appointments, and chores to do. Staff members including clinicians can evoke their motivation to engage in treatment by use of MI.

19.4.2 Ambivalence About Change and Therapist's Response to Client's Ambivalence

Women at shelters are characterized by ambivalence. For instance, they desire to be independent of the spouse psychologically as well as financially, and at the same time they desire to continue being dependent. They feel responsible for the children, and at the same time they feel burdened. They want connection and emotional support from family, and at the same time they want disconnection due to guilty feeling. Their ambivalence already existed during abuses from the spouse. While abused, they wanted separation, and at the same time they did not want permanent separation, hoping that their spouses change. They wanted to flee with children, and at the same time they wanted to stay with children. They wanted help from family, and simultaneously they did not want to seek help.

Prolonged ambivalence leads to depression and helplessness. While staying at shelters, the pattern of their ambivalence makes their depression and somatic symptoms continue.

By expressing empathy, developing discrepancy, and supporting self-efficacy, the clinician can help the client go through decision-making process to take necessary actions: reuniting with the spouse, getting a divorce, implementing a legal action, child fostering, getting employed, pursuing a separation, and looking for family counseling, which are all for the change in the course of life.

19.4.3 Motivation for Change

According to TTM, people evaluate alternatives on validity and make a final decision to take actions in the preparation stage of change. Women at shelters are noted with low self-esteem, low level of self-efficacy, and limited support system. MI can evoke their desire, concerns, aspirations, values, and goals of life so that they become motivated for change in action.

19.5 MI Application

MI helps women at shelters be motivated for change in life; depressed women seem resistant, but MI considers resistance as ambivalence. Women feel ambivalent about changing their life and pattern of behavior, and MI helps them be motivated to challenge for change.

MI principles are the basis in using MI skills. The following examples of client-clinician dialogue illustrate the use of some of MI skills mentioned above. The clients below are women at shelters.

19.5.1 Expressing Empathy

When they feel that the clinician empathizes their inner feelings, they become motivated to talk about their fears and frustration. Empathy is best expressed when counselors listen to what clients try to convey in a reflective way. Simple reflection, amplified reflection, and double-sided reflection are basic types of reflection, and these are essential in expressing empathy.

Simple reflection is repeating what the client says exactly or slightly differently; it occasionally brings client to think in the other perspective and gain insight into their way of seeing things.

Client: I worry a lot how my kids are doing at home with their father.
Clinician: You worry their father might not care them well. (simple reflection)

Amplified reflection is reading what the client feels or thinks but he or she does not say straight; it helps a client feel not alone but supported emotionally. Then he or she becomes motivated to do something in action.

Client: I have to wait till I get a full-time job before I get my kids away from their father.
Clinician: You worry if it will not happen soon to support your kids financially. (amplified reflection)

Double-sided reflection is reflecting a client's contradiction or inner conflict; it also helps the client make a decision and take it to action.

Client: I miss my kids so badly; I don't think I can stand any longer. No meaning to live here without my kids. I will go back home tonight.
Clinician: You feel like it would be better being with your kids now, but on arrival at this shelter, you said your kids are better at home with their father till you are ready to support your kids financially. (double-sided reflection)

19.5.2 Building Discrepancy

It helps clients see contradiction in their thoughts and help motivating them to change. Discrepancy between their goal and their present behavior is what they should be aware of.

Client: I got no energy to go out for a walk like other residents at this place. I lay down most of time thinking about many different things, and then thoughts spin around in my head, and it gives headache again.
Clinician: You have headache again, with no energy to move around like others but some energy to think about many things. (double-sided reflection)

19.5.3 Roll with Resistance

Resistance is a signal for the clinician to change strategies from confrontation to reflection which is reframing the client's statement in a new perspective.

Client: I expected something helpful for my life when I admitted myself to this shelter. But I have found no differences from those shelters I stayed before. No more need to stay here. I want to pack and leave today.
Clinician: Not much help you have found since arrival. (simple reflection) You wanted to make some kind of changes in your life this time. (reframing amplified reflection) What could have helped you to make changes? (evoking open-ended question)

19.5.4 Support Self-Efficacy

Affirming what the client has achieved even if trivial is empowering the client to be motivated for change.

Client: I am afraid that I am a failure, defeated after all, throughout my life. I don't see any alternatives but this feeling.

Clinician: This time of your life makes you feel hopeless. (amplified reflection) Admitting this painful feeling tells that you are a courageous woman. (affirmation)

19.5.5 Eliciting Change Talk

The more change talk, the higher a possibility of behavior change; evoking questions as well as reflection can elicit the client's concerns, needs, desire, reasons, and confidence for change. Change talk leads to commitment for change in action.

Clinician: What do you think your inner strengths are to help your life going under such stressful marriage? (evoking open-ended question)

19.6 Conclusions

Domestic violence victims are reported to have various kinds of psychosomatic symptoms with a high level of depression, anxiety, and PTSD. Women at shelters are found with a chronic ambivalence about change, and the ambivalence prolongs their psychological problems and worsens their somatic symptoms.

MI is a supportive communication style, expressing empathy for clients, building discrepancy between where they are and where they want to be, rolling with resistance by reflection, and supporting their self-efficacy to make a decision and take an action. MI elicits the client's motivation for change by asking open-ended questions, affirming the inner strengths of the client, reflective listening, and summarizing.

MI is found to be a cost-effective, short-term, evidence-based, and culturally sensitive approach. It can be effectively implemented within the services provided by shelters for domestic violence victims and can help women at shelters alleviate their psychosomatic symptoms.

More research should be made to find the effectiveness of MI in alleviating psychosomatic symptoms of clients with psychological problems such as depression, anxiety, and PTSD. MI combined with other therapies needs to be studied to examine its effectiveness in psychosomatic population. Also, some multicultural studies are to be made to find out the cultural influence in applying MI to psychosomatic population. In addition, MI training for clinicians, staff, and graduate students in psychosomatic medicine on regular basis is suggested.

References

1. Miller, W. R. (1983). Motivational interviewing with problem drinkers. *Behavioural Psychotherapy, 11*, 147–172.
2. Miller, W. R., & Rollnick, S. (2002). *Motivational interviewing preparing people to change*. New York: Guilford Press.
3. Arkowitz, H., Westra, H. A., Miller, W. R., et al. (2008). *Motivational interviewing in the treatment of psychological problems*. New York: Guilford Press.
4. Rollnick, S., Miller, W. R., & Butler, C. C. (2008). *Motivational interviewing in health care: Helping patients change behavior*. New York: Guilford Press.
5. Koh, K. B. (2002). *Stress and psychosomatic medicine*. Seoul: Ilchokak.
6. Arkowitz, H., & Burke, B. L. (2008). Motivational interviewing as an integrative framework for the treatment of depression. In H. Arkowitz, H. A. Westra, W. R. Miller, et al. (Eds.), *Motivational interviewing in the treatment of psychological problems*. New York: Guilford Press.
7. Zuckoff, A., Swartz, H. A., & Grote, N. K. (2008). Motivational interviewing as a prelude to psychotherapy of depression. In H. Arkowitz, H. A. Westra, W. R. Miller, et al. (Eds.), *Motivational interviewing in the treatment of psychological problems*. New York: Guilford Press.
8. Kang, H. S. (2006). The effect of psychodrama on depression for battered women. *The Korean Journal of Psychodrama, 9*, 1–11.
9. Cho, S. H. (2011). Preliminary studies to enhance the need for reducing psychosomatic disorder by psychodrama. *The Korean Journal of Psychodrama, 14*, 139–146.
10. Nixon, R. D. V., Resick, P. A., & Nishith, P. (2004). An exploration of comorbid depression among female victims of intimate partner violence with posttraumatic stress disorder. *82*, 315–320.
11. Stein, M. B., & Kennedy, C. (2001). Major depressive and post-traumatic stress disorder comorbidity in female victims of intimate partner violence. *Journal of affective disorders, 66*, 133–138.
12. Rasmussen, L. A., Hughes, M. J., & Murray, C. A. (2008). Applying motivational interviewing in a domestic violence shelter: A pilot study evaluating the training of shelter staff. *Journal of Aggression, Maltreatment & Trauma, 17*, 296–317.
13. Hughes, M. J., & Rasmussen, L. A. (2010). The utility of motivational interviewing in domestic violence shelters: A qualitative exploration. *Journal of Aggression, Maltreatment & Trauma, 19*, 300–322.
14. Prochaska, J. O., & DiClemente, C. C. (1983). Stages and processes of self-change of smoking: Toward an integrative model of change. *Journal of Consulting and Clinical Psychology, 51*, 390–395.
15. Amrhein, P. C., Miller W. R., Yahne C. E, et al. (2000, September). *Committing language emergent from a motivational interview predicts behavioral change in drug-addicted clients*. Paper presented at the International Conference on Treatment of Addictive Behaviors, Cape Town, South Africa.
16. Bohart, A. C., Elliot, R., Greenberg, L. S., et al. (2002). Empathy. In J. C. Norcross (Ed.), *Psychotherapy relationship that work*. New York: Oxford University Press.
17. Burns, D., & Nolen-Hoeksma, S. (1992). Therapeutic empathy and recovery from depression: A structural equation model. *Journal of Consulting and Clinical Psychology, 92*, 441–449.
18. Miller, W. R., Benefield, R. G., & Tonigan, J. S. (1993). Enhancing motivation for change in problem drinking: A controlled comparison of two therapist styles. *Journal of Consulting and Clinical Psychology, 61*, 455–461.
19. Patterson, G., & Chamberlain, P. (1994). A functional analysis of resistance during parent training. *Clinical Psychology Research and Practice, 1*, 53–70.

Chapter 20
Wisdom and Wisdom Psychotherapy in Coping with Stress

Michael Linden

20.1 Introduction

Stress and burdens are part of everyday life. When asking people on the street or when riding a train using the Different Burdens in Life Scale (DBL Scale) [1], one finds relevant numbers which indicate problems in various areas of their lives. If one takes a cutoff score of 48 on the scale, which signals a general negative judgment on one's situation in life, 21.5 % of the interviewed feel bad about their lives (money, work, friends, partnership, politics or environment, etc.).

Such burdens can cause pathological and psychosomatic reactions if a person is overtaxed and unable to adjust to or cope with given demands. In the ICD-10 [2], there is a separate chapter on reactions to severe burdens. It includes acute stress reaction, posttraumatic stress disorder (PTSD), and adjustment disorders. PTSD is defined as a persisting reaction to an extraordinary and life-threatening event, which will cause almost everybody to react excessively, though not necessarily enduring. In contrast, adjustment disorders occur in the context of normal and everyday events of all kinds. They are characterized by a multitude of unspecific symptoms like depression, anxiety, and psychosomatic complaints. They cannot be explained by the eliciting event or situation but rather by a maladjustment to the stressor. A clinical syndrome, which gives a good example of how daily problems can turn into severe and persistent mental disorders, is the posttraumatic embitterment disorder (PTED) [3, 4]. It is seen in the aftermath of events which are experienced by many persons like losing one's job, being divorced, being insulted by someone, being treated unfairly, or being humiliated. People react with feelings of embitterment,

M. Linden, M.D. (✉)
Research Group Psychosomatic Rehabilitation at der Charité University Medicine Berlin

Department of Behavioral and Psychosomatic Medicine at the Rehabilitation Center Seehof, Lichterfelder Allee 55, 14513 Teltow/Berlin, Germany
e-mail: michael.linden@charite.de

K.B. Koh (ed.), *Somatization and Psychosomatic Symptoms*,
DOI 10.1007/978-1-4614-7119-6_20,

lowered mood, aggressive reactions to third parties, withdrawal from social encounters, sleep problems, somatoform symptoms, or even suicidal ideation. Adjustment disorders can cause impairment in a person's life to a considerable degree. Epidemiological data show that they are rather frequent, can take a chronic course, and lead to negative social consequences [5–8].

As adjustment disorders cannot be explained by the extraordinary feature of the eliciting event, the coping repertoire of the person is at the heart of the negative development. Some people react to the same situation with maladjustment, while others are able to cope well with it; the same event can cause "eustress" or "distress."

There is an old saying, "per aspera ad astra" (only by hardship you can reach the stars). Likewise, stress can also induce "posttraumatic growth," i.e., it can lead to positive development like better appreciation of life as it is, better personal relationship, acceptance of one's own capacities, or development of new perspectives in life [9–11]. The core issue is the balance between the burden on one side and vulnerability or resilience of the person on the other side. A diathesis-stress model can help to understand adjustment disorders. There are many psychological processes which decide how a person reacts to negative life events and which act as mediators between burdens and reactions. Therapists must take such factors into account in the diagnosis and treatment of persons with stress and adjustment disorders. This chapter will focus on wisdom and wisdom-related psychological processes as one dimension of resilience and in coping with stress in healthy individuals as well as patients with adjustment disorders.

20.2 Cognitive and Emotional Intelligence

It is scientifically not decided whether cognitive intelligence helps to cope with negative life events. Intelligence can be divided into "fluid intelligence" and "crystalline intelligence" [12–14]. Fluid intelligence is the global capacity to adjust to new problems and situations without reference to earlier experience or learning. It is independent of education, mostly inherited, and needed in new situations which require flexibility and creativity. Crystalline intelligence is dependent on education and experience. This term is used when problems arise for which there are some kind of standard solutions. The measurement of these two types of intelligence is well established in psychology. No firm correlations have been found between such general cognitive capacities and the ability to master life. This is somewhat different for special subtypes of intelligence such as the ability to solve complex problems. Persons with good problem-solving skills (a) use systemic knowledge, (b) learn from past experiences, and (c) always look for alternatives before doing the next step [15, 16]. Such problem-solving skills can also help to cope with burdens in life.

Emotional intelligence is different from cognitive intelligence. It comprises social and practical intelligence which has been described as "hot intelligence" [17]. Mayer and Salovey [18, 19] described several components: (a) to recognize one's own emotions, (b) to control them, (c) to translate them into expression and action, (d) to be empathetic towards emotions of others, and (e) to be able to relate emotionally to others. This is in some part similar to "emotional creativity" or interpersonal and intrapersonal intelligence [20]. Emotional and cognitive intelligence are independent of each other [21]. While cognitive intelligence is negatively correlated with age, emotional intelligence is to some degree positively correlated with age. Although the concept of emotional intelligence has been criticized due to some vagueness [22], it is interesting in the context of coping with negative life events as it combines several dimensions which are most important in terms of control over emotions and relating to others.

20.3 Control Attributions, Sense of Coherence, and Moral

While concepts of intelligence focus on how to solve problems, concepts of attribution focus on how to evaluate and interpret events. According to the "transactional stress model" [23], stress is not caused by the event per se but by anticipations of negative consequences because of a discrepancy between demand and means of coping. Anticipations, interpretations, and attributions, especially control attributions, are at the core of the problem [23–26]. No control creates helplessness. One way of gaining control is to give events a sense, which makes them explainable in a certain way and thereby predictable. It has been shown that "psychological preparedness" and giving a sense to negative events or psychological trauma have preventive as well as therapeutic effects [27, 28].

Giving a sense to life is the same as what Antonovsky has described in his model of "sense of coherence" [29]. The model of sense of coherence has three components: (a) sense of comprehensibility, i.e., the ability to understand and integrate new events in a structured frame of reference; (b) sense of manageability, i.e., the feeling that there are personal or other resources, like God, to cope with whatever will come; and (c) sense of meaningfulness, i.e., to see life as full of sense and that it is worth to invest in solving given problems.

In the context of attributional concepts, moral is of special importance when it comes to problem-solving and coping with negative life events [30, 31]. It is a system of rules for guiding persons in life. Developmental psychology has described moral as the ability to discriminate between what is good or bad and the ability to act accordingly even in the presence of seduction. It therefore includes self-control. Moral is not only the acceptance of some social norms but the ability to make sound judgments on what is socially acceptable, what is just, and what will have the best outcome in the long run. Moral is of special importance in situations which are ambiguous and pose severe dilemma. There are several levels in the development of moral: (a) the preconventional niveau, with a hedonistic orientation towards external consequences of actions; (b) the conventional-conformist niveau, oriented towards important partners in primary groups like the family; and (c) the postconventional niveau, oriented towards principles and rules which form kind of a social contract and are based on fundamental rules of justice. The higher the development of moral, the better a person can put negative life events in a more general frame of reference and find problem solutions of a more general nature. This includes the ability to forgive. This is an important dimension in positive psychology. Forgiveness does not mean to accept injustice, to subdue to an aggressor, to ignore bad things, to forget, or to reconcile. Instead it is a form of coping, which allows a person to close up with what has happened, stop ruminations, leave feelings of revenge behind, free oneself from bad emotions, and look forward again [32–35].

20.4 Wisdom

An even more complex level of coping with stressors is described by wisdom psychology. Wisdom has been defined as expertise in coping with difficult problems in life for which there is no simple solution. It is the ability to solve unsolvable life problems [36–39].

Unsolvable and ambiguous problems and situations in life are rather the rule than the exception: Am I going to marry or not, this partner or another? Is it the best choice to accept this or that job? Is it better to leave my sick child at home and go to work or stay there and not go to work? Should I spend money and buy this robe or rather give it to charity? While intelligence or attributions try to find specific and rational solutions for problems, wisdom is the capacity to accept contradictions and ambiguities and to start actions in the presence of uncertainty. Wisdom is a complex multidimensional psychological capacity, which summarizes important dimensions of cognitive and emotional intelligence, sense of coherence and moral, and further capacities which help to deal with severe and complex problems in life. Persons with higher scores in wisdom do not remember bad things so much, do not so often look back but more to the future, can overcome negative experiences more quickly, learn better from past experiences, and have better relations with other persons and a better feeling of well-being [39–41]. Core dimensions are the following: (a) factual and procedural knowledge, (b) long-term perspective, (c) contextualism, (d) value relativism, (e) change of perspective, (f) empathy, (g) recognition and acceptance of one's own emotions, (h) emotional serenity, (i) distance from oneself, (j) uncertainty tolerance, and (k) control over one's own levels of aspiration. Detailed definitions are given in Table 20.1. In spite of the fact that some people see wisdom as some secret ability which is only given to special persons, wisdom psychology has shown that everybody has and needs these abilities.

20.5 Wisdom Psychotherapy

It has been shown that wisdom capacities can be trained and learned [3, 40–43]. In order to achieve higher scores in wisdom while dealing with a problem, it is enough to take 5 min for consideration, to consult with another person in reality or in sensu,

Table 20.1 Dimensions of wisdom

1. Factual and procedural knowledge General and specific knowledge on how the world or specific situations are set up and functioning
2. Long-term perspective Knowledge about positive and negative consequences, in the short term and the long term, and the ability to act according to the optimal outcome
3. Contextualism Ability to see that present problems are relative to the context, be it time, situation, or persons.
4. Value relativism Ability to accept that there are different and possibly contradictory values, which does not mean to abandon one's own values nor to fight and belittle the other values
5. Change of perspective Ability to look at problems from different sides and the perspective of other persons
6. Empathy Ability to feel how other persons feel
7. Recognition and acceptance of one's own emotions Ability to see, accept, and endure how one feels
8. Emotional serenity Ability to control one's own emotions and not allow them to overflow oneself
9. Distance from oneself Ability to see oneself through the eyes of others and to accept that one is not the center of the world
10. Uncertainty tolerance Ability to tolerate that nothing is for sure in life and that everything can have unexpected courses and outcomes, while this does not hinder from acting
11. Control over one's own levels of aspiration Ability to control one's own aspirations and not make judgments relative to what others have, or one had, or desires, instead of to what is necessary

From Linden [3, 45], Baumann and Linden [39]

or to actively think about the problem from the perspective of another person or under other circumstances.

Based on such findings, a specific training for wisdom capacities can be applied to persons who have difficulties in overcoming negative life events. If wisdom is a capacity which can help to cope with or "to solve unsolvable life problems" and if wisdom can be learned and taught, it also should be useful in a therapeutic context. Wisdom psychotherapy [3, 39, 44–46] is a form of cognitive behavioral therapy which can be applied to patients with adjustment or posttraumatic stress disorders as individual or group psychotherapy. The core of the treatment is to teach wisdom competence. A special intervention is to use the "method of unsolvable problems," in which fictitious life problems are presented for which there is no "correct" solution, but different solutions depending on who is asked. The problems in training are short descriptions of unjust and difficult yet common events that are mostly irreversible and can cause embitterment. All problems include three persons, the offender, the victim, and a third person who is involved without being a driving actor (Table 20.2). The descriptions leave room for speculation and interpretation.

Table 20.2 Fictitious life problems for the training of wisdom

Conflicts at workplace
Mrs. Miller has been working in a small company side to side with the owner for 28 years with high commitment. The company is in financial trouble. One day she receives a letter which tells that she is dismissed. She learns that a young girl has been hired at the same time
Partnership conflicts
In 20 years of marriage, Mrs. Miller took care of her children, the household, and the family's social activities, in order to support her husband's career. Her husband leaves her for his younger assistant who is, he says, the love of his life

Fictitious problems allow a general "problem-solving training" instead of trying to solve the specific problem of the patient, which could bear the danger of uncontrollable reactions. It is advisable to start the training with a problem that differs from the personal problem of the patient (e.g., a relationship conflict, if the patient's problem is at the workplace).

To stimulate a learning process, the patient has to deal with the problem in a structured way. He or she is asked the following: (a) To describe the feelings and thoughts that come up when thinking that this negative life event had happened to him or her and that he or she is the victim. What would he or she do? (b) To describe the feelings and thoughts that come up when thinking that he or she was the acting person (offender). What would he or she do? (c) To describe the feelings and thoughts that come up when thinking that he or she was the third person. What would he or she do? (d) To describe what reactions would be harmful. Which "solutions" could add insult to injury? (e) To describe what reactions to solve the problem would be reasonable and appropriate for the current situation. Which reactions would be reasonable and appropriate in the long run? (f) To describe what positive outcomes could come from the negative life event. (g) To describe what the person might think about the event and how he or she would like to describe it when writing a biography many years later. (h) To describe what a psychologist (manager, priest, grandmother with much life experience, etc.) who may be an expert in solving problems would recommend.

In this way, negative and positive emotions are recognized, and a change of perspective is stimulated including empathy towards the other involved persons (especially towards the "offender" and his/her possible motives). General knowledge relevant to problem-solving is activated; value relativism (different values, motives, and life goals of the involved persons can be distinguished and result in different perspectives and behaviors) as well as contextualism (the temporal and situational embedding of the problem may be reflected). Functional and dysfunctional strategies are identified (e.g., self-harm by suicide or alcohol, acts of revenge, long-lasting social and occupational adversities caused by embitterment) which help to clarify goals and can activate a reorientation and development of new perspectives. By contrasting short-term and long-term consequences, the patient becomes aware that complex life problems always have negative as well as positive consequences and that it is important to accept these ambiguities. Empirical data suggest that this approach can help to teach patients new approaches to deal with negative life events which cannot be reversed and to improve symptoms of stress and strain [46, 47].

20.6 Conclusions

There are many ways to deal with stressors in life, especially negative life events which may vary across cultures. If no solution can be found, stress reactions persist, causing multiple psychosomatic complaints, depression, aggression, or embitterment. There are a lot of problems that are too difficult or impossible for anyone to solve, such as infidelity of a beloved one, severe humiliation, or death. Therefore, skills are needed to solve such unsolvable problems. Intelligence and coping skills in general, attributions and sense of coherence, moral, and wisdom can be problem-solving approaches which can help in such situations. Wisdom is the most comprehensive concept. It has preventive properties as it is more closely related to the quality of life and well-being than socioeconomic status or health. Wisdom can also be trained in a systematic way to patients who are stuck in negative life events. Wisdom therapy is indicated especially when the goal is not to solve problems but to accept what cannot be changed, to forgive what cannot be undone, and to move on to new perspectives regardless of whatever may have happened in the past. It is an approach to strengthen resilience rather than to improve symptoms.

References

1. Linden, M., & Ritter, K. (2007). Differentielle lebensbelastetheit. *Psychiatrie und Psychotherapie, 4*, 140–147.
2. WHO. (1992). *International statistical classification of diseases and related health problems* (10th ed.). Geneva: WHO.
3. Linden, M. (2003). The posttraumatic embitterment disorder. *Psychotherapy and Psychosomatics, 72*, 195–202.
4. Linden, M., Rotter, M., Baumanna, K., et al. (2007). *The Post-Traumatic Embitterment (PTED)*. Bern: Hogrefe & Huber.
5. Snyder, S., Strain, J. J., & Wolf, D. (1990). Differentiating major depression from adjustment disorder with depressed mood in the medical setting. *General hospital psychiatry, 12*, 159–165.
6. Bronisch, T., & Hecht, H. (1989). Validity of adjustment disorder, comparison with major depression. *Journal of Affective Disorders, 17*, 229–236.
7. Despland, J. N., Monod, L., & Ferrero, F. (1995). Clinical relevance of adjustment disorder in DSM-III-R and DSM-IV. *Comprehensive Psychiatry, 36*, 454–460.
8. Strain, J. J., Smith, G. C., Hammer, J. S., et al. (1998). Adjustment disorder. A multisite study of its utilization and interventions in the consultation-liaison psychiatry setting. *General Hospital Psychiatry, 20*, 139–149.
9. Selye, H. (1977). *Streß*. Rowohlt, Reinbeck.
10. Tedeschi, R. G., & Calhoun, L. G. (2004). Posttraumatic growth, conceptual foundations and empirical evidence. *Psychological Inquiry, 15*, 1–18.

11. Zöllner, T., Calhoun, L. G., & Tedeschi, R. G. (2006). Trauma und persönliches Wachstum. In A. Maercker & R. Rosner (Eds.), *Psychotherapie der Posttraumatischen Belastungsstörungen*. Stuttgart: Thieme.
12. Cattell, R. B. (1963). Theory of fluid and crystallized intelligence. *Journal of Educational Psychology, 54*, 1–22.
13. Cattell, R. B. (1971). *Abilities - their structure, growth and action*. Boston: Houghton Mifflin.
14. Conrad, W. (1983). Intelligenzdiagnostik. In K. J. Groffmann & L. Michel (Eds.), *Enzyklopädie der Psychologie*. Göttingen: Hogrefe.
15. Dörner, D., Kreuzig, H. W., Reither, F., et al. (1983). *Vom Umgang mit Unbestimmtheit und Komplexität*. Bern: Huber.
16. Dörner, D., & Schölkopf, J. (1991). Controlling complex systems: Or Expertise als "grandmother's know-how. In K. A. Ericsson & J. Smith (Eds.), *Toward a general theory of expertise: Prospects and limits*. New York: Cambridge University Press.
17. Mayer, J. D., Salovey, P., & Caruso, D. R. (2004). Emotional intelligence: Theory, findings, and implications. *Psychological Inquiry, 3*, 197–215.
18. Mayer, J. D., & Salovey, P. (1995). Emotional intelligence and the construction and regulation of feelings. *Applied and Preventive Psychology, 4*, 197–208.
19. Mayer, J. D., & Salovey, P. (1997). What is emotional intelligence? In P. Salovey & D. Sluyter (Eds.), *Emotional development and emotional intelligence: Implications for educators*. New York: Basic Books.
20. Averill, J. R. (1999). Creativity in the domain of emotion. In T. Dalgleish & M. Power (Eds.), *Handbook of cognition and emotion*. Chichester: Wiley.
21. Gardner, H. (2001). *Die Rahmen-Theorie der vielfachen Intelligenzen*. Stuttgart: Klett-Cotta.
22. Matthews, G., Roberts, R. D., & Zeidner, M. (2004). Seven myths about emotional intelligence. *Psychological Inquiry, 3*, 179–196.
23. Lazarus, R. S. (1966). *Psychological stress and the coping process*. New York: McGraw-Hill.
24. Six, B. (1987). Attribution. In D. Frey & S. Greif (Eds.), *Sozialpsychologie*. München: Psychologie Verlags Union.
25. Seligman, M. E. P. (1995). *Helplessness*. San Francisco: Freeman.
26. Horowitz, M. J. (1976). *Stress response syndromes*. Northvale, NJ: Aronson.
27. Becerra, H. (1995). Solidarität Gefolterter im Gefängnis in Perren-Klingler, Trauma Bibel in der Einheitsübersetzung. Daniel 3:51.
28. Basoglu, M., & Mineka, S. (1992). The role of uncontrollable and unpredictable stress in posttraumatic stress responses in torture survivors. In M. Basoglu (Ed.), *Torture and first consequences: Current treatment approaches*. Cambridge: Cambridge University Press.
29. Antonovsky, A. (1997). *Salutogenese – Zur Entmystifizierung der Gesundheit*. Tübingen: Deutsche Gesellschaft für Verhaltenstherapie.
30. Trautner, H. M. (1997). *Lehrbuch der Entwicklungspsychologie*. Göttingen: Hogrefe.
31. Kohlberg, L. (1973). The claim of moral adequacy of a highest stage of moral judgment. *Journal of Philosophy, 70*, 630–646.
32. Wade, N. G. (2005). In search of a common core: A content analysis of interventions to promote forgiveness. *Psychotherapy, 42*, 160–177.
33. Wade, N. G., Post, B. C., & Cornish, M. A. (2011). Forgiveness therapy to treat embitterment: A review of relevant research. In M. Linden & A. Maercker (Eds.), *Embitterment: Societal, psychological, and clinical perspectives*. Wien: Springer.
34. Bradfield, M., & Aquino, K. (1999). The effects of blame attributions and offender likeableness on forgiveness and revenge in the workplace. *Journal of Management, 25*, 607–631.
35. Lin, W., Mack, D., Enright, R. D., et al. (2004). Effects of forgiveness therapy on anger, mood, and vulnerability to substance abuse among inpatient substance-dependent clients. *Journal of Consulting and Clinical Psychology, 72*, 1114–1121.
36. Baltes, P. B., & Smith, J. (1990). Weisheit und Weisheitsentwicklung: Prolegomena zu einer psychologischen Weisheitstheorie. *Zeitschrift für Entwicklungspsychologie und Pädagogische Psychologie, 22*, 95–135.

37. Staudinger, U. M., & Glück, J. (2011). Psychological wisdom research: Commonalities and differences in a growing field. *Annual Review of Psychology, 62*, 215–241.
38. Sternberg, R. J., Jarvin, L., & Grigorenko, E. L. (Eds.). (2009). *Teaching for wisdom, intelligence, creativity, and success*. Thousand Oaks, CA: Corwin.
39. Baumann, K., & Linden, M. (2008). *Weisheitskompetenzen und Weisheitstherapie*. Lengerich: Pabst Verlag.
40. Linden, M., Rotter, M., Baumann, K., et al. (2007). *Posttraumatic embitterment disorder*. Bern: Huber & Hogrefe.
41. Clayton, V. (1982). Wisdom and intelligence: The nature and function of knowledge in the later years. *International Journal of Aging & Human Development, 15*, 315–323.
42. Böhmig-Krumhaar, S. A. (1998). *Leistungspotentiale wert-relativierenden Denkens: Die Rolle einer wissensaktivierenden Gedächtnisstrategie*. Berlin: Max-Planck-Institut für Bildungsforschung, Studien und Berichte.
43. Baltes, P. B., Glück, J., & Kunzmann, U. (2002). Wisdom: Its structure and function in regulating successful life span development. In C. R. Snyder & S. J. Lopez (Eds.), *Handbook of positive psychology* (pp. 327–347). Oxford: Oxford University Press.
44. Schippan, B., Baumann, K., & Linden, M. (2004). Weisheitstherapie - kognitive Therapie der posttraumatischen Verbitterungsstörung. *Verhaltenstherapie, 14*, 284–293.
45. Linden, M. (2008). Posttraumatic embitterment disorder and wisdom therapy. *Journal of Cognitive Psychotherapy, 22*, 4–14.
46. Linden, M., Baumann, K., Lieberei, B., et al. (2011). Treatment of posttraumatic embitterment disorder with cognitive behaviour therapy based on wisdom psychology and hedonia strategies. *Psychotherapy and Psychosomatics, 80*, 199–205.
47. Linden, M. (2012). Embitterment in a cultural context. In S. Barnow (Ed.), *Cultural Variations in emotion regulation and treatment of psychiatric patients*. Göttingen: Hogrefe.

Chapter 21
Current Advances in the Psychopharmacology of Psychosomatic Medicine

Amarendra N. Singh

21.1 Introduction

Psychosomatic medicine is a way of approaching health problems, and psychosomatic disorders in general are pathological expression of biological, psychological, and socioecological parameters of human health.

Psychopharmacology, on the other hand, is one of the rapidly developing disciplines and has become a widely used therapeutic tool in psychosomatic medicine or consultation-liaison psychiatry [1]. Psychopharmacology is moving rapidly from empirical to practical approach. Psychopharmacological treatment in psychosomatic medicine or consultation-liaison psychiatry has expanded greatly in the past decade. A variety of new psychotropic drugs helps to meet patients' specialized needs and enhances the quality of care and then the quality of life [2–5].

Psychopharmacological agents most used in psychosomatic medicine or consultation-liaison psychiatry are antidepressants, anxiolytic agents, hypnotics, antipsychotics, beta-blockers, and mood stabilizers. In particular, this chapter will focus on the use of psychopharmacological agents in (a) anxiety disorders, (b) depressive disorders, (c) primary insomnia, (d) somatization, (e) eating disorders, (f) migraine, and (g) fibromyalgia.

A.N. Singh, M.D. (✉)
Psychopharmacology, Department of Psychiatry, Pharmacology and Neurosciences, Queen's University, Kingston, ON, Canada
e-mail: singha@queensu.ca

K.B. Koh (ed.), *Somatization and Psychosomatic Symptoms*,
DOI 10.1007/978-1-4614-7119-6_21, © Springer Science+Business Media New York 2013

21.2 Anxiety Disorders

Recent research has confirmed the need of diagnostic subtyping for the appropriate treatment of anxiety disorders. Pharmacotherapy with antianxiety drugs remains the mainstay of treatment, but concomitant nonpharmacological treatment should be considered for all anxiety sufferers.

21.2.1 Panic Disorder

The goal here is to control panic attacks in the short term and then continue long-term maintenance treatment if needed. Recent advances in this area are the utilization of (a) selective serotonin reuptake inhibitor (SSRI) [6] agents, (b) serotonin and noradrenergic reuptake inhibitor (SNRI) [7] agents, and (c) buspirone [8] and atypical antipsychotics such as risperidone [9] and quetiapine.

Venlafaxine XR, paroxetine, sertraline, Cipramil, escitalopram, and fluvoxamine are effective drugs for panic disorder patients. The side effects of SSRI and SNRI in many panic disorder patients necessitate that the starting dose should be usually half of the normal range of dosage. Sexual side effects are one of the most common side effects of the above drugs, particularly on maintenance therapy; hence in these patients, Viagra, if not contraindicated, should be used. These drugs should be gradually tapered to avoid the occurrence of serotonin withdrawal syndrome when they are discontinued. Buspirone has not been successful in panic disorders [8]. However, risperidone, olanzapine, and Seroquel as augmentors of SSRI [9, 10] have shown better results. Carbamazepine and valproic acid have been found to be effective in case reports [11]. 5-Hydroxytryptamine (5HT)2 or also receptor antagonists such as mirtazapine [12] or ondansetron can be used, and reboxetine, a selective noradrenaline reuptake inhibitor (NARI) drug in the dosage of 6–8 mg a day, is known to be markedly effective in this disorder [13].

In acute and moderately severe panic disorder, combined pharmacotherapy of benzodiazepines with SSRI or SNRI should be started. After 4 weeks, the benzodiazepine should be tapered and discontinued within 6 weeks because antidepressant therapy will continue to be effective in the long term. This kind of regimen will prevent the abuse potential of benzodiazepines [14].

21.2.2 Generalized Anxiety Disorder

Venlafaxine XR, paroxetine, escitalopram, sertraline, fluvoxamine, and mirtazapine are the recent drugs known to be significantly effective in generalized anxiety disorder. Partial benzodiazepine receptor agonists such as bretazenil and abecarnil are also effective while possessing a low risk for dependence. Riluzole, a presynaptic glutamate release inhibitor in a dose of 100 mg, has shown promising results [15].

21.2.3 Obsessive-Compulsive Disorder (OCD)

Drugs that have been significantly effective in OCD are fluoxetine, paroxetine, sertraline, and fluvoxamine [16]. Recent studies on therapeutic effects of SSRIs have revealed that OCD symptoms may improve in 2–3 weeks but their improvement may be delayed after 4–6 weeks; hence, the duration of treatment for control of symptoms usually should be at least 10–12 weeks. The effective doses of SSRIs are in the higher range of 40–60 mg in fluoxetine and paroxetine and 150–200 mg in fluvoxamine and sertraline.

Clomipramine, a tricyclic drug, still remains the drug of choice in difficult and refractory OCD, while fluoxetine is one of the most popular SSRIs for therapeutic use in OCD patients. Augmentation and combination of antidepressants are also worth trying in OCD patients. OCD is a chronic illness; hence, the duration of treatment depends on the clinical condition of individual patients.

21.2.4 Posttraumatic Stress Disorder (PTSD)

SSRIs have been effective in controlling the positive symptoms of PTSD, such as re-experiencing the events and arousal, but not responsive to negative symptoms, such as withdrawal and avoidance [17]. Beta-blockers (e.g., propranolol, pindolol) can be effectively used in controlling persistent symptoms of automatic arousal. Carbamazepine [18] and valproate [19] improve irritability, anger, and aggressive outbursts in PTSD patients.

SSRIs (sertraline and fluoxetine), SNRIs (venlafaxine XR and duloxetine) and NaSSA (mirtazapine) have also shown significant improvement, but long-term treatment (up to 15 months) and gradual reduction of dose are required for controlling arousal, depressive, and withdrawal symptoms. Prazosin, α-1-adrenergic antagonist, has been effective in controlling nightmares and daytime intrusions in PTSD patients.

21.2.5 Social Phobia or Social Anxiety Disorder

SSRIs and SNRIs have replaced benzodiazepines as a first-line treatment in social phobia. Paroxetine [20, 21], fluvoxamine [22], sertraline [23], and venlafaxine

XR [21] are the drugs of choice in this disorder. Gabapentin and pregabalin have also shown significant therapeutic benefit. Atypical antipsychotics, in limited studies, have shown benefits but further studies are needed for defining their future role in social phobia. Long-term treatment for more than 18 months is needed for this chronic disorder.

21.2.6 Specific Phobia

Pharmacotherapies in this disorder need long-term research but at present SSRI drugs have shown significant therapeutic benefits, particularly from paroxetine combined with exposure therapy.

SSRI, SNRI, and noradrenergic and specific serotonergic antidepressant (NaSSA) drugs have shown significant therapeutic benefits and have established a primary role in most anxiety disorder categories and also offer some protection against relapse. However, their side effects limit widespread use of these drugs. The side effects include sexual dysfunction, nausea, vomiting, headache, agitation, insomnia, bleeding, and vivid dreams. Rare side effects are syndrome of inappropriate secretion of antidiuretic hormone, apathy, serotonin syndrome, and discontinuation syndrome.

Medical illnesses such as Parkinson's disease, cancer, seizures, stroke, and thyroid and gastric diseases usually produce symptoms of anxiety disorders, and these patients respond very well to pharmacotherapy. Hence, the suitable medications described above should be used to relieve their suffering. In all anxiety disorder patients, the therapeutic results are enhanced with the addition of cognitive therapy and oriental therapies such as meditation, yoga, Zen therapy, Niakan, acupuncture, bioenergic therapy, Monko therapy, Kenpo therapy, Mo-hezhiguan therapy, transcendental therapy, and Morita therapy [24, 25]. Future success of psychopharmacotherapy will depend on finding a genetic risk factor which coexists with environmental factors, thereby gaining further insight into the epigenetic process.

21.3 Depressive Disorders

Recent advances in the treatment of depression have demonstrated wider therapeutic activities, improved safety, tolerability, selectivity and reduced adverse reaction profiles [26, 27]. These newer antidepressants can be classified as (1) SSRIs, (2) SNRIs, (3) NARIs, (4) NaSSA, and (5) norepinephrine and dopamine modulator (bupropion).

21.3.1 Selective Serotonin Reuptake Inhibitor (SSRI)

The SSRIs are chemically distinct from traditional antidepressants, such as tricyclic, tetracyclic, and monoamine oxidase inhibitors (MAOIs), but share the common route of selective and potent inhibition of neuronal reuptake of serotonin and have none or little effect on neuronal reuptake of norepinephrine, acetylcholine, and histamine. Thus, these drugs have less sedative, anticholinergic, and cardiovascular effects than other antidepressants of tricyclic and tetracyclic class.

Fluoxetine, fluvoxamine, sertraline, indalpine, paroxetine, citalopram alaproclate, escitalopram, and femoxetine belong to the SSRI group of drugs. Overall, SSRIs have equal therapeutic efficacy but possess a better side effect profile, thus becoming more acceptable to patients. The common side effects of SSRIs are diarrhea, nausea, dry mouth, anorexia, sweating, weight gain or loss, agitation, headache, sexual disorders, insomnia, tremor, and dizziness, whereas the rare side effects are hyponatremia, bruising and bleeding due to platelet dysfunction, and inappropriate secretion of antidiuretic hormone. In addition, physicians should keep discontinuation syndrome in mind while using SSRIs except fluoxetine.

21.3.2 Serotonin and Noradrenergic Reuptake Inhibitor (SNRI)

This new class of drugs acts on both noradrenergic and serotonergic neurotransmitters and may have more advantages compared to other antidepressants. They lack actions on adrenergic, muscarinic, or histamine receptors, which are responsible for many of the adverse effects of older antidepressants. This group consists of venlafaxine, duloxetine, and milnacipran. Duloxetine has equal effects on both noradrenergic and serotonergic neurotransmitters, whereas venlafaxine has more serotonergic action and milnacipran more noradrenergic action. The side effect profile of SNRIs is similar to that of SSRIs and discontinuation syndrome should also be taken into account during the use of SNRIs.

21.3.3 Selective Noradrenaline Reuptake Inhibitor (NARI)

Reboxetine belongs to this group and is the first nontricyclic selective noradrenaline reuptake inhibitor. It mediates its therapeutic effect by increasing the action of noradrenaline in the brain without significant interaction with muscarinic, alpha1-adrenergic, and H1-histaminergic receptors that mediate the classic side effects of the tricyclic antidepressant (TCAs). The side effect profile of reboxetine is consistent with a noradrenergic agent that possesses weak anticholinergic and serotonergic activity.

21.3.4 Noradrenergic and Specific Serotonergic Antidepressant (NaSSA)

Mirtazapine represents this group. The antidepressant effect of the drug is a result of increased neurotransmission of both noradrenergic and serotonergic neurotransmitters. Its efficacy has been reported to be similar to that of older antidepressants. Mirtazapine develops reversible type of neutropenia which is nonprogressive in nature and dose-related. The adverse effects related to the anticholinergic system and cardiac effects are low. It does not usually cause nausea, sexual dysfunction, or anorexia. Its side effects include weight gain and sedation.

21.3.5 Norepinephrine and Dopamine Modulator (e.g., Bupropion)

Bupropion is not a drug causing sedation or sexual dysfunction. It has little cardiotoxicity and is a stimulating drug for retarded depression or fatigue. It is also used for augmentative purposes with SSRIs, SNRIs, and NaSSA. Its side effects are agitation in some cases and seizures in higher doses. The usual dose range is 150–300 mg a day.

21.3.6 Cautions in the use of SSRIs and Genetic Tests

An increase of suicidal ideation in patients who use SSRIs has been cautioned by the FDA. They advised that children and adolescents should avoid the use of paroxetine. On the whole, since 2004, a label of this drug has warned that pediatric and adolescent patients should be closely observed due to worsening depression or suicidality.

Recent genetic researchers have helped us to develop the concept of drug therapy tailored to patients' genetic makeup [5, 27], thereby finding the best treatment on an individual basis for depressed patients [28]. At the present time, genetic tests are commercially available to screen for allelic variation in the CYP-450 gene which gives a clue to individual variation of drug metabolism. However, these tests have limitations due to factors such as smoking, diet, and genetic makeup. Other tests are with the help of variation in the gene for spermine/spermidine *N* (1)-acetyltransferase (SSAT) and variation in corticotropin-releasing hormone (CRH) [29]. However, of all the tests available, the most widely studied test is 5-HTT (serotonin transporter) [28–31], which is used to choose the class of antidepressant to start treatment. Besides, this test helps in determining the patients' vulnerability to side effects of antidepressants.

21.4 Primary Insomnia

Therapeutic use of benzodiazepine hypnotics for insomnia has become limited due to the development of tolerance, dependence, and rebound phenomenon. Recent advances in the treatment of insomnia lie in the discovery of "non-benzodiazepine hypnotics" [32].

21.4.1 Non-benzodiazepine Hypnotics

This group of drugs is non-benzodiazepine receptor agonists and chemically unrelated to benzodiazepines. However, these drugs act through benzodiazepine receptors. Three drugs belonging to this group are changing the pharmacotherapy of insomnia. These drugs are as follows: (1) cyclopyrrolone (zopiclone, eszopiclone), (2) imidazopyridine (zolpidem), and (3) pyrazolopyrimidine (zaleplon).

21.4.1.1 Zopiclone

Zopiclone modulates the action of the neurotransmitter, GABA, to produce its hypnotic effect. It also binds only to a distinct site on the GABA/chloride ion channel complexes located in the cerebral cortex, cerebellum, and hippocampus and not to peripherally located complexes. The efficacy of this drug is to enhance sleep induction and maintenance, reduce sleep latency and nocturnal awakening, and enhance the quality of stage 3 and 4 sleep and produce sleep which mimics natural sleep. The therapeutic advantages of zopiclone over benzodiazepine hypnotics are as follows:

(i) Predominantly primary action-orientated drug; no significant secondary action (no receptor affinities to serotonin, dopamine, peripheral benzodiazepine sites, α-1, α-2 adrenergic receptors)
(ii) Markedly reduced activity for amnesia or memory disturbance
(iii) Reduced affinities for tolerance and dependence
(iv) Markedly reduced effect on psychomotor activities and cognition
(v) Absence of confusion in the elderly
(vi) Lack of accumulation
(vii) Stage 3 of sleep is increased; thus, the only hypnotic which increases the total duration of deep sleep
(viii) No effect on stage 4 and little or no effect on REM sleep

These drugs require no reduction of dose for elderly patients. Eszopiclone is a newer cyclopyrrolone agent approved by the FDA for primary insomnia without limitation of the duration of use which is different from other approved non-benzodiazepine hypnotics. Individual testing for 5HT7 genetic variation may help us to know the patients' vulnerability to side effect of the drugs.

21.4.1.2 Zolpidem

This drug is active at omega-1 benzodiazepine receptor. This drug shortens the sleep latency, prolongs total sleep time, but has little or no effect on sleep stages. The development of tolerance and physical dependence has rarely been observed.

Absorption of zolpidem with food shows lower oral bioavailability in comparison to that taken without food; about 70 % of oral bioavailability is found. Its elimination half-life is 1.5–2.4 h, but unlike zopiclone, zolpidem has a longer half-life in the elderly and a shorter half-life in children. Zolpidem ER has no limitation in the duration of use like eszopiclone and has a slightly longer half-life than zolpidem. Discontinuation of this drug often causes rebound insomnia and infrequently produces daytime sedation or amnesia.

21.4.1.3 Zaleplon

Zaleplon is chemically unrelated to benzodiazepines and binds differently to the benzodiazepine type I site on the gamma-aminobutyric acid (GABA) subtype A/chloride ion channel complex. Zaleplon is rapidly absorbed and reaches peak plasma concentration in about 1 h, which is also its half-life. The adverse reactions of this drug are minimal; no rebound insomnia and no psychomotor retardation in daytime. Neither tolerance nor dependence has been observed after discontinuation of this drug. The sleep latency is decreased by the use of this drug, which enhances the quality of sleep.

The other newer drug released by the FDA is ramelteon, a melatonin MT_1 and MT_2 receptor agonist. Ramelteon influences homeostatic sleep signaling mediated by suprachiasmatic nucleus. It is mostly used in elderly patients in a dose of 4–8 mg. Gaboxadol as elective extrasynaptic $GABA_A$ has a mechanism of action different from other GABA agents. This drug also involves $GABA_A$ receptor in thalamus.

21.5 Somatization

In recent years, the number of somatizing patients is increasing. These patients complain of many physical symptoms, but no organic basis is found, thus leaving the physician to investigate the presence of psychosocial stressors [33]. Somatoform disorders are frequently comorbid with depressive and anxiety disorders [34]. Somatization is regarded as a general process by which bodily symptoms may be used as a culturally sanctioned idiom of distress to implicate problems of family, work, school, financial, or other problems [33].

Pharmacotherapy is an adjunct treatment for somatization. Illness behaviors are to be addressed with psychotherapy such as insight-orientated psychotherapy and cognitive therapy.

Family therapy and behavior therapy can be also used. However, ruling out medical conditions with nonspecific symptoms and planning to care rather than cure should be the objective of the therapy. Establishing a primary therapist with regular visits to educate, to remove the coexisting anxiety and depression, and finally to enhance effective coping is the first step for success of the treatment of somatizing patients.

However, SSRI (e.g., fluoxetine) improves the presenting symptoms in patients with body dysmorphic disorder [35, 36]. Hypochondriasis also improves markedly with SSRIs. However, psychopharmacological intervention has been unsuccessful in conversion disorder. In pain disorder, tricyclic, SSRI, and SNRI agents augment analgesic effects. SSRIs are also beneficial to the obsessional cluster of somatoform disorders, but in the somatic cluster, less is known about the response of pharmacotherapy [36]. Further studies are needed for improving the horizon of success in somatoform disorders.

21.6 Eating Disorders

21.6.1 Anorexia Nervosa

In anorexia nervosa, the main therapeutic goals are threefold: (1) to stimulate appetite and increase weight, (2) dietary advice, and (3) treating underlying disorders which precipitate anorexic tendencies such as depression, obsessive-compulsive disorder, personality disorder, and substance abuse.

Drugs chosen for the treatment of anorexia nervosa promote weight gain and also resolve underlying precipitating causes. Tricyclic antidepressants, such as amitriptyline, clomipramine, trimipramine, and Norpramin, and tetracyclic antidepressants, such as maprotiline, remain the favored drugs, while antipsychotics such as olanzapine, risperidone, and quetiapine (Seroquel) have shown significant improvement; the most convincing result came from the use of olanzapine [37].

Benzodiazepines in small doses during the weight gain are beneficial to controlling reactive anxiety. The benzodiazepines most appropriate for this phase are sublingual lorazepam and alprazolam but should be used in the short term, e.g., 4–6 weeks, with antidepressants which will then continue for a long-term treatment. SSRIs and SNRIs have therapeutic effects for controlling relapses in anorexia nervosa. Cyproheptadine, a serotonin antagonist, which increases weight, has also been used in daily doses of 12–32 mg with a significant result.

NaSSA agent, mirtazapine [2, 3], has shown significant therapeutic efficacy in patients with anorexia nervosa. Individual psychotherapy and family therapy have also been tried with success. Overall, the recent trend for better management of anorexia nervosa has been the combination of pharmacotherapy with individual psychotherapy, family therapy, and dietary advice.

21.6.2 Bulimia Nervosa

In the treatment of bulimia nervosa, antidepressants [38, 39], particularly fluoxetine, have been remarkably and significantly successful. In Canada, the Health Protection

Branch has approved fluoxetine as an antibulimic agent. Other newer SSRI drugs, such as fluvoxamine, sertraline, and paroxetine, are also beneficial to bulimia. Naltrexone, a long-acting oral narcotic antagonist, has also been found to be effective in reducing binge eating and vomiting in patients refractory to antidepressants. The dosage of this drug ranges from 200 to 300 mg a day.

In recent studies, topiramate [40] has been found to be an effective drug for bulimia nervosa. In bulimia nervosa, in addition to pharmacotherapy, cognitive behavioral therapy either individually or in group helps to improve eating behavior as well as attitude toward body shape and weight. Recent studies have shown the superiority of combined drug and cognitive behavioral therapy over behavior therapy alone. Thus, the management of bulimia in the future will have to focus on combined therapies which include pharmacotherapy, cognitive behavioral therapy, and dietary advice.

21.6.3 Binge Eating Disorder

Fluoxetine, sertraline, and citalopram have shown significant efficacy in binge eating disorder. Sibutramine, an SNRI [41] in a daily dose of 15 mg, and reboxetine, an NARI drug [42] in a daily dose of 8 mg, are also effective in this disorder.

Night eating syndrome, characterized by morning anorexia, insomnia, and evening hyperphagia, is less studied for treatment purposes, but the drugs used for binge eating disorder are also therapeutically beneficial. On the whole, anorexia nervosa has not responded to psychopharmacotherapy, but relapses are definitely controlled, once weight is recovered in these patients with the use of SSRI and SNRI agents. On the other hand, psychopharmacological management of bulimia nervosa and binge eating disorder has resulted in very satisfactory outcomes.

21.7 Migraine

Recent advances in migraine therapy have been the development of sumatriptan, which is a 5-hydroxytryptamine (5HT)-like receptor agonist [2–5]. Sumatriptan mediates selective vasoconstriction within carotid arterial circulation supplying intracranial and extracranial tissues such as brain and meninges. Mechanism of antimigraine activity could, thus, involve vasoconstriction of dura blood vessels. This drug has remarkable activity in controlling the acute pain of migraine. Imitrex can be given orally in a dose of 100 mg or by subcutaneous injection in a dose of 6 mg. Patients who do not respond to the oral dose should not have any more tablets. The maximum oral dose in 24 h is 300 mg or by injection 12 mg a day. This drug should not be used in patients suffering from heart diseases, cerebrovascular diseases, and hemiplegic and basilar migraine and in patients receiving MAOIs, selective 5-HT reuptake inhibitors, and lithium. Intravenous route causes coronary vasospasm; hence, the route should not be used.

Newer serotonin agonists, triptans, rizatriptans, almotriptans, eletriptans, and frovatriptan, have been shown to be very effective in reducing migraine pain.

21.7.1 Prophylactic Management

Prophylaxis of migraine is still covered by six groups of drugs: beta-blockers (e.g., atenolol, metoprolol, and propranolol), calcium channel blockers (e.g., verapamil and flunarizine), serotonin antagonists (e.g., cyproheptadine and pizotifen), antidepressants (e.g., amitriptyline, doxepin, and phenelzine), antiepileptics (e.g., sodium valproate), and nonsteroidal anti-inflammatory drugs (e.g., naproxen). Recent research has shown that enalapril, an angiotensin-converting enzyme (ACE) inhibitor, may also be effective in preventing migraine. The prophylactic treatment should be on a long-term basis and should be tapered in the light of improvement.

21.8 Fibromyalgia

The following are the main psychopharmacological agents found to be therapeutically beneficial to fibromyalgia.

21.8.1 Tricyclic Antidepressants

Amitriptyline – 10–25 mg to start and titrate up to 100 mg; Nortriptyline – start at 10–25 mg and titrate up to 100 mg.

21.8.2 SNRI

Venlafaxine, duloxetine, and milnacipran possess analgesic effects and have much fewer adverse reactions than TCA. The FDA has approved duloxetine for the treatment of fibromyalgia. However, SSRIs have not produced significant improvement of symptoms in patients with fibromyalgia.

21.8.3 Cyclobenzaprine

Cyclobenzaprine, a muscle relaxant medication, is chemically related to TCA and might be the basis of effectiveness in TCA. In doses of 10–40 mg, this drug is effective for fibromyalgia.

21.8.4 $\alpha_2\delta$-Ligand Anticonvulsants (e.g., Pregabalin, Gabapentin)

In particular, pregabalin is effective for fibromyalgia. The dose range of pregabalin is from 150 to 300 mg a day, while the dose for gabapentin ranges from 1,200 to 2,400 mg a day.

21.8.5 Tramadol

It is given 25–250 mg a day in divided doses. The combination of acetaminophen and tramadol (Tramacet) is more effective than tramadol alone. Pregabalin and duloxetine are considered the first line of treatment in fibromyalgia, and tramadol could be considered the second-line drug of choice.

21.9 Psychopharmacotherapy for Physically Ill Patients

Patients who are physically ill and present with depression or anxiety can be treated successfully with psychopharmacotherapy.

21.9.1 Cardiac Diseases

In coronary artery disorder, depression can be treated with SSRI, NaSSA, and bupropion. The drugs of choice are fluoxetine, paroxetine, sertraline, bupropion, and mirtazapine. Antipsychotics, especially quetiapine, olanzapine, and risperidone, are preferred in schizophrenic patients with cardiac diseases. In the treatment of anxiety disorder patients with cardiac diseases, benzodiazepine anxiolytics are being replaced by SSRIs and buspirone.

21.9.2 Renal Diseases

Most SSRIs can be used in depressive patients with renal diseases. However, paroxetine should be given half of the adult dose, while the other SSRIs do not need a dose adjustment. Bupropion should be avoided in these patients because water-soluble active metabolite may accumulate, whereas mirtazapine and venlafaxine should be used in less than half of the adult dose because renal clearance of both drugs is decreased by 30–50 %, and particularly the half-life of venlafaxine is prolonged in renal insufficiency. For the use of antipsychotics, quetiapine and olanzapine are preferred, whereas risperidone should be avoided [43]. For the use of anxiolytics and sedatives, most benzodiazepine anxiolytics except chlordiazepoxide can be used, and zolpidem is the drug of choice among hypnotics. Most antidepressants are metabolized by the liver and excreted by the kidneys; thus, reduction of initial doses of antidepressant is a reasonable way to avoid the possibility of potentially active metabolite accumulation.

21.9.3 Cerebrovascular Diseases

In cerebrovascular diseases, antidepressants such as fluoxetine and citalopram are recommended, because other newer antidepressants have not been studied in the diseases. Most antipsychotics, especially atypical antipsychotics, should be avoided in the elderly [44] because of increased cerebrovascular accidents in the elderly by exposure to atypical antipsychotics but lower doses of low-potency drugs such as quetiapine can be used with caution.

21.9.4 Seizure Disorders

Most psychotropic drugs have a lower seizure threshold in a normal dose; hence, lower doses of psychotropic drugs should be tried with caution. Haloperidol, quetiapine, and olanzapine pose lower risks for seizure than other antipsychotics.

21.9.5 Hepatic Diseases

Most of the psychotropic drugs are metabolized in the liver; hence, all psychotropics should be used in lower doses with caution in patients with hepatic diseases.

21.9.6 Gastrointestinal Diseases

A recent report on the association between SSRIs and bleeding has raised concern for its use in patients with peptic ulcer or any other diseases causing bleeding from the gut.

21.9.7 Respiratory Diseases

SSRIs are the preferred drugs of choice for treating depression in patient with respiratory diseases. Atypical antipsychotics except clozapine can be used, if needed, in psychotic patients with respiratory diseases. Buspirone is the safest anxiolytic drug, because it does not depress respiration. However, SSRI with anxiolytic properties can be a better choice.

21.10 Conclusions

Psychopharmacological advances in psychosomatic medicine or consultation-liaison psychiatry have been in the area of anxiety disorders, depressive disorders, insomnia, somatization, eating disorders, migraine, and fibromyalgia. The ultimate goal of psychopharmacological management remains to bring optimal benefits to patients along with minimal adverse reactions which will enhance the quality of care. However, it should be kept in mind that for holistic management of patients with mental disorders including psychosomatic disorders in consultation-liaison psychiatry, nonpharmacological therapies, such as cognitive therapy, behavior therapy, and somatopsychic approaches, are necessary and vital.

References

1. Singh, A. N. (2006). Psychosomatic medicine and psychopharmacology, symbiosis of present future. *International Congress Series, 1287*, 12–16. Elsevier BV, Amsterdam.
2. Singh, A. N. (2006). Recent advances in the psychopharmacology of psychosomatic medicine. *International Congress Series, 1287*, 206–212. Elsevier BV, Amsterdam.
3. Singh, A. N., & Nagata, K. (2003). Recent advances in the psychopharmacology of psychosomatic medicine. *Pyschiatria et Neurologia Japonica, 105*, 441–447.
4. Singh, A. N. (1992). Pharmacological therapy in psychosomatic medicine. *Japanese Journal of Psychosomatic Medicine, 32*, 589–598.
5. Singh, A. N. (2010, September 10–12). *Recent advances in the psychopharmacology of psychosomatic medicine*. Paper presented at the 14th Congress of the Asian College of Psychosomatic Medicine, Beijing, China.
6. Boyer, W. (1995). Serotonin uptake inhibitors are superior to imipramine and alprazolam in alleviating panic attacks: A meta-analysis. *International Clinical Psychopharmacology, 10*, 45–49.
7. Bradwejn, J., Ahokas, A., Stein, D. J., et al. (2005). Venlafaxine extended release capsules in panic disorder: Flexible-dose, double-blind, placebo-controlled study. *The British Journal of Psychiatry, 187*, 352–359.
8. Sheehan, D. V., Raj, A. B., Sheehan, K. H., et al. (1990). Is buspirone effective for panic disorder? *Journal of Clinical Psychopharmacology, 10*, 3–11.
9. Simin, N. M., Hoge, E. A., Fischman, D., et al. (2006). An open-label trial of risperidone augmentation for refractory anxiety disorders. *The Journal of Clinical Psychiatry, 67*, 381–385.
10. Sepede, G., de Berardis, D., Gambi, F., et al. (2006). Olanzapine augmentation in treatment-resistant panic disorder: A 12-week, fixed-dose, open-label trial. *Journal of Clinical Psychopharmacology, 26*, 45–49.

11. Keck, P. E., Jr., McElroy, S. L., Tugrul, K. C., et al. (1993). Anti-epileptic drugs for the treatment of panic disorder. *Neuropsychobiology, 27*, 150–153.
12. Sarchiapone, M., Amore, M., De Risio, S., et al. (2003). Mirtazapine in the treatment of panic disorder: An open-label trial. *International Clinical Psychopharmacology, 18*, 35–38.
13. Bertani, A., Perna, G., Migliarese, G., et al. (2004). Comparison of the treatment with paroxetine and reboxetine in panic disorder: A randomized, single-blind study. *Pharmacopsychiatry, 37*, 206–210.
14. Singh, A. N. (1983). *A clinical picture of benzodiazepine dependence and guidelines for reducing dependence* (pp. 14–18). Princeton, NJ: Excerpta Medica Office.
15. Matthew, S. J., Amiel, J. M., Coplan, J. D., et al. (2005). Open-label trial of riluzole in generalized anxiety disorder. *The American Journal of Psychiatry, 162*, 2379–2381.
16. Jefferson, J. W., & Greist, J. H. (1996). The pharmacotherapy of obsessive-compulsive disorder. *Psychiatric Annals, 26*, 202–209.
17. Silver, J. M., Sandberg, D. P., & Hales, R. E. (1990). New approaches in the pharmacotherapy of post-traumatic stress disorder. *The Journal of Clinical Psychiatry, 51*(Supp. 10), 33–38.
18. Lipper, S., Davidson, J. R., Grady, T. A., et al. (1986). Preliminary study of carbamazepine in post-traumatic stress disorder. *Psychosomatics, 27*, 849–854.
19. Fesler, F. A. (1991). Valproate in combat-related post-traumatic stress disorder. *The Journal of Clinical Psychiatry, 52*, 361–364.
20. Baldwin, D., Bobes, J., Stein, D. J., et al. (1999). Paroxetine in social phobia/social anxiety disorder: Randomised, double-blind, placebo-controlled study. *The British Journal of Psychiatry, 175*, 120–126.
21. Baldwin, D., DeMartinis, N., Mallick, R. (2004, February 9–13). *Patient-reported functioning in SAD and improvement with treatment: A comparison of venlafaxine XR, paroxetine and placebo*. Program and abstracts of the International Congress of Biological Psychiatry, Sydney, Australia.
22. Stein, M. B., Fyer, A. J., Davidson, J. R., et al. (1999). Fluvoxamine treatment of social phobia: A double-blind, placebo-controlled study of fluvoxamine. *115*, 128–134.
23. Van Ameringan, M. A., Lane, R. M., Walker, J. R., et al. (2001). Sertraline treatment of generalized social phobia: A 20 week, double-blind, placebo-controlled study. *The American Journal of Psychiatry, 158*, 275–281.
24. Singh, A. N. (2006). Therapeutic uses of oriental approaches in psychosomatic medicine. *International Congress Series, 1287*, 91–96. Elsevier BV, Amsterdam.
25. Singh, A. N. (1992). Non-pharmacological approaches of Hindu Buddhist medicine in psychosomatic disorders. *Japanese Journal of Psychosomatic Medicine, 32*, 417–425.
26. Singh, A. N., & Janier, A. K. (1999). Recent advances in the treatment of depression. *Journal of the Indian Medical Association, 1*, 19–24.
27. Perlis, R. H. (2007). Pharmacogenetic studies of antidepressant response: How far from the clinic? *The Psychiatric Clinics of North America, 30*, 125–138.
28. Smits, K. M., Smits, L. J., Schouten, J. S., et al. (2007). Does pretreatment testing for serotonin transporter polymorphisms lead to earlier effects of drug treatment in patients with major depression? A decision-analytic model. *Clinical Therapeutics, 29*, 691–702.
29. Liu, Z., Zhu, F., Wang, G., et al. (2007). Association study of corticotrophin-releasing hormone receptor 1 gene polymorphisms and antidepressant response in major depressive disorder. *Neuroscience Letters, 414*(2), 155–158. Elsevier, Ireland.
30. Smits, K., Smits, L., Peeters, F., et al. (2007). Serotonin transporter polymorphisms and the occurrence of adverse events during treatment with selective serotonin reuptake inhibitors. *International Clinical Psychopharmacology, 22*, 137–143.
31. Hu, X. Z., Rush, A. J., Charney, D., et al. (2007). Association between a functional serotonin transporter polymorphism and citalopram treatment in adult outpatients with major depression. *Archives of General Psychiatry, 64*, 783–792.
32. Singh, A. N. (2004). Recent advances in the pharmacotherapy of insomnia. *WHO Lecture Series, 6*(1), 46–55.
33. Ikemi, Y. (1966). *Integration of occidental and oriental psychosomatic treatment in integration of Eastern and Western psychosomatic medicine* (pp. 37–46). Kyushu: Kyushu University Press.

34. Lieb, R., Meinschmidt, G., & Aryaya, R. (2007). Epidemiology of the association between somatoform disorders and anxiety and depressive disorders: An update. *Psychosomatic Medicine, 69*, 860–863.
35. Phillips, K. A., Albertini, R. S., & Rasmussen, S. A. (2002). A randomized placebo-controlled trial of fluoxetine in body dysmorphic disorder. *Archives of General Psychiatry, 59*, 381–388.
36. Fallon, B. A. (2004). Pharmacotherapy of somatoform disorders. *Journal of Psychosomatic Research, 56*, 455–460.
37. Mitchell, J. E., de Zwaan, M., & Roerig, J. L. (2003). Drug therapy for patients with eating disorders. *Current Drug Targets. CNS and Neurological Disorders, 2*(1), 17–29. Bentham Science Publishers, Oak Park, IL.
38. Yager, J. (2008). Binge eating disorder: The search for better treatments. *The American Journal of Psychiatry, 165*, 4–6.
39. Advokat, C., & Kutlesic, V. (1995). Pharmacotherapy of the eating disorders: A commentary. *Neuroscience and Biobehavioural Reviews, 19*(1), 59–66. Elsevier, USA.
40. Nickel, C., Tritt, K., Muehlbacher, M., et al. (2005). Topiramate treatment in bulimia nervosa patients: A randomized, double-blind, placebo-controlled trial. *International Journal of Eating Disorders, 38*, 295–300.
41. Appolinario, J. C., Bacaltchuk, J., Sicheri, R., et al. (2003). A randomized double-blind placebo-controlled study of sibutramine in the treatment of binge eating disorder. *Archives of General Psychiatry, 60*, 1109–1116.
42. Silviera, R. O., Zanatto, V., Appolinario, J. C., et al. (2005). An open trial of reboxetine in obese patients with binge eating disorder. *Eating and Weight Disorders, 10*, e93–e96.
43. Snoeck, E., Peer, A., Mannens, G., et al. (1995). Influence of age, renal and liver impairment on the pharmacokinetics of risperidone in man. *Journal of Biomedical Life Science - Psychopharmacology, 122*, 223–229.
44. Percudani, M., Barbui, C., Fortino, I., et al. (2005). Second-generation antipsychotics and risk of cerebrovascular accidents in the elderly. *Journal of Clinical Psychopharmacology, 25*, 468–470.

Chapter 22
Emotion, Interventions, and Immunity

Kyung Bong Koh

22.1 Introduction

Psychological stress can alter one's immune function and increase susceptibility to physical disease [1–3]. It can be assumed that negative life events (stressors) lead to negative affective states (distress), producing alterations in human immunity [4]. For example, an individual's emotional states, such as anxiety or depression, can be key factors in triggering immune alterations [4, 5].

Anxiety and depression are associated with disease recurrence in patients with genital and oral herpes [6]. Emotional factors are also thought to play roles in numerous diseases, including Graves' disease, rheumatoid arthritis, systemic lupus erythematosus, asthma, and diabetes [7]. Immunosuppression has been reported in human subjects who experience symptoms of anxiety and depression in response to situations such as examinations, bereavement, separation, and divorce [8–14]. In animals, immunosuppression has also been demonstrated in response to a variety of stressors [8, 15, 16].

Stress-reducing interventions such as relaxation may enhance immune function [17]. However, little is known about the effects on immune function of different coping styles or interventions in healthy individuals or in patients with emotional disorders. Herein, the author is going to review the effects of coping methods and interventions such as relaxation, meditation, cognitive behavioral therapy, psychotherapy, and pharmacotherapy on immune function, as well as the relationship between stress or emotion and immunity.

K.B. Koh, M.D., Ph.D. (✉)
Department of Psychiatry, Yonsei University College of Medicine,
50 Yonsei-ro, Seodaemun-gu, Seoul 120-752, Korea
e-mail: kbkoh@yuhs.ac

K.B. Koh (ed.), *Somatization and Psychosomatic Symptoms*,
DOI 10.1007/978-1-4614-7119-6_22, © Springer Science+Business Media New York 2013

22.2 Stress and Immunity

Academic stress, such as an examination period for medical students, has long been used as a model for investigating the interaction between stress and immunity. A number of studies using this model have indicated that examination stress downregulates immune functions such as lymphocyte proliferation, natural killer (NK) cell activity, salivary immunoglobulin A (IgA), latency of herpes virus and Epstein-Barr virus, production of interferon-γ (IFN-γ), interleukin-2 (IL-2) receptor gene expression, and mucosal wound healing [18–27]. In contrast, immune activation has been reported in response to examination stress in other studies. For example, salivary immunoglobulin A (IgA) levels were reported to be enhanced in students during an acute stress of an imminent examination [28]. The levels of phytohemagglutinin (PHA)-stimulated IL-2 production and lymphocyte proliferative responses to PHA were also shown to be significantly higher during an examination period than during a non-examination period [29–31]. Similarly, in another study, students with reactions to examination stress had significantly higher numbers of leukocytes, neutrophils, and monocytes during the examination period than those without stress reactions [32]. Such activated immune response may be associated with the intensity and/or duration of stress [15]. Mild, brief, and controllable states of challenged homeostasis may actually be perceived as pleasant or exciting, which could be positive stimuli for emotional and intellectual growth and development. Immune response may also be enhanced when the stressful condition is mild to moderate in intensity [15]. In contrast, more severe, protracted, and uncontrollable situations of psychological and physical distress are likely to lead to overt disease states [33], apparently resulting from immunosuppression. Therefore, immune activation can be considered to be a transient phenomenon that occurs prior to the downregulation of the immune function, which reflects the body's defensive response to stress [34]. It is also possible that arousal/hypervigilance associated with examinations play a role in activating immunity. From these perspectives, immune activation may be a biological signal warning an impending danger to health, as well as the body's physiological defense against stress.

Stress also modulates inflammatory responses [35, 36]. Previous research has suggested that psychological stressors or perceived stress levels are associated with increased production of proinflammatory cytokines, such as IL-1, IL-6, tumor necrosis factor-α (TNF-α), and IFN-γ [37–40]. In addition, a meta-analytic study found that brief stressors such as academic examinations changed the profile of cytokine production via a decrease in levels of IFN-γ and increases in levels of IL-6 and IL-10 [41]. However, one previous study reported reduced lipopolysaccharide (LPS)-stimulated expression of proinflammatory cytokines, such as IL-6 and TNF-α [42]. This is in line with the finding of Koh et al.'s study [43] in which only PHA was used to stimulate lymphocytes and reduced IL-6 production levels were found during an academic stress period. These differences might depend on cognitive stress appraisals such as the perceived levels of challenge or threat, control expectancy [42], and the intensity and duration of stressors or coping ability [31, 44]. Koh et al. [43] also reported that vacation associated with low stress is more likely to have a counterstress effect on proinflammatory cytokines (e.g., IL-6 and TNF-α production) than on an anti-inflammatory cytokine (e.g., IL-10 production) and that a stressor may affect changes in immune function independently of self-reported stress.

22.3 Emotion and Immunity

22.3.1 Depression and Immunity

Many studies have suggested that depressed patients exhibit decreased immune functions in a variety of immune measures when compared to nondepressed controls [45–48]. Examinations of the impact of depression on T cell responses in humans found that, in the context of bereavement or severe major depressive disorder, proliferation of peripheral blood mononuclear cells in response to the T cell mitogens, PHA and concanavalin A (Con A), was significantly reduced [8, 45, 49–51]. The degree of immunosuppression may be related to the severity of the depression in depressive disorders [48]. Lymphocyte responses to PHA and pokeweed mitogen (PWM) in patients with melancholic and psychotic depression were significantly lower than those with minor depression [52]. Compared to patients with non-melancholic depression, patients with melancholia demonstrated reduced in vivo cell-mediated immunity as assessed by delayed-type hypersensitivity skin responses [53].

Although there have been both successful and unsuccessful replication attempts, meta-analyses in this area have reached a consensus that reliable decreases in T cell responses are observed in depressed individuals [54, 55]. In addition, in vivo measures of cell-mediated immune function including skin responses to commonly encountered antigens have suggested decreased T cell activity in depressed patients [53].

The mechanisms of T cell alterations in depression in humans have yet to be established. However, a number of possibilities have been identified. Interestingly, flow cytometric assessments revealed that CD4+ T cells from depressed patients exhibit evidence of accelerated spontaneous apoptosis as well as increased expression of the receptor for Fas (CD95), which mediates apoptotic signaling by Fas ligand [56–58]. One possibility that might explain increased T cell apoptosis in depression, especially in the context of increased immune activation, is tryptophan depletion. A number of cytokines and cytokine signaling pathways have been known to activate the enzyme, indoleamine 2,3-dioxygenase (IDO), which breaks down tryptophan into kynurenine, thus depleting serotonin [59, 60]. Activations of both IDO and kynurenine have in turn been associated with the development of depression [59, 61, 62]. Relevant to T cell apoptosis, tryptophan is an essential proliferative stimulus for effector T cells, and in a tryptophan-deprived environment, T cells undergo apoptosis [63, 64].

Another mechanism that has been considered regarding T cell responses in major depressive disorder is inhibition of T cell function by glucocorticoids. Glucocorticoids have multiple effects on immune responses including inhibition of inflammation, mediation of cell trafficking, and induction of apoptosis in multiple immune cell types including T cells [65]. In addition, increased peripheral blood concentrations of the glucocorticoids (cortisol) are a hallmark of major depressive disorder [66]. Nevertheless, no relationships have been found between increased cortisol secretion and decreased in vitro proliferative responses to T cell mitogens in depressed patients [67]. Moreover, several studies demonstrated that peripheral blood lymphocytes from depressed patients exhibit decreased responsiveness to the in vitro inhibitory effects of glucocorticoids on T cell proliferation [66, 68, 69]. Such decreased responsiveness of peripheral blood lymphocytes, including T cells, to glucocorticoids in depressed patients may be related to decreased expression of glucocorticoid receptors [66, 69].

An additional potential mechanism whereby T cell function may be impaired in patients with depression is the disruption of T cell function by inflammatory cytokines, such as tumor necrosis factor-α (TNF-α), which is elevated in depressed patients [70]. For example, both in vitro and in vivo studies demonstrated that chronic exposure of T cells to TNF-α decreases T cell proliferation and cytokine production [71, 72]. In addition, depression enhances the production of proinflammatory cytokines, including IL-6 [73–75]. There is growing evidence that the production of proinflammatory cytokines stimulated by depression can influence a spectrum of conditions associated with aging, including cardiovascular disease, osteoporosis, arthritis, type 2 diabetes, certain cancers, periodontal disease, frailty, and functional decline [76]. Therefore, depression can downregulate the cellular immune response; as a consequence, processes such as prolonged infection and delayed wound healing that fuel sustained proinflammatory cytokine production may be promoted by depression [76].

Several genes that play roles in T cell function are associated with major depressive disorder and responses to antidepressants [77]. Single nucleotide polymorphisms (SNPs) in the genes PSMB4 (proteasome beta4 subunit, which is important for antigen processing) and TBX21 (T bet, which is important in T cell differentiation) are associated in a dose-dependent fashion with the likelihood of being diagnosed with depression [77].

On the other hand, activated T cells may play an important neuroprotective role in the context of stress and inflammation [78–80]. For example, generation of autoreactive T cells through immunization with central nervous system (CNS)–specific antigens reverses stress-induced decreases in hippocampal neurogenesis as well as depressive-like behavior in rodents. T regulatory cells may also play a role in depression through the downregulation of chronic inflammatory responses. Based on the hypothesis that T cells may subserve neuroprotective and anti-inflammatory functions during stress and inflammation, impaired T cell function may directly contribute to the development of depression. Further elucidation of T cell pathology may lead to new insights into immune system contributions to depression. Moreover, enhancement of T cell function may represent an alternative strategy to treat depression [81].

22.3.2 Anxiety and Immunity

It was observed that a group of subjects with generalized anxiety disorder, panic disorder, or both had a higher frequency of upper respiratory infection compared with controls [82]. Recurrent lesions of genital herpes were preceded by higher levels of anxiety and concomitant blunting of T cell blastogenesis [24]. In another study, lymphocyte response was negatively correlated with anxiety among hospitalized patients [83]. A 72-h stimulation with anti-CD3+ induced significantly lower expression of CD25+ in generalized anxiety disorder patients compared to controls [84]. In addition, patients with panic disorder had significantly lower levels of CD4+ than healthy controls and depressive disorder patients [85]. Koh et al.'s study [86] found a reduced cell-mediated immune function (e.g., lymphocyte proliferative response to PHA and IL-2 production) in patients with anxiety disorders compared to normal controls. However, lymphocyte proliferative response to mitogens varies within a wide range; decreased, normal, and increased responses have been observed in panic disorder patients compared with normal controls [87–91]. IgA levels are increased in panic disorder patients compared to normal controls [92].

Patients with obsessive-compulsive disorder do not differ from normal controls in plasma concentration of IL-1β, IL-6, soluble IL-6 receptor, sIL-2R, or transferrin receptor [93]. Subjects suffering from posttraumatic stress disorder (PTSD) after a hurricane had lower NK cell activity when compared to normal controls [94]. In another study, however, combat veterans with PTSD had enhanced cell-mediated immunity compared with healthy civilians and servicemen in a test of cell-mediated immunity [95]. Such unexpected findings suggest that the arousal/hypervigilance associated with PTSD may be more influential on immune functioning than the anxiety symptoms which often accompany PTSD.

Anxiety disorders such as panic disorder are accompanied by activation of the hypothalamic-pituitary-adrenal (HPA) axis, which seems to be correlated with the degree of anxiety experienced by patients. On the other hand, decrease of anxiety after alprazolam therapy occurs in concert with normalization of the HPA axis function [89]. In panic disorder, however, there may be dissociations between the HPA axis and immune systems. This hypothesis is supported by the observation that administration of corticotrophin-releasing hormone (CRH) with the ensuing adrenocorticotropic hormone (ACTH)-cortisol hypersecretion failed to modify the lymphocyte proliferative response to PHA [89].

As opposed to a clinical level of anxiety, subclinical anxiety seen in people suffering from familial traumatic injury [96] or medical students during examination stress [97] may be associated with increased immune function (e.g., mitogen-induced lymphocyte proliferation, NK cell activity). Such immune enhancement in subclinical anxiety may be considered a transient phenomenon occurring prior to the downregulation of immune function, reflecting the body's defense against a stressor. Thus, immune alteration depends on clinical or subclinical levels of anxiety and the levels of hypervigilance [34]. In addition, it was reported that subclinical anxiety during an examination period was associated with reduction in proinflammatory cytokines such as TNF-α production [98].

22.4 Coping Strategies and Immunity

Coping responses or strategies represent specific actions that people take in order to deal with a given problem or stressor [99]. An individual's coping strategies are known to affect the stress responses [100] such as endocrine and immune functions. A significant negative correlation was reported between an individual's coping style of "comforting cognition" and cortisol response during mental stress [101]. Coping by accepting the reality of stressful situations proved protective for patients with hepatitis B, whereas coping by substance use increased the risk of having an inadequate count of hepatitis B antibody [102]. In the context of personal relationships and immune function, lonelier medical students had lower NK cell activity than students who were not as lonely [103]. Medical students who reported greater social support showed stronger immune response to hepatitis B vaccine than those with less support [104]. In an experimental study, expressing emotionally traumatic events that had not previously been disclosed to others was associated with increased proliferative response to PHA [24].

A few studies reported relationships between coping and immunity in different stress situations and at different perceived stress levels. Law students who were optimistic showed higher numbers of CD4+ cells in less conflictual situations and lower numbers of CD4+ cells in more conflictual situations [105]. However, in another study, higher levels of active coping were significantly related to greater increases in proliferative response to PHA and Con A at high stress levels. In contrast, at low stress levels, active coping was not significantly related to proliferative responses, whereas avoidance was associated with greater proliferative response to Con A [106]. Positive reappraisal and seeking social support were associated with alteration of immune function during chronic stress periods in another previous study; in particular, positive reappraisal was found to reverse stress-induced immune responses [31].

22.5 Interventions and Immunity

22.5.1 Stress Reduction Interventions and Immunity

Stress management techniques such as relaxation and meditation may affect immune function. It was reported that biofeedback-assisted relaxation training was associated with reductions in tension and anxiety and improvement in phagocytic abilities, such as enhanced neutrophil activation [107]. In another study, a single 20-min session of relaxation training resulted in significant increases in salivary IgA concentrations from the prerelaxation period to the postrelaxation period, in contrast to a non-relaxation control group [108]. Stress reduction has also been shown to diminish inflammatory responses [109, 110]. Koh et al. [111] reported that significant reductions in the change (stress period value minus baseline period value) in

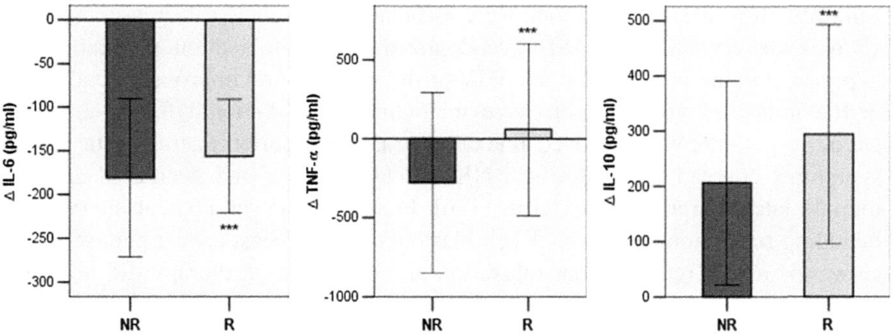

Fig. 22.1 Effects of relaxation on the changes in proinflammatory and anti-inflammatory cytokine production. *R* relaxation group, *NR* non-relaxation group. ***Significant reductions in the change (stress period value minus baseline period value) in the levels of IL-6 and TNF-α production, but significant enhancement in the change in the level of the IL-10 production in a relaxation group compared with a non-relaxation group (From Koh et al. [111])

the total Global Assessment of Recent Stress score, systolic and diastolic blood pressure, levels of IL-6, and TNF-α production and significant enhancement in the change in the level of the IL-10 production were found in a relaxation group of medical students compared with a non-relaxation group (Fig. 22.1). These results suggest that relaxation is associated with reduction in stress-induced psychological or physiological responses and proinflammatory cytokine alterations but with enhancement in stress-induced anti-inflammatory cytokine alteration. Therefore, relaxation is more likely to have counterstress effect on proinflammatory cytokines than on anti-inflammatory cytokine.

Healthy individuals experiencing job-related stress who participated in mindfulness meditation showed greater antibody responses to the influenza vaccine when compared to a control group [112]. Within the meditation group, increased meditation practice was correlated with decreased stress-induced IL-6. These data suggest that engagement in compassion meditation may reduce stress-induced immune responses [113]. However, one study found that stress reduction techniques such as relaxation did not affect IL-6 levels in healthy individuals [114].

Telomerase activity is a predictor of long-term cellular viability, which decreases with chronic psychological distress [115]. In a study investigating the effects of a 3-month meditation retreat on mononuclear cell telomerase activity, telomerase activity was significantly greater in retreat participants than in controls at the end of the retreat [116].

Stress management techniques may affect immune function in patients with physical diseases. One study of the effects of relaxation on immunity in males at high risk for human immunodeficiency virus (HIV)-1 infection found positive correlations between the frequency of relaxation practice and numbers of T helper cells, T inducer cells, the T helper/T suppressor ratio, and the number of NK cells during the high-stress week of serostatus determination [117]. A study of the effects of relaxation on immunity in HIV-positive men showed that lower stress levels achieved after relaxation practice were associated with greater decreases in herpes simplex virus type 2 IgG [118]. A randomized study of relaxation, meditation, and hypnosis training in asymptomatic HIV-positive men found improved T cell counts in the treatment group which were maintained at a 1-month follow-up [119]. Geriatric patients who received relaxation training reported decreases in distress symptoms coupled with increased NK cell cytotoxicity and decreased antibody titers to latent herpes simplex virus [120]. In addition, psychological intervention, including relaxation, improved T cell blastogenesis in breast cancer patients [121]. However, it was reported that relaxation and visualization therapy did not affect lymphocyte proliferation in breast cancer patients undergoing radiotherapy [122].

A mindfulness-based stress reduction (MBSR) program that incorporated relaxation, meditation, gentle yoga, and daily home practice also increased NK cell activity in HIV-positive men [123] and buffered CD4+ T lymphocyte declines in HIV-1-infected adults [124]. Over time, women with breast cancer showed enhanced NK cell activity and reduced levels of IL-4 and IL-10 production in the MBSR group compared with the non-MBSR group [125]. In breast and prostate cancer patients, the post-MBSR intervention level of NK cell production of IL-10 and T cell production of IFN-λ were also reduced, whereas T cell production of IL-4 increased when compared to the pre-intervention level [126].

A combined program of light- to moderate-intensity aerobic and resistance exercise offsets the apparent decrement in NK cell activity with weight loss in obese women [127].

On the other hand, Koh and Lew [128] examined the effect of vitamin B complex on academic stress-induced immune alteration in medical students and found that vitamin B complex reduced anxiety levels, but did not affect cell-mediated immunity, such as lymphocyte proliferative response to PHA and PHA-stimulated IL-2 production.

22.5.2 Therapeutic Interventions and Immunity

There is consistent support for the efficacy of cognitive behavioral treatment (CBT) to aid the successful discontinuation of benzodiazepine medication in patients with panic disorder and to help maintain treatment gains while not taking medication [129]. However, there are very few studies on the effects of pharmacotherapy and CBT on immune function. One study reported that there was no significant effect of alprazolam therapy on lymphocyte proliferative response to PHA in patients with panic disorder [89]. Patients in the CBT plus paroxetine condition had significantly improved agoraphobic behavior and anxiety discomfort, whereas patients in the CBT plus placebo condition did not [130]. However, the differential efficacy of psychopharmacological treatment versus the combination of this drug with CBT on immunity remains unclear. One study examined the relationship between the reduced anxiety level by therapeutic interventions, such as CBT with an antianxiety agent, and cell-mediated immunity (CMI) in patients with panic disorder. This study revealed that the reduced level of self-reported anxiety by the combined therapeutic intervention was associated with increased blastogenic response [91].

However, another study reported little effect of psychotherapy in patients with anxiety or depression on immunity. The CD4+/CD8+ ratio remained elevated in a small number of patients with anxiety disorders, but there were no significant changes in this parameter over the 8-week course of inpatient psychotherapy. In addition, no difference in the CD4+/CD8+ ratio was found between depressive patients and healthy controls nor in this parameter over the course of inpatient psychotherapy [131]

Symptom remission may abrogate reduced NK cell activity associated with major depressive disorder [132]. On the other hand, antidepressants such as selective serotonin reuptake inhibitors (SSRIs) appear to promote a return of NK cell number to control levels. However, it is likely that effectiveness is related to the subtype of depressive disorder. It is particularly interesting that although both major depressive disorder and dysthymic disorder were successfully treated with these antidepressants, dysthymic patients required a more prolonged duration of treatment for NK cell numbers to return to control values than major depressive disorder patients. Thus, when assessing the relationship between depression and immune status, it is necessary to recognize not only the severity of illness but also the duration of illness and age of onset.

T cell proliferation in response to PHA and Con A remained stable or increased after psychological intervention (strategies to reduce stress, improve mood, alter health behaviors, and maintain adherence to cancer treatment and care) in patients with breast cancer [133]. In addition, breast cancer patients receiving cognitive behavioral stress management showed greater Th1 cytokine IL-2 and IFN-γ production than the control group [134]. Breast cancer patients who received experiential-existential group psychotherapy also showed lower percentages of NK cells, CD8+ cells, and CD4+ cells and lower proliferative response to PWM when compared to patients in the waiting list control group [135].

22.6 Future Directions

Studies that have examined immune activity in somatoform disorder patients are sparse in comparison with those in depressive disorder and anxiety disorder patients. In Koh et al.'s study [136], patients with undifferentiated somatoform disorder as a group showed reduced cell-mediated immunity (e.g., blastogenic responses to PHA) when compared with healthy controls. Moreover, alteration of proinflammatory cytokines can be anticipated in patients with somatoform disorders who often show sickness behavior, because proinflammatory cytokines may trigger a brain-cytokine system that organizes the sickness response [137]. Therefore, further studies are needed to evaluate immunity in somatoform disorder patients.

In order to elucidate the relationship between stress or emotion and immunity, it is necessary to integrate the data related to immune, endocrine, autonomic nervous

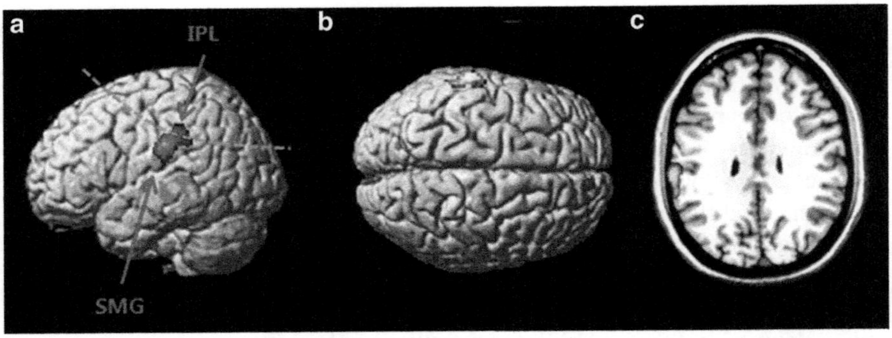

Fig. 22.2 Hypoperfused brain areas in more immune-suppressed group compared with less immune-suppressed group in surface projection (**a**, **b**) and transaxial plane (**c**). Hypoperfusion was significant at the left inferior parietal lobule (*IPL*) and the left supramarginal gyrus (*SMG*) in more immune-suppressed group compared with less immune-suppressed group (FDR, $p<0.05$). *FDR* false discovery rate (From Koh et al. [136])

system, and brain activity measured at the same time, because bodily homeostasis can be maintained by interaction between these variables [138]. In particular, these interactions should be examined in a clinical sample including somatoform disorder patients. In a previous study [139], changes in lymphocyte proliferation and NK activity have been associated with negative life events only among individuals with greater left frontal cortical activation. In a recent study on neural activity in patients with undifferentiated somatoform disorder, Koh et al. [136] reported that hypoperfusion was significant at the left inferior parietal lobule and the left supramarginal gyrus in the more immune-suppressed subgroup compared to the less immune-suppressed subgroup (Fig. 22.2). These results also suggest the role of cerebral asymmetry in altered immunity in the patients.

On the other hand, there have been few studies on the relationship between depression and cytokine-related genes, in contrast with a number of studies on the relationship between depression and inflammation-related cytokines or between depression and serotonin-related genes. Therefore, the interaction between depression, cytokines, and genes should be included in the future studies.

In addition, to confirm the interaction between emotion and immune function, the effectiveness of a variety of treatment modalities on immunity should be investigated in a clinical sample of mental disorder or physical disease patients.

22.7 Conclusions

Meta-analyses showed statistically reliable decreases in T cell responses in depressed individuals. Patients with anxiety disorders, especially panic disorder, are likely to show reduced immune function, although several studies showed contradictory findings. This literature review reveals evidence that relaxation, mindfulness-based stress reduction, and cognitive behavioral therapy are effective interventions to counter the effects of stress on immunity. The ability of such interventions to improve immunity has been demonstrated for patients with panic disorder, for HIV-infected men, and for breast cancer patients, as well as for healthy individuals experiencing stress. These results provide a rationale for clinical applications to improve immunity in patients with immune-related disorders. Further studies are needed to examine the effects of a variety of therapeutic interventions on immunity in a larger variety of mental disorders or physical diseases, as well as the long-term effects of treatment on immune function. Research efforts in this area will also add to the body of literature regarding the interactions between emotion and immune function. In particular, the interaction between immune, endocrine, autonomic nervous system, and brain activity should be examined in a clinical sample including somatoform disorder patients. In addition, the interaction between depression, cytokines, and genes should be included in the future studies.

References

1. Elliot, G. R., & Eisengdorfer, C. (1982). *Stress and human health: Analysis and implications of research*, A Study by the Institute of Medicine and the National Academy of Sciences, New York: Springer.
2. Herberman, R. B. (1982). *NK cells and other natural effector cells*. New York: Academic Press.
3. Levy, L. (1974). Psychosocial stress and disease: A conceptual model. In E. K. Gunderson & R. H. Rahe (Eds.), *Life stress and illness*. Springfield, MA: Thomas.
4. Herbert, T. B., & Cohen, S. (1993). Depression and immunity: A meta-analytic review. *Psychological Bulletin, 113*, 472–486.
5. Weisse, C. S. (1992). Depression and immunocompetence: A review of the literature. *Psychological Bulletin, 111*, 475–489.
6. Locke, S. E., & Gorman, J. R. (1989). Behavior and immunity. In H. I. Kaplan & B. J. Sadock (Eds.), *Comprehensive textbook of psychiatry*. Baltimore, MD: Williams & Wilkins.
7. Camara, E. G., & Danao, T. C. (1989). The brain and the immune system: A psychosomatic network. *Psychosomatics, 30*, 140–146.
8. Bartrop, R. W., Luckhurst, E., & Lazarus, L. (1977). Depressed lymphocyte function after bereavement. *Lancet, 1*, 834–836.
9. Tecoma, E. S., & Huey, L. Y. (1985). Psychic distress and the immune response. *Life Sciences, 36*, 1799–1812.
10. Calabrese, J. R., Skwerer, R. G., Barna, B., et al. (1986). Depression, immunocompetence, and prostaglandins of the E series. *Psychiatry Research, 17*, 41–47.
11. Perez, M., & Farrant, J. (1988). Immune reactions and mental disorders (editorial). *Psychosomatic Medicine, 18*, 11–13.
12. Hickie, I., Silove, D., & Hickie, C. (1990). Is there immune dysfunction in depressive disorders? *Psychological Medicine, 20*, 755–761.
13. Khansari, D. N., Murugo, A. H., & Faith, R. E. (1990). Effects of stress on the immune system. *Immunology Today, 11*, 170–175.
14. Kiecolt-Glaser, J. K., & Glaser, R. (1992). Stress and the immune system: Human studies. In A. Tasman & M. B. Riba (Eds.), *American psychiatric press review of psychiatry* (Vol. 11). Washington, DC: American Psychiatric Press.

15. Weiss, J. M., & Sundar, S. (1992). Effects of stress on cellular immune responses in animals. In A. Tasman & M. B. Riba (Eds.), *American psychiatric press review of psychiatry* (Vol. 11). Washington, DC: American Psychiatric Press.
16. Kelley, K. W. (1985). Immunological consequences of changing environmental stimuli. In G. Moberg (Ed.), *Animal stress*. Bethesda, MD: American Psychological Society.
17. Kiecolt-Glaser, J. K., & Glaser, R. (1986). Psychological influences on immunity. *Psychosomatics, 27*, 621–624.
18. Glaser, R., Rice, J., Speicher, C. E., et al. (1986). Stress depresses interferon production and natural killer (NK) cell activity in humans. *Behavioral Neuroscience, 100*, 675–678.
19. Glaser, R., Rice, J., Sheridan, J., et al. (1987). Stress-related immune suppression: Health implications. *Brain, Behavior, and Immunity, 1*, 7–20.
20. Marchesi, G. F., Cotani, P., Santone, G., et al. (1989). Psychological and immunological relationships during acute academic stress. *New Trends in Experimental and Clinical Psychiatry, 5*, 5–22.
21. Glaser, R., Kennedy, S., Lafuse, W. P., et al. (1990). Psychological stress-induced modulation of interleukin-2 receptor gene expression and interleukin-2 production in peripheral blood leukocytes. *Archives of General Psychiatry, 47*, 702–712.
22. Dobbin, J. P., Harth, M., Mccain, G. A., et al. (1991). Cytokine production and lymphocyte transformation during stress. *Brain, Behavior, and Immunity, 5*, 339–348.
23. Glaser, R., Pearson, G. R., Jones, J. F., et al. (1991). Stress-related activation of Epstein-Barr virus. *Brain, Behavior, and Immunity, 5*, 219–232.
24. Fawzy, F. I. (1995). Behavior and immunity. In H. I. Kaplan & B. J. Sodock (Eds.), *Comprehensive textbook of psychiatry*. Baltimore, MD: Willams & Wilkins.
25. Deinzer, R., & Schuller, N. (1998). Dynamics of stress-related decrease of salivary immunoglobulin A (sIgA): Relationship to symptoms of the common cold and studying behavior. *Behavioral Medicine, 23*, 161–169.
26. Marucha, D. T., Kiecolt-Glaser, J. K., & Favagehi, M. (1998). Mucosal wound healing is impaired by examination stress. *Psychosomatic Medicine, 60*, 362–365.
27. Rojas, I. G., Padgett, D. A., Sheridan, J. F., et al. (2002). Stress-induced susceptibility to bacterial infection during cutaneous wound healing. *Brain, Behavior, and Immunity, 16*, 74–84.
28. Bosch, J. A., Brand, H. S., Ligtenberg, A. J. M., et al. (1998). The response of salivary protein levels and S-IgA to an academic examination are associated with daily stress. *Journal of Psychophysiology, 4*, 170–178.
29. Kang, D., Coe, C. L., & McCarthy, D. O. (1996). Academic examinations significantly impact immune responses, but not lung function, in healthy and well-managed asthmatic adolescents. *Brain, Behavior, and Immunity, 10*, 164–181.
30. Koh, K. B. (2001). The relationship of stress-induced hypothalamic-pituitary-adrenal axis function with cell-mediated immunity. *Journal of Korean Neuropsychiatric Association, 40*, 857–866.
31. Koh, K. B., Choe, E., Song, J. E., et al. (2006). Effect of coping on endocrinoimmune functions in different stress situations. *Psychiatry Research, 143*, 223–234.
32. Maes, M., van Bockstaele, D. R., Gastel, A. V., et al. (1999). The effects of psychological stress on leukocyte subset distribution in humans: Evidence of immune activation. *Neuropsychobiology, 39*, 1–9.
33. Chrousos, G. P. (1992). The concept of stress and stress system disorders. *Journal of the American Medical Association, 267*, 1244–1252.
34. Koh, K. B. (1998). Emotion and immunity. *Journal of Psychosomatic Research, 45*, 107–115.
35. Chrousos, G. P. (1995). The hypothalamic-pituitary-adrenal axis and immune-mediated inflammation. *The New England Journal of Medicine, 332*, 1351–1362.
36. Sternberg, E. M., Chrousos, G. P., Wilder, R. L., et al. (1992). The stress response and the regulation of inflammatory disease. *Annals of Internal Medicine, 117*, 854–866.

37. Maes, M., Song, C., Lin, A., et al. (1998). The effects of psychological stress on humans: Increased production of pro-inflammatory cytokines and a Th1-like response in stress-induced anxiety. *Cytokine, 10*, 313–318.
38. Maes, M., Song, C., Lin, A., et al. (1998). Immune and clinical correlates of psychological stress-induced production of interferon—γ and IL-10 in humans. In N. P. Plotnikoff, R. E. Faith, A. J. Murgo, & R. A. Good (Eds.), *Cytokines, stress and immunity*. Boca Raton, FL: Raven Press.
39. Goebel, M. U., Mills, P. J., Irwin, M. R., et al. (2000). Interleukin-6 and tumor necrosis factor-α production after acute psychological stress, exercise, and infused isoproterenol: Differential effects and pathways. *Psychosomatic Medicine, 62*, 591–598.
40. Steptoe, A., Willemsen, G., Owen, N., et al. (2001). Acute mental stress elicits delayed increases in circulating inflammatory cytokine levels. *Clinical Science, 101*, 185–192.
41. Segerstrom, S. C., & Miller, G. E. (2004). Psychological stress and the human immune system: A meta-analytic study of 30 years of inquiry. *Psychological Bulletin, 130*, 601–630.
42. Wirtz, P. H., von Kanel, R., Emini, L., et al. (2007). Variations in anticipatory cognitive stress appraisal and differential proinflammatory cytokine expression in response to acute stress. *Brain, Behavior, and Immunity, 21*, 851–859.
43. Koh, K. B., Lee, Y., Beyn, K. M., et al. (2012). Effects of high and low stress on proinflammatory and antiinflammatory cytokines. *Psychophysiology, 49*, 1290–1297.
44. Koh, K. B. (2011). *Stress and psychosomatic medicine*. Seoul: Ilchokak.
45. Kronfol, A., Silva, J., Gredin, J., et al. (1983). Impaired lymphocyte function in depressive illness. *Life Sciences, 33*, 241–247.
46. Kronfol, Z., & House, J. D. (1984). Depression, cortisol, and immune function. *Lancet, 1*, 1026–1027.
47. Krueger, R. B., Levy, E. M., & Cathcart, E. S. (1984). Lymphocyte subsets in patients with major depression: Preliminary findings. *Advances, 1*, 5–9.
48. Stein, M., Keller, S. E., & Schleifer, S. J. (1985). Stress and immunomodulation: The role of depression and neuroendocrine function. *Journal of Immunology, 135*, 827–833.
49. Schleifer, S. J., Keller, S. E., Camereno, M., et al. (1983). Suppression of lymphocyte stimulation following bereavement. *Journal of the American Medical Association, 250*, 374–377.
50. Schleifer, S. J., Keller, S. E., Meyerson, A. T., et al. (1984). Lymphocyte function in major depressive disorder. *Archives of General Psychiatry, 41*, 484–486.
51. Stein, M., Miller, A. H., & Trestman, R. L. (1991). Depression, the immune system, and health and illness. *Archives of General Psychiatry, 48*, 171–177.
52. Maes, M., Bosmans, E., Suy, E., et al. (1989). Impaired lymphocyte stimulation by mitogens in severely depressed patients. *The British Journal of Psychiatry, 155*, 793–798.
53. Hickie, I., Hickie, C., Lloyd, A., et al. (1993). Impaired in vivo immune responses in patients with melancholia. *The British Journal of Psychiatry, 162*, 651–657.
54. Irwin, M. R., & Miller, A. H. (2007). Depressive disorders and immunity: 20 years of progress and discovery. *Brain, Behavior, and Immunity, 21*, 374–383.
55. Zoriller, E. P., Luborsky, L., McKay, J. R., et al. (2001). The relationship of depression and stressors to immunological assays: A meta-analytic review. *Brain, Behavior, and Immunity, 15*, 199–226.
56. Eilat, E., Mendlovic, S., Doron, A., et al. (1999). Increased apoptosis in patients with major depression: A preliminary study. *Journal of Immunology, 163*, 533–534.
57. Ivanova, S. A., Semke, V. Y., Vetlugina, T. P., et al. (2007). Signs of apoptosis of immunocompetent cells in patients with depression. *Neuroscience and Behavioral Physiology, 37*, 527–530.
58. Szuster-Ciesielska, A., Slotwinska, M., Stachura, A., et al. (2008). Accelerated apoptosis of blood leukocytes and oxidative stress in blood of patients with major depression. *Progress in Neuro-Psychopharmacology & Biological Psychiatry, 32*, 686–694.
59. Dantzer, R., O'Connor, J. C., Freund, G. G., et al. (2008). From inflammation to sickness and depression: When the immune system subjugates the brain. *Nature Reviews Neuroscience, 9*, 46–56.

60. Schwarcz, R., & Pellicciari, R. (2002). Manipulation of brain kynurenines: Glial targets, neuronal effects, and clinical opportunities. *Journal of Pharmacology and Experimental Therapeutics, 303*, 1–10.
61. Bonaccorso, S., Marino, V., Puzella, A., et al. (2002). Increased depressive ratings in patients with hepatitis C receiving interferon-alpha-based immunotherapy are related to interferon-alpha-induced changes in the serotonergic system. *Journal of Clinical Psychopharmacology, 22*, 86–90.
62. Capuron, L., Ravaud, A., Neveu, P. J., et al. (2002). Association between decreased serum tryptophan concentrations and depressive symptoms in cancer patients undergoing cytokine therapy. *Molecular Psychiatry, 7*, 468–473.
63. Beisssert, S., Schwarz, A., Schwarz, T., et al. (2006). Regulatory T cells. *The Journal of Investigative Dermatology, 126*, 15–24.
64. Mellor, A. L., Munn, D., Chandler, P., et al. (2003). Tryptophan catabolism and T cell responses. *Advances in Experimental Medicine and Biology, 527*, 27–35.
65. McEwen, B. S., Biron, C. A., Brunson, K. W., et al. (1997). The role of adrenocorticoids as modulators of immune function in health and disease: Neural, endocrine and immune interactions. *Brain Research Reviews, 23*, 79–133.
66. Pariante, C. M., & Miller, A. H. (2001). Glucocorticoid receptors in major depression: Relevance to pathophysiology and treatment. *Biological Psychiatry, 49*, 391–404.
67. Kronfol, Z., House, J. D., Silva, J., Jr., et al. (1986). Depression, urinary free cortisol excretion and lymphocyte function. *The British Journal of Psychiatry, 148*, 70–73.
68. Bauer, M. E., Papadopoulos, A., Poon, L., et al. (2003). Altered glucocorticoid immunoregulation in treatment resistant depression. *Psychoneuroendocrinology, 28*, 49–65.
69. Raison, C. L., & Miller, A. H. (2003). When not enough is too much: The role of insufficient glucocorticoid signaling in the pathophysiology of stress-related disorders. *The American Journal of Psychiatry, 160*, 1554–1565.
70. Miller, A. H., Maletic, V., Raison, C. L., et al. (2009). Inflammation and its discontents: The role of cytokines in the pathophysiology of major depression. *Biological Psychiatry, 65*, 732–741.
71. Cope, A. P., Liblau, R. S., Yang, X. D., et al. (1997). Chronic tumor necrosis factor alters T cell responses by attenuating T cell receptor signaling. *The Journal of Experimental Medicine, 185*, 1573–1584.
72. Cope, A. P., Londei, M., Chu, N. R., et al. (1994). Chronic exposure to tumor necrosis factor (TNF) in vitro impairs the activation of T cells through the T cell receptor/CD3 complex; reversal in vivo by anti-TNF antibodies in patients with rheumatoid arthritis. *The Journal of Clinical Investigation, 94*, 749–760.
73. Dentino, A. N., Pieper, C. F., Rao, K. M. K., et al. (1999). Association of interleukin-6 and other biologic variables with depression in older people living in the community. *Journal of American Geriatrics Society, 47*, 6–11.
74. Maes, M., Bosmans, E., Jongh, D., et al. (1995). Increased serum IL-6 and IL-1 receptor antagonist concentrations in major depression and treatment resistant depression. *Cytokine, 9*, 853–858.
75. Maes, M., Lin, A., Delmeire, L., et al. (1999). Elevated serum interleukin-6 (IL-6) and IL-6 receptor concentrations in posttraumatic stress disorder following accidental man-made traumatic events. *Biological Psychiatry, 45*, 833–839.
76. Kiecolt-Glaser, J. K., & Glaser, R. (2002). Depression and immune function: Central pathways to morbidity and mortality. *Journal of Psychosomatic Research, 53*, 873–876.
77. Wong, M. L., Dong, C., Maestre-Mesa, J., et al. (2008). Polymorphisms in inflammation-related genes are associated with susceptibility to major depression and antidepressant response. *Molecular Psychiatry, 13*, 800–812.
78. Lewitus, G. M., & Schwartz, M. (2009). Behavioral immunization: Immunity to self-antigens contributes to psychological stress resilience. *Molecular Psychiatry, 14*, 532–536.

79. Lewitus, G. M., Wilf-Yarkoni, A., Ziv, Y., et al. (2009). Vaccination as a novel approach for treating depressive behavior. *Biological Psychiatry, 65*, 283–288.
80. Rook, G. A., & Lowry, C. A. (2008). The hygiene hypothesis and psychiatric disorders. *Trends in Immunology, 29*, 150–158.
81. Miller, A. H. (2010). Depression and immunity: A role for T cells? *Brain, Behavior, and Immunity, 24*, 1–8.
82. La Via, M. F., Workman, E. W., & Lydiard, R. B. (1992). Subtype response to stress-induced immunodepression. *Functional Neurology, 7*(Supp. 3), 19–22.
83. Linn, B. S., Linn, M. W., & Jensen, J. (1981). Anxiety and immune responsiveness. *Psychological Reports, 49*, 969–970.
84. La Via, M. F., Munno, I., Lydiard, R. B., et al. (1996). The influence of stress intrusion on immunodepression in generalized anxiety disorder patients and controls. *Psychosomatic Medicine, 58*, 138–142.
85. Marazziti, D., Ambrogi, F., Vanacore, R., et al. (1992). Immune cell imbalance in major depressive and panic disorders. *Neuropsychobiology, 26*, 23–26.
86. Koh, K. B., & Lee, B. K. (1998). Reduced lymphocyte proliferation and interleukin-2 production in anxiety disorders. *Psychosomatic Medicine, 60*, 479–483.
87. Schleifer, S. J., Keller, S. E., Scotte, B. J., et al. (1990). Lymphocyte function in panic disorder. *Biological Psychiatry, 27*(suppl.), 66A.
88. Surman, O. S., Williams, J., Sheehan, D. V., et al. (1986). Immunological response to stress in agoraphobia and panic attacks. *Biological Psychiatry, 21*, 768–774.
89. Brambilla, F., Bellodi, L., Perna, G., et al. (1992). Psychoimmunoendocrine aspects of panic disorder. *Neuropsychobiology, 26*, 12–22.
90. Andreoil, A., Keller, S. E., Taban, C., et al. (1990). Immune function in major depressive disorder: Relation to panic disorder comorbidity. *Biological Psychiatry, 27*(suppl. 9A), 95A.
91. Koh, K. B., & Lee, Y. (2004). Reduced anxiety level by therapeutic interventions and cell-mediated immunity in panic disorder patients. *Psychotherapy and Psychosomatics, 73*, 286–292.
92. Ramesh, C., Yeragani, V. K., & Balon, R. (1991). A comparative study of immune status in panic disorder patients and controls. *Acta Psychiatrica Scandinavica, 84*, 396–397.
93. Maes, M., Meltzer, H. Y., & Bosmans, E. (1994). Psychoimmune investigation in obsessive-compulsive disorder: Assays of plasma transferrin, IL-2 and IL-6 receptor, and IL-1β and IL-6 concentrations. *Neuropsychobiology, 30*, 57–60.
94. Ironson, G., Wynings, C., Schneiderman, N., et al. (1997). Posttraumatic stress symptoms, intrusive thoughts, loss, and immune function after Hurricane Andrew. *Psychosomatic Medicine, 59*, 128–141.
95. Watson, P. B., Muller, H. K., Jones, I. H., et al. (1993). Cell-mediated immunity in combat veterans with post-traumatic stress disorder. *The Medical Journal of Australia, 159*, 513–516.
96. Schleifer, S. J., Keller, S. E., Scott, B. J., et al. (1989). *Familial traumatic injury and immunity*. San Francisco, CA: American Psychiatric Association New Research. May (Abstract).
97. Koh, K. B. (1995). The Relationship between stress and natural killer-cell activity in medical college students. *Korean Journal of Psychosomatic Medicine, 3*, 3–10.
98. Chandrashekara, S., Jayashree, K., Veeranna, H. B., et al. (2007). Effects of anxiety on TNF-α levels during psychological stress. *Journal of Psychosomatic Research, 63*, 65–69.
99. Menaghan, E. G. (1982). Measuring coping effectiveness: A panel analysis of marital problems and coping efforts. *Journal of Health and Social Behavior, 23*, 220–234.
100. Holroyd, K. A., & Lazarus, R. S. (1982). Stress, coping and somatic adaptation. In L. Goldberger & S. Breznitz (Eds.), *Handbook of stress: Theoretical and clinical aspects*. New York: Free Press.
101. Bohnen, N., Nicolson, N., Sulon, J., et al. (1991). Coping style, trait anxiety and cortisol reactivity during mental stress. *Journal of Psychosomatic Research, 35*, 141–147.
102. Burns, V. E., Carroll, D., Ring, C., et al. (2002). Stress, coping, and hepatitis B antibody status. *Psychosomatic Medicine, 64*, 287–293.

103. Kiecolt-Glaser, J. K., Garner, W., Speicher, C., et al. (1984). Psychosocial modifiers of immunocompetence in medical students. *Psychosomatic Medicine, 46*, 7–14.
104. Glaser, R., Kiecolt-Glaser, J. K., Bonneau, R., et al. (1992). Stress-induced modulation of the immune response to recombinant hepatitis B vaccine. *Psychosomatic Medicine, 54*, 22–29.
105. Segerstrom, S. C. (2001). Optimism, goal conflict, and stressor-related immune change. *Journal of Behavioral Medicine, 24*, 441–467.
106. Stowell, J. R., Kiecolt-Glaser, J. K., & Glaser, R. (2001). Perceived stress and cellular immunity: When coping counts. *Journal of Behavioral Medicine, 24*, 323–339.
107. Peavey, B. S., Lawlis, G. F., & Goven, A. (1985). Biofeedback-assisted relaxation: Effects on phagocytic capacity. *Biofeedback and Self-Regulation, 10*, 33–47.
108. Green, R. G., & Green, M. L. (1987). Relaxation increases salivary immunoglobulin A. Psychological *Reports, 61*, 623–629.
109. Laidlaw, T. M., Booth, R. J., & Large, R. G. (1996). Reduction in skin reactions to histamine after a hypnotic procedure. *Psychosomatic Medicine, 58*, 242–248.
110. Kabat-Zinn, J., Wheeler, E., Light, T., et al. (1998). Influence of a mindfulness meditation-based stress reduction in patients with moderate to severe psoriasis undergoing phototherapy (UVB) and photochemotherapy (PUVA). *Psychosomatic Medicine, 60*, 625–632.
111. Koh, K. B., Lee, Y., Beyn, K. M., et al. (2008). Counter-stress effects of relaxation on proinflammatory and anti-inflammatory cytokines. *Brain, Behavior, and Immunity, 22*, 1130–1137.
112. Davidson, R. J., Kabat-zinn, J., Schumacher, J., et al. (2003). Alterations in brain and immune function produced by mindfulness meditation. *Psychosomatic Medicine, 65*, 564–570.
113. Pace, T. W., Negi, L. T., Adame, D. D., et al. (2009). Effect of compassion meditation on neuroendocrine, innate immune and behavioral responses to psychosocial stress. *Psychoneuroendocrinology, 34*, 87–98.
114. Lutgendorf, S. K., Logan, H., Costanzo, E., et al. (2004). Effects of acute stress, relaxation, and a neurogenic inflammatory stimulus on interleukin-6 in humans. *Brain, Behavior, and Immunity, 18*, 55–64.
115. Epel, E. S., Blackburn, E. H., Lin, J., et al. (2004). Accelerated telomere shortening in response to life stress. *Proceedings of the National Academy of Sciences of the United States of America, 101*, 17312–17315.
116. Jacob, T. L., Epel, E. S., Lin, J., et al. (2011). Intensive meditation training, immune cell telomerase activity, and psychological mediators. *Psychoneuroendocrinology, 36*, 664–681.
117. Baggett, H. L., Antoni, M. H., & August, S. M. (1990). The effects of frequency of relaxation practice on immune markers in an HIV-1 high risk group. *Psychosomatic Medicine, 52*, 243.
118. Cruess, S., Antoni, M., Cruess, D., et al. (2000). Reductions in herpes simplex virus type 2 antibody titers after cognitive behavioral stress management and relationships with neuroendocrine function, relaxation skills, and social support in HIV-positive men. *Psychosomatic Medicine, 62*, 828–837.
119. Taylor, D. N. (1995). Effects of a behavioral stress-management program on anxiety, mood, self-esteem, and T-cell count in HIV positive men. *Psychological Reports, 76*, 451–457.
120. Kiecolt-Glaser, J. K., Glaser, R., & Williger, D. (1985). Psychosocial enhancement of immunocompetence in a geriatric population. *Health Psychology, 4*, 25–41.
121. Andersen, B. L., Golden-Kreutz, D., Emery, C. F., et al. (2007). Distress reduction from a psychological intervention contributes to improved health for cancer patients. *Brain, Behavior, and Immunity, 21*, 953–961.
122. Nunes, D. F., Rodriguez, A. L., da Silva Hoffmann, F., et al. (2007). Relaxation and guided imagery program in patients with breast cancer undergoing radiotherapy is not associated with neuroimmunomodulatory effects. *Journal of Psychosomatic Research, 63*, 647–655.
123. Robinson, F. P., Mathews, H. L., Witek-Janusek, L., et al. (2003). Psycho-endocrine-immune response to mindfulness-based stress reduction in individuals infected with the human immunodeficiency virus: a quasiexperimental study. *Journal of Alternative and Complementary Medicine New York, 9*, 683–694.

124. Creswell, J. D., Myers, H. F., Cole, S. W., et al. (2009). Mindfulness meditation training effects on CD4+ T lymphocytes in HIV-1 infected adults: A small randomized controlled trial. *Brain, Behavior, and Immunity, 23*, 184–188.
125. Witek-Janusek, L., Albuquerque, K., Chroniak, K. R., et al. (2008). Effect of mindfulness based stress reduction on immune function, quality of life and coping in women newly diagnosed with early stage breast cancer. *Brain, Behavior, and Immunity, 22*, 969–981.
126. Carlson, L. E., Speca, M., Patel, K. D., et al. (2003). Mindfulness-based stress reduction in relation to quality of life, mood, symptoms of stress, and immune parameters in breast and prostate cancer outpatients. *Psychosomatic Medicine, 65*, 571–581.
127. Scanga, C. B., Verde, T. J., Paolone, A. M., et al. (1998). Effects of weight loss and exercise training on natural killer cell activity in obese women. *Medicine & Science in Sports & Exercise, 30*, 1666–1671.
128. Koh, K. B., & Lew, S. H. (1999). The effect of vitamin B-complex on stress-induced immune alteration. *Korean Journal of Psychosomatic Medicine, 7*, 196–202.
129. Otto, M. W., Hong, J. J., & Safren, S. A. (2002). Benzodiazepine discontinuation difficulties in panic disorder: Conceptual model and outcome for cognitive behavioral therapy. *Current Pharmaceutical Design, 8*, 75–80.
130. Kampman, M., Keijsers, G. P., Hoogduin, C. A. L., et al. (2002). A randomized, double-blind, placebo-controlled study of the effects of adjunctive paroxetine in panic disorder patients unsuccessfully treated with cognitive-behavioral therapy alone. *The Journal of Clinical Psychiatry, 63*, 772–777.
131. Atanackovic, D., Kroger, H., Serke, S., et al. (2004). Immune parameters in patients with anxiety or depression during psychotherapy. *Journal of Affective Disorders, 81*, 201–209.
132. Irwin, M., Lacher, U., & Caldwell, C. (1992). Depression and reduced natural killer cytotoxicity: A longitudinal study of depressed patients and control subjects. *Psychological Medicine, 22*, 1045–1050.
133. Andersen, B. L., Farrar, W. B., Golden-Kreutz, D. M., et al. (2004). Psychological, behavioral, and immune changes after a psychological intervention: A clinical trial. *Journal of Clinical Oncology, 22*, 3570–3580.
134. Antoni, M. H., Lechner, S., Diaz, A., et al. (2009). Cognitive behavioral stress management effects on psychosocial and physiological adaptation in women undergoing treatment for breast cancer. *Brain, Behavior, and Immunity, 23*, 580–591.
135. van der Pompe, G., Duivenvoorden, H. J., Antoni, M. H., et al. (1997). Effectiveness of a short-term group psychotherapy program on endocrine and immune function in breast cancer patients: An exploratory study. *Journal of Psychosomatic Research, 42*, 453–466.
136. Koh, K. B., Sohn, S.-H., Kang, J. I., et al. (2012). Relationship between neural activity and immunity in patients with undifferentiated somatoform disorder. *Psychiatry Research: Neuroimaging, 202*, 252–256.
137. Dantzer, R. (2005). Somatization: A psychoneuroimmune perspective. *Psychoneuroendocrinology, 30*, 947–952.
138. Daruna, J. H., & Morgan, J. E. (1990). Psychosocial effects on immune function: Neuroendocrine pathways. *Psychosomatics, 31*, 4–12.
139. Liang, S.-W., Jemerin, J. M., Tschann, J. M., et al. (1997). Life events, frontal electroencephalogram laterality, and functional immune status after acute psychological stressors in adolescents. *Psychosomatic Medicine, 59*, 178–186.

Index

K.B. Koh (ed.), *Somatization and Psychosomatic Symptoms*,
DOI 10.1007/978-1-4614-7119-6, © Springer Science+Business Media New York 2013

R

S

Z

9781461471189